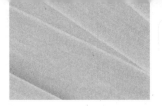

W9-CEM-368

Spirituality:
Living Our Connectedness

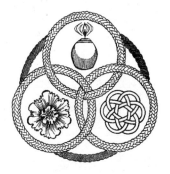

Margaret A. Burkhardt PhD, RN, MNC
Mary Gail Nagai-Jacobson MSN, RN

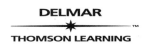

DELMAR

™

THOMSON LEARNING

Australia Canada Mexico Singapore Spain United Kingdom United States

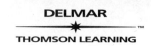

DELMAR

THOMSON LEARNING

Spirituality: Living Our Connectedness

Margaret A. Burkhardt
and
Mary Gail Nagai-Jacobson

Health Care Publishing Director:
William Brottmiller

Executive Marketing Manager:
Dawn F. Gerrain

Product Development Manager:
Marion S. Waldman

Production Editor:
James Zayicek

Product Development Editor:
Jill Rembetski

Library of Congress Cataloging-in-Publication Data:
Burkhardt, Margaret A.
  Spirituality : living our connectedness / Margaret A. Burkhardt, Mary Gail Nagai-Jacobson.
  p. cm.
  Includes bibliographical references and index.
  ISBN 0-7668-2082-3
  1. Nurse and patient.
2. Nurses—Religious life.
3. Spiritual life. 4. Healing—Religious aspects. I. Nagai-Jacobson, Mary Gail. II. Title.
  RT85.2 .B87 2001
  610.73'06'99—dc21
                  2001037124

NOTICE TO THE READER

To the One who is unnameable yet closer than our own breath,
in Whom we live, move, and have our being.
To all who support, challenge, guide, and inspire us
as companions on our journeys.
To all who embrace the journey.

Contents

Chapter 4
Healing Presence, Spiritual Presence   86

PART 2   CARING FOR THE NURSE'S SPIRIT   115

Chapter 5
Connecting with the Physical Self   117

Chapter 6
Connecting with Inner Self and Sacred Source   147

Illuminating the Spiritual Journey: Jean Watson's Story   181

Chapter 7
Connecting through Cycles of Rest and Re-Creation   187

Chapter 8
Connecting with Nature   207

Chapter 9
Connecting Through Ritual   234

PART 3 SHARING SACRED JOURNEYS   263

Chapter 12
Attending to Spirit 319

Chapter 13
Considerations for the Journey 348

List of Self-Nurture Boxes

Preface

Some books are never finished. This is one of them. No matter how much we write about any subject in this book, there is more to explore and share. Volumes have been written about the topics in this book. We trust that you will seek out resources that call to you. The spiritual journey, too, is always unfolding and, in this sense, is never finished. There is always more to explore and to reflect upon as you journey. We have written this book as a resource and companion for the journey—an invitation to delve deeper into your own spiritual journey. Knowing and attending to ourselves as spiritual beings grounds our spiritual caregiving with others. This book is for anyone who seeks to integrate spirituality more intentionally into his or her life and work, especially professional nurses, students, and other health care professionals. We trust this book will help you to recognize the spiritual in all life—the mundane, everyday events as well as experiences of the deep valley and the lofty mountaintop—through the cycles, seasons, and transitions of life.

This book is grounded in an understanding that all persons are spiritual beings for whom care of the spirit is an integral part of healing and wholeness. Although we know that spirituality influences health and that people express the desire for their health care providers to address spiritual concerns, nurses and other health professionals often hesitate to address or overlook this important health consideration. Nurses cite discomfort surrounding issues of spirituality, fear of imposing their beliefs on another, limited educational preparation regarding spiritual matters, and constraints of time as some of the barriers to integrating spirituality into healthcare. This book is designed to address many of these concerns, assisting you in becoming more skilled in and comfortable with integrating care of the spirit into healthcare practice.

Spirituality is a broad concept, transcending religious boundaries. By virtue of being human, all people are spiritual, regardless of whether or how they participate in religious observance. Spirituality as discussed here is understood to be the essence of our being, the animating spirit or soul through which we know and experiences connectedness with all of life: with our Self, with Others, with Nature/Cosmos, and with the Divine or Sacred Source. Thus, spirituality is ultimately about relationships. Both giving and receiving care occurs in the context of relationship. We illuminate the significance of these connections through examples from the laboratory of the lived experience, and through the questions and insights that derive from these experiences. Each of our stories is unique, and, at the same time, each story belongs to all of us.

FEATURES

This book is designed to engage you in personal exploration and reflection as you travel your spiritual path. To assist you, we include questions for reflection, suggestions for nurturing your own spirituality, and stories illuminating the spiritual journey. Reflection, a way of looking beneath and beyond the apparent, helps us to grow, stretch, discover meaning, and gain wisdom. Suggestions for self-nurture offer encouragement for incorporating meaningful spiritual practice into your life. This book is enriched by the stories, poetry, and psalms of people who were willing to share their journeys for our reflection and learning. Many of these stories belong to nurses. Where they have given permission, the names of the storytellers are included. Some stories are woven through several chapters, particularly that of Esber Tweel, who graciously shares reflections from his personal journal as he confronts living with debilitating illness. Give yourself the gift of time and space to *be* with yourself as you use this book. Use the features in ways that are personally meaningful to you. You can also adapt reflective questions and self-nurture activities for use with patients and others.

Living in and caring for others in a world of many traditions impels us to provide holistic care for persons whose spiritual grounding might be different from our own. Although we cannot know the substance of each religious or spiritual perspective, we can approach each person as a spiritual being, honor that which is important to them on the road to healing, and learn from them how to provide support on their spiritual path. Although we have attempted to be mindful and respectful of many traditions, our language might not fit your expression. If you find our language troublesome, honor yourself and your expression by translating it into words that fit for you. Because we have used different translations for the various citations from the Judeo-Christian scriptures, we reference only book, chapter, and verse. We trust that you will use the translation of your choice if you wish to explore these citations further. We appreciate that expressions of spirituality in different spiritual traditions are shaped by many factors, including social and cultural context. This book discusses cultural considerations and ways to facilitate spiritual care within the context of culture, particularly when a person's spiritual expression flows from an explanatory model that is different from our own. We may speak of cultures and geographical locations broadly as in "Native American traditions" or "African religions," but we recognize that these broad categories contain numerous groups and sub-groups that can differ greatly from each other. We encourage you to continue learning about people and cultures—not only from books but also from the people for whom you care. We encourage you as well to continue to grow in the knowledge and experience of your own tradition. As we live in the authenticity of our own spirituality we are able to bring to others the strengths and resources of our spirituality while honoring each person's unique path.

ORGANIZATION

Part 1 presents spirituality as the heart of caring for the whole person in the context of the connectedness that defines us. These chapters provide an opportunity to reflect on the nature of healing, the art of being present in the midst of questions of mystery and suffering, and the place of faith, hope, forgiveness, grace, and gratitude in our spiritual unfolding. Part 2 focuses on the necessity of caring for the nurse's spirit. Seeing ourselves as whole body-mind-spirit persons and caring for ourselves within the context of our connectedness, we become more effective instruments of healing and wholeness. Part 3 focuses on sharing sacred journeys that are a part of life and nursing care. Approaching persons as ongoing stories is discussed as one means of seeing the whole person. We offer approaches to nurturing personal spirituality through prayer, meditation, and mindfulness; through attending to our physical self, touch, and movement; through rest and re-creation; through ritual and creativity; through sharing our stories; and through nurturing important connections with Self, Others, God or Sacred Source, and Nature. Throughout this book, we encourage you to be mindful and to reflect. By pausing to do just that, you will give life to the words and make them your own.

Integrating spirituality into health care requires us to translate our knowledge about spirituality into skillful assessment, planning, and intervention. With spiritual care, the process of assessment is often an intervention as well. Attentive listening, especially for a person's story, and intentional presence, which are essential processes for spiritual caregiving, are described in this book. Appreciating that spirituality defies quantification, we include examples of a variety of guides and instruments that can help facilitate spirituality assessment, with discussion of how to use them appropriately and effectively.

The spiritual path is a life journey with many turns, both expected and unexpected. The way leads through charted and uncharted territory, traversing all manner of terrain. Sometimes we feel a sense of being exactly where we are supposed to be, but sometimes we feel lost and afloat. We find ourselves struggling up a mountain, putting one foot in front of the other across an arid desert, resting in a meadow, racing the wind at the water's edge. We find ourselves on our knees in gratitude and bent over in despair, raising a fist in anger or our hands in a song of praise. A major element of spiritual caregiving is that of authenticity, acting from the essence of our being, living our relationships authentically. As in a hologram, starting with any facet of spirituality leads to the whole. Each chapter of this book is written to stand on its own so that you can begin with the aspect that your particular needs and interests draw you to. You may choose to read from beginning to end, but you may also choose particular chapters and stories and appreciate the full flavor of the book.

As you expand your own comfort and competence in spiritual caregiving for others and yourself, we trust this book will be both an ever-new beginning and a companion along the way, offering food for thought and reflection, nurturing for your soul, and encouragement for the journey. May you journey well!

ABOUT THE AUTHORS

Our life stories began to intertwine 20 years ago when we both joined the faculty of the Charleston Division of West Virginia University School of Nursing. As we recognized and resonated with the spiritual seeker in each other, we began sharing with others through classes and workshops, and writing about our growing recognition of the importance of attending to the spiritual within ourselves and others. Our lives and nursing experience continued to teach us that the spiritual dimension of our being, which is not addressed well in conventional health care, is an integral part of our wholeness and an essential aspect of our health and healing. Mary Gail has worked in oncology, mental health, hospice, and community settings in both urban and rural areas. Peggy (Margaret) has worked in community health and primary care in rural and urban areas. We have had the privilege of working with and learning from people of many walks of life and various cultural and spiritual traditions. Each has enriched our own lives and broadened our understanding of the spiritual nature in all of us. Attention to personal spiritual practices, academic courses, workshops, spiritual retreats, shared prayer and worship, study about and sharing spiritual experiences of other traditions, reading and study, observations and reflections on Life, and sharing within family and communities and with those who come into our lives have all been part of our spiritual journeys. As we write this book, Mary Gail continues to find new dimensions to her beliefs in, understandings of, and relationship with the living God, the risen Christ, and the presence of the Holy Spirit. Her experience of the Judeo-Christian tradition grounds her seeing in the life of Jesus, a life lived in full and right relationship to God and in right relationship to all of life. Peggy's Catholic heritage and relationship to Christ and the Spirit continues to be enriched by exploring the roots and wisdom of her husband's Jewish tradition, the wisdom of Native American spirituality, the spiritual teachings of Eastern traditions, and spiritual practices that open awareness to God's presence in all of life. While living in the truth that we are each given in our spiritual journey, we honor the Mystery and Truth that embraces us all, in Love, on the journey.

ACKNOWLEDGMENTS

In reflecting on our lives we are aware of persons who, from our earliest memories, offered nurture to our spirits. A concept such as *healing presence* has meaning for us because we have experienced such presence. Our lives teach us that relationships are at the heart of life as spiritual journey. We recognize that our relationships with family, friends, colleagues, and patients/clients have all contributed to our work and writing. To communities of friendship and faith in which we have been nurtured and challenged, and by which we are shaped, our deepest gratitude. Our inspiration has come as well from many whom we have never met and who may no longer be in earthly form. And so, we are aware that persons too numerous to name are a part of this book as they have shared life with us, offering challenge, inspiration, love, and the gifts of their presence. We are grateful to them all.

This book, which has been taking shape in our lives and friendship for many years, has been a co-creative effort among many. We are grateful to all who have partnered with us in bringing this project into form. We offer particular thanks to Lynn Keegan for inviting us to undertake this adventure and for her vision, her support, and her commitment to encouraging nurses to honor their role as instruments of healing. We are grateful as well to Barbara Dossey for her ongoing mentoring, encouragement, and support of our work in the area of spirituality and healing. We offer deep appreciation to Floyd Beer, Tammy Campbell, Jude Fleming, Beth Gwynn, Nancy Hendrickson, Sandra Bauer Melville, Cricket Rose, Scott Thompson, Esber Tweel, Penny Unger, Joni Walton, Jean Watson, and Lisa Wayman whose generous sharing of their personal stories enriches all of us. Our thanks also goes to the editorial staff at Delmar Thomson Learning, particularly Jill Rembetski, for support and guidance in bringing this book into being.

And finally, we express our gratitude to our families:

—to the families to which we were born and the families into which we married, for the sacrifices made, challenges undertaken, adventures dared, lessons offered, examples lived, support given, and caring in many forms—these legacies of everyday and extraordinary courage and faithfulness are given to us across the generations over time and space;

—for the families being created and yet to come we add to these legacies our stories in the trust that their lives, too, will be strengthened and enlivened by the gifts of their past as they carry us all into the future;

—to Joe Golden and Ray Jacobson in whose lives we see authenticity of being and integrity of doing, and through whose presence in our lives we understand more deeply the gift of companionship on the journey.

Without you, this book would not have come into being.

We would also like to thank the following reviewers:

Joanne Bonicelli
Director of Complementary Therapy
Pikes Peak Hospice
Colorado Springs, CO 80903-5607

Julia Byrd, RN, BA, L-MT, C-AT
Director, School of Wholistic Nursing
Syosset, NY 11791

Lynn Keegan, RN, PhD, HNC, FAAN
Director Holistic Health Consultants
Port Angeles, Washington

Dr. Karilee Halo Shames
Assistant Professor
Florida Atlantic University
Boca Raton, FL 33486

John Nash
Social/Bereavement Counselor
The Community Hospice
Albany, NY 12205

Lizzie Teichler, RN-C, FNP, AHNC, MSN, PhD(C)
Instructor, School of Nursing
University of Colorado Health Sciences Center
Louisville, CO 80027

Spirituality: Essence and Connection

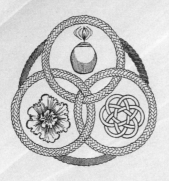

*S*pirituality is at the heart of caring for the whole person. This section discusses spirituality as the core or essence of our being, and the role of the spiritual in healing across time and traditions. Being a healing presence is the most essential element of spiritual care giving for ourselves and others as we live our connectedness with God or Sacred Source, Self, Others, and Nature. The spiritual path is a life journey of discovering ever more that our wholeness, grounded in our connectedness, encompasses mystery and meaning, joy and suffering, indeed, all of our life experiences.

The Spiritual Core

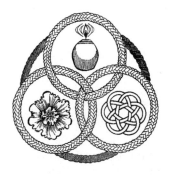

We join spokes together in a wheel

but it is the center hole that makes the wagon move.

We shape clay into a pot,

but it is the emptiness inside that holds whatever we want.

We hammer wood for a house,

but it is the inner space that makes it livable.

We work with being,

but non-being is what we use.

LAO TSU, 1988

Spirituality is the inherent aspect of our human *beingness*. The spiritual core is the place that is closer than our own breath, yet unlimited in its expansiveness. Spirituality impels us to seek and to discover the *more* of who we are and calls us to enter the depths of our own being, where we discover our intrinsic connectedness with all of life and with the eternal Oneness and Sacred Source of our being. Spirituality enables us to wonder and reflect as we see the light in the darkness, discover meaning, see beauty, experience love, and know that we are made for Love. Spirituality, connecting us with the source of our being, infuses our knowing, being, and doing.

Like a diamond, spirituality has many facets and is packaged with different wrappings. As you explore spirituality throughout this book, listen to what rings true for you at this time and place in your journey. We offer various understandings and expressions of spirituality for your reflection, with the trust that you will take from this what you need to more deeply experience the living of your own spirituality.

REFLECTION 1–1

Spirituality is a life-filled path, a spirit-filled way of living . . . to choose one path is to reject another . . . what is common to all paths that are spiritual is, of course, the Spirit-breath, life, energy . . . It belongs to none of us and all of us. We all share it. Spirituality does not make us otherworldly; it renders us more fully alive (Fox, 1991).

Spirituality is being awake. Getting rid of illusions. Spirituality is never being at the mercy of any event, thing, or person. Spirituality means having found the diamond mine inside yourself. Religion is intended to lead you there (deMello, 1998).

Spirituality is a brave search for the truth about existence, fearlessly peering into the mysterious nature of life, an attitude toward everything-a daily choosing of a way to approach the different textures of life, both the big questions and events and the daily happenings and concerns (Lesser, 1999).

- How do you feel as you read these different descriptions of spirituality? What thoughts come to mind? What rings true for you and what feels incomplete? What would you add to any of these? What questions do these prompt for you?

- Describe your experience of spirituality and what spirituality means to you.

- Where and how does spirituality fit into your view of life and of human experience?

HOLISTIC PERSPECTIVE

Spirituality is perhaps the most basic—yet least understood—aspect of who we are as human beings. The discussion of spirituality and healing in this book is grounded in a holistic view of persons and life. The holistic paradigm appreciates that humans are whole, integral, body-mind-spirit beings in continual interaction within an environment. The linear, analytical mind often speaks of body, mind, and spirit as though they are separate parts of a person. This artificial distinction, the illusion of separation, is a creation of the mind. Rather than separate parts, the body-mind-spirit being is in essence an intertwined and interpenetrating unity. Thus, every human experience has body-mind-spirit components, while being experienced by the whole person. Understanding the wholeness of persons is basic to providing care that includes concerns related to each of these spheres. Within the holistic perspective, spirituality cannot be separated from our lives and experiences as physical, emotional, social, and thinking persons. Indeed, spirituality infuses all of who we are, and we come to know our spiritual selves as we embrace all the spheres of our being. Because spirituality permeates all of life, we can access our spiritual core through every sphere of our being.

The metaphor of a hologram helps us understand the unitary nature of spirituality. A hologram is a type of transparent picture, created by using lasers, in which the image is multidimensional rather than two-dimensional. Holograms often seem to be flat when approached through the sense of touch. When beholding the hologram visually, however, the image appears multidimensional and can exhibit movement. Though the image that is seen is nonmaterial, we see it nonetheless. Within a hologram, the information of the whole is contained in every part. If any place of a hologram is illuminated with coherent light, an image of the entire hologram is provided, although the clarity of the image is reduced slightly and oriented differently as the piece of the hologram becomes smaller (Dossey, 1982). The whole image is there, but the ability to see it depends on the size of the window. Similarly, spirituality is a phenomenon that is understood differently depending on the perspective from which it is viewed. If viewed from only one perspective, some parts of the image might not be seen. Its many facets form something like an image that, although real, is no "thing." It is possible to retrieve a sense of the whole by illuminating a particular element or facet of spirituality, although the clarity could be slightly diminished.

NURSING'S HERITAGE:
NIGHTINGALE'S SPIRITUAL CORE

Where shall I find God? In myself. That is the true Mystical Doctrine. But then I myself must be in a state for Him to come and dwell in me. This is the whole aim of the Mystical Life; and all Mystical Rules in all times and countries have been laid down for putting the soul into such a state (Nightingale, quoted in Dossey [2000], p. 325).

Care of the spirit has been an imperative for nursing from the beginning. The efforts of contemporary scholars give us renewed insight into the spiritual core of nursing's founder, Florence Nightingale, and the profound influence of her spirituality on her life and legacy of nursing. This discussion is drawn particularly from the works of Calabria & Macrae (1994), Macrae (1995), and Dossey (1998; 2000).

The spiritual life was an ever-present reality for Florence Nightingale. At an early age, she experienced a clear sense of God's calling her to be of service. Her belief that serving God meant serving humanity ultimately led to her work in nursing and in hospital reform, and her deep spirituality grounded her views of both nursing practice and social reform. Nightingale believed that spirituality is intrinsic to human nature, extending beyond the bounds of religion. Although her spirituality was clearly grounded in Christianity and she deepened her own self-knowledge through intensely studying the Bible, Nightingale felt that, to more fully know God, we must explore and understand the beliefs and practices of the world's major religious and spiritual traditions. Her writings reflect her exploration of both Western and Eastern religious and mystic traditions. Indeed, we can see through her life and writings that Nightingale herself was a mystic (Dossey, 1998; 2000). Central to her spiritual philosophy is the belief that the universe is the incarnation or embodiment of a transcendent God, and that, through a shift in consciousness, humans have the potential for and possibility of experiencing their inner divinity. Her spirituality reflects the unitive nature found in all mystical traditions; that is, a pervading awareness of intimate connection with a higher reality and intelligence that creates, organizes, and sustains the universe. Julian of Norwich, a 14th century mystic, describes this intimacy of connection, this oneness with the higher reality, or God in these words: "Our soul is oned to God, unchangeable goodness, and therefore between God and our soul . . . there is no between" (Doyle, 1983). Nightingale believed that, in the divine plan, "human consciousness is tending to become what God's consciousness is— to become one with the consciousness of God" (Calabria & Macrae, 1994, p. 58) and that humans would eventually realize their inner spiritual nature. This inner spiritual nature is the source of our yearning for and being drawn toward union with God. In Nightingale's understanding, mysticism is the attempt to draw near to God, not so much by the rites and ceremonies of religious practice, as by inward disposition. She noted that the foundation of all real mystical traditions is "that for all our actions, all our words, all our thoughts, the food upon which they are to live and have their being is to be the indwelling Presence of God, the union with God; that is, with the Spirit of Goodness and Wisdom" (Dossey, 2000, p. 343).

Nightingale was a practical mystic and a scientist. She saw no conflict between spirituality and science; rather, she believed that science was necessary for developing a mature concept of God. In *Suggestions for Thought* (Calabria & Macrae, 1994), Nightingale included extensive commentaries on both Universal Law and Divine Law. She believed that we gain knowledge of and become closer to God by observing and attending to the laws of the universe and that even spiritual development is subject to law. She also believed that our inner connection with God is a source of creativity, insight, and knowledge that helps us understand life events and experiences such as illness. Although she acknowledged that there is much to learn from the Bible and other spiritual and inspirational texts, she held that the source of religious knowledge ultimately comes through our capabilities of observation, thought, and feeling, applied to the universe, past, present, and to come. She wrote that "whatever contributes to the advance of man's nature from the imperfect towards the perfect, whatever helps ignorance to knowledge, helps us to know and feel the Father, to enrich His Holy Spirit as existing within each of us" (Calabria & Macrae, 1994, p. 116). In whatever ways one helped to improve conditions for another or bring about greater awareness and knowledge was, for Nightingale, an expression of spirituality and a way of connecting with God.

Dossey (1998) comments that, in the manner of mystics in the Western religious tradition, Nightingale's spirituality compelled her toward and infused her social action. Her work, then, was an expression of her experience of the God within, or her union with God. Her writings reflect a deep personal consciousness of and ability to connect with her inner core and Sacred Source. She derived guidance and strength for her work from the Divine Presence within her. She wrote, "I am conscious of a voice that I can hear, telling me more truth and good than I *am*. As I rise to *be* more truly and more rightly, this voice is ever beyond and above me, calling me to more and more good" (Calabria & Macrae, 1994, p. 127). This statement reflects the importance of *being* most truly and authentically who we are, so that our *doing* flows from this spiritual core. Nightingale believed that God intends us to be responsible for each other, working to identify and address that which will promote a better existence for others and ourselves. We must respond to the circumstances around us, being cognizant of Natural Law and God's Law, so we can promote that which is good. In *Notes on Nursing* (1859/1992), Nightingale directs nurses to observe patients and their environments and to take appropriate action regarding that which will save lives and increase health and comfort. In this regard, she notes the folly of not attending to what we can do to alleviate illness and suffering, while expecting God to take it away.

SELF-NURTURE: Explore Another Spiritual Perspective

With an open heart and mind, explore a religious or spiritual perspective that is different from your own. You might read about another tradition, talk to someone about his or her tradition, or attend a ceremony, service, or ritual of another tradition. Consider how both your perspective and the other tradition lead to deeper awareness of the spiritual core. What insights into your own spiritual journey emerge from this exploration?

SPIRITUALITY IS NATURAL

*In this life the search for the spiritual begins with the longing
of the soul for nourishment (Vardey, 1995, p. xvii).*

As we have noted, our deepest core is spirit. Spirituality and spiritual expression have been evident among *Homo sapiens* from the earliest traces of our existence. Although creation stories from around the world give different accounts of the origins of the world and its creatures and offer various insights into why we are here, these stories all link us in one way or another to spiritual influences or greater forces that brought us into being. A sense of the sacred manifests in different ways at different times—perhaps in the worship of the sun or of fire, honoring the earth for her bounty, acknowledging the sacred in all life, standing in awe of the power, goodness, love of a Divine Being or Life Force. The experience of living with the known and unknown within the world prompted people to develop beliefs about and codes of conduct for relating to each other, to the sacred, and to the natural world. These beliefs and codes were often expressed within spiritual rituals and practices reflecting awe, wonder, fear, gratitude, petition for guidance, support, healing and for meeting other needs.

Armstrong's (1993) extensive study, *The History of God,* indicates that humans are essentially spiritual animals. By virtue of being human, all persons, at all ages, in all cultures, whether or not they are religious, are biopsychosocialspiritual beings. Awareness of and ways of expressing spirituality can vary with age and developmental levels. Although we are always spiritual, awareness of and ability to access and trust our spiritual core can grow and change over time and in relation to life experiences. The spiritual journey is a process. Fowler (1981) notes that we may begin and even spend much of our life with a spirituality that relies solely or primarily on the beliefs, experience, and judgments of others. He also suggests that we have the potential for moving beyond this into a spirituality grounded in openness to and trust of our own inner knowing of the imperatives of absolute love and justice and personal experiences of a transcendent actuality that is inclusive of all. Spiritual maturity, however, is not necessarily consistent with chronological age.

The Buddhists define spirituality as shamatha,
or "tranquil abiding." (Lesser, 1999)

As the essence of who we are and how we are in the world, spirituality, like breathing, is essential to our human existence. Within many traditions, the spiritual sphere is considered the source or life-giving principle for human existence. The Hebrew Scriptures describe the spirit or breath of God as that which gives life to the first human. In the English language, the words *spirit* and *spirituality* derive from the Latin *spiritus*, which means breath. The Greek word for breath, *pneuma*, refers to the vital spirit or soul. The soul animates all that we are and do. Indeed, Emerson (1983) suggests that the soul, though not organ, function, faculty, intellect, or will, "is the background of our being, in which they lie,—an immensity not possessed and that cannot be possessed" (p. 387). He describes the soul as a light that animates and exercises all our organs, uses our memory and analytical abilities as hands and feet, and is master of our intellect and will. In essence, Emerson considers the person to be an organ of the soul or, stated another way, we are embodied souls.

Embodied Soul

In the manner in which the soul permeates the body with its energy,
it causes and consummates all human action
(Hildegard of Bingen, in Uhlein, 1983, p. 54).

Carol Picard (1997) reminds us that there is a deep spiritual tradition regarding soul that crosses millennia and cultures. She writes that the nature of the person as embodied soul was a belief held within both Western and Eastern traditions in pre-Hellenic times and by early Greek philosophers. She notes that writings of later Greek philosophers, although considering the body to be distinct from the soul, described the soul as the moving principle or essential character of the body. Although the ancient Hebrew understanding of embodied soul is still found in the gospels of the Christian Scriptures, Picard comments that the concept of body and soul as connected yet separate was established in the Christian tradition by about the 8th century. In the 17th century, the chasm widened as Descartes' proposition that the properties of soul and body are mutually exclusive became generally accepted in the West. The concept of duality provided philosophical underpinnings that enabled the development of Western biomedicine. The body became the domain of science, and matters of the soul belonged to the church.

While the view of body as separate from soul became the dominant belief in most Western religious traditions, mystics, in their direct experiences of God, continued to express the soul/body unity. Julian of Norwich, wrote "God does not despise creation, nor does God disdain to serve us in the simplest function that belongs to our bodies in nature because God loves the soul, and the soul is made in the image of God" (Doyle, 1983, p. 28). Julian also stated that we cannot be whole until our sensuality is connected to our substance, writing that "both our Substance and Sensuality together may rightly be called our Soul. That is because they are both oned in God" (Doyle, 1983, p. 97).

Nursing theory reflects appreciation of the person as embodied soul. Jean Watson (1985; 1999) describes soul as a core aspect of person. Margaret Newman (1994) discusses nursing's obligation within the new paradigm to care for persons as embodied consciousness, embodied souls, noting that this care is a moral imperative for nursing. Picard (1997) reflects that "embodied soul is the human form of possibility in all unique expressions . . . the mystery, an expression of the capacity for growth and expansion, with the need for nurturance" (pp. 47, 50). The more authentically we connect with our spiritual core, the more we come to recognize soulfulness as the source of our connection to and sense of communion with all aspects of our planetary life. We see this, not only in the lives of mystics but in the experiences of scholars and scientists as well (Dossey, 1989; Benson, 1997; Berry, 1998; Ornish, 1998; Watson, 1999).

Within the soul's aliveness resides our source of creativity, potential, resource, and possibility (Kollmar, 1998; 1999). As the essence of who we are, the soul is the sphere of our being that is whole and complete and wherein we are most authentically our Self. Soul is a vehicle for, rather than a state of, consciousness and is not limited to space and time, as is the body. Soul is where we know and experience our oneness with God or the Sacred Source within us and beyond. Soul expresses in and through us in many ways. Emerson (1983) notes that, although soul is subtle, undefinable, and unmeasurable, we know that it pervades and contains us. Similar to how the heart is always sending nourishment to the body, the "soul is unrelenting in providing life at the core of our being" (Dolan, 2000, p. 2). As a quality or a dimension of experiencing life and ourselves, soul has to do with depth, relatedness, value, heart, and personal substance (Moore, 1992).

Spirituality, an expression of soul, is awareness of who we are and how to be our most authentic Selves. As embodied souls, there is no way to behave or act outside our spiritual selves, although we can act outside of our personal religious perspective. Because it is intangible in many ways and defies quantification, spirituality often eludes the cognitive mind. Our language is lacking when we try to express the experience of spirit or soul. It is like trying to describe the taste of honey to one who has never savored it. Yet, because our very essence is spirit or soul, we speak about it however we can, often with symbols, metaphor, and story.

RELATIONSHIP BETWEEN SPIRITUALITY AND RELIGION

People often speak of spirituality in terms of religious beliefs and practices. Some people consider that they or others are not spiritual if they do not attend religious services or believe in God. We see this in health-care settings when nurses and other practitioners identify spiritual care-giving with determining a patient's religious affiliation or with understanding health related beliefs, norms, and taboos of different religions. Such knowledge is important and can provide insight into a person's spirituality. However, spiritual care-giving is more effective when grounded in the understanding that spirituality is broader than religion and awareness that, even though we are all spiritual, some people might not be religious.

> *Religions are like cookbooks and guidebooks: they are not the food or the foreign country; rather, they suggest ingredients and point us in the right direction . . . You can walk a wonderful spiritual path with or without adhering to a religion. All paths are available; none are exclusively right or wrong or even required. (Lesser, 1999, p. 28-98)*

Knowledge of the histories, symbols, beliefs, practices, and languages of various religious traditions increases the nurse's ability to hear, recognize, and address religious needs of patients. Nurses are often more comfortable discussing spiritual concerns when they present within an identifiable religious context than when they occur within a broader perspective of spirituality. However, seeking information about religious affiliation and practices alone offers little more than a glimpse into a person's spiritual self, particularly if the person is only nominally affiliated with the religious tradition. When nurses and other practitioners routinely assume that spiritual needs are met by satisfying the rites and rituals of a particular religion, interventions can become standardized rather than individualized to the patient's needs (Mansen, 1993). This is of special concern when a person's spirituality is not expressed through an affiliation or alignment with a particular religion.

Spiritual journeys reflect the reality of our experience within and beyond religious traditions. Some journeys are shaped by the experience of living with two or more religious traditions and involve what Habito (1993) names "intrareligious dialogue," an "encounter of two religious traditions within the same individual" (p. 4). He describes this experience as one in which the person is "invited to place herself *within* the differing religious traditions being considered and let those traditions meet and discover mutual resonances and throw light upon one another, as well as mutually challenge one another from the perspective of the core message of each" (p. 4). Reflecting on his personal spiritual path, he writes

> In the course of my Zen journey over the years, I myself have had to struggle and come to grips with the Christian faith in which I was born and raised . . . Zen practice has invited me to listen with renewed fervor and attention to the Good News brought by Jesus, proclaiming the reign of God in our midst. If anything, Zen practice has enabled me to appreciate and reaffirm the dynamism and the possibilities of the Christian Gospel message, while at the same time becoming more critical of the ways in which many of us who profess adherence to it have sanitized, distorted, muffled, or institutionalized it, or have used it for our own egoistic purposes, whether consciously or unconsciously (p. 3-4).

Although many people express and experience their spirituality within the context of religion, many find their spirituality nurtured only partially or not at all within the constructs of religion. Appreciating that spirituality and religion, though related, are not synonymous, is well documented in nursing and healthcare literature (Burkhardt, 1989; Emblen, 1992; Engebretson, 1996; Fehring, Miller, & Shaw, 1997; Goddard, 1995; Hall, 1997; Mansen, 1993; Meraviglia, 1999; Nagai-Jacobson & Burkhardt, 1989; Nolan & Crawford, 1997; Sussman, Nezami, & Mishra, 1997). Religion as an expression of spirituality is not, per se, part of our essential nature. We choose a religious perspective. The integral essence and manifestation of each person's wholeness and being that we call spirituality is not subject to choice, but simply is. Borysenko (1999) suggests that religion is like a train whose destination is spirituality, cautioning us not to mistake the vehicle for the destination. She notes that even though religions have words to describe themselves, spirituality is a deep experience that has no words that do it justice. Vardey (1995) reminds us of Swiss psychologist Carl Jung's words that the living spirit is eternally renewed and "pursues its goal in manifold and inconceivable ways throughout the history of mankind. Measured against it, the names and forms which men [humans] have given it means very little; they are only the changing leaves and blossoms on the stem of the eternal tree" (p. xviii).

The word *religion* derives from the Latin *re-ligare,* meaning to re-tie or reconnect. Interestingly we find the same root for the word *ligament,* the tissue that helps to bind together or connect the structural components of the body. Religion provides a structure and process that connects people anew through shared beliefs, values, and practices. Taylor (1982) expands this understanding, suggesting that religion's truest purpose is to promote, celebrate, and give evidence of the deep, organic connection of self with others and all of life. This is echoed by de Mello (1998), who holds that good religion is intended to bring us to awareness.

Religion refers to an organized system of beliefs regarding the cause, purpose, and nature of the universe that is shared by a group of people and to the practices, including worship and ritual, related to that system. Various religions offer different frameworks for relating to the unseen Mystery; moral codes that guide living with and relating to each other; insights regarding the meaning and purpose of life; directives that facilitate connecting with our own spirit; and perspective about our place in and relationship with the natural world. Because culture influences our values and beliefs, religious and other spiritual expressions often relate to personal culture. This is particularly evident when religion pervades all aspects of a culture, including political, educational, and social institutions, such as among cultural groups like the Amish in the United States and in countries such as Israel and Iran. Mbiti (1975) gives an example of this in his discussion of African religions. Noting that religion is one of the richest parts of African cultural heritage, he writes that "religion is found in all areas of human life. It has dominated the thinking of African peoples to such an extent that it has shaped their cultures, their social life, their political organizations and economic activities" (p. 9). Looking at the cultural heritage of African religions, Mbiti further reflects that, contrasted with religions like Islam and Christianity that were started by or based on the teachings of a particular person, African religions "evolved slowly, over many centuries, as people lived their lives responding to situations and reflecting on them" (p. 9). Because African religions, as with many indigenous spiritual traditions, have no sacred scriptures like the Koran in Islam or the Bible in Judaism and Christianity, they have, in the words of Mbiti, "been written in hearts and lives and shared in the oral tradition" (p. 9).

Although religions reflect particular understandings of spirituality, there are many ways of understanding or accessing spirituality that transcend religion. Although many people find that adherence to religious precepts and practices assists in attending to their spiritual selves, some religious beliefs, structures, and practices could limit full expression of spirituality. Borysenko (1999) speaks of religious dropouts, those people who no longer find spiritual nurture in the traditions in which they were raised. These people might feel a lack of spiritual community, that their tradition does not help them connect with the spiritual, or a general sense of betrayal by the institution or anger at God for injustices that have been done under the guise of religion. She notes that many such dropouts are women who feel excluded by a patriarchal system, leading to anger and frustration at not finding a place for their spiritual expression.

THE YIN AND YANG OF SPIRITUAL EXPRESSION AND EXPERIENCE

Within all human experience, we find the juxtaposition of contrasts, of complementary opposites—joy and sadness, hot and cold, light and dark, yin and yang, feminine and masculine. This holds true as well for spirituality, which is expressed and experienced in stillness and through movement, alone and with others, through silence and with words, with the cognitive mind and through intuitive knowing, through the perspective of our feminine or of our masculine nature (remembering that whether by gender we are female or male, we all have both feminine and masculine qualities). In various religious and spiritual traditions, the Sacred Source can be viewed as having masculine qualities, feminine characteristics, or both. For some, the Divine is experienced as a transcendent being or force existing above and apart from creation, but for others, the Divine is immanent, residing within our own being and in all of creation. The masculine part of our being tends to be more cognitive, perceiving the spiritual journey as a linear process, in which we move upward from that which is considered less sacred toward that which is viewed as more sacred. From the perspective of our feminine being, which is more intuitive and comprehends the wholeness of life, the spiritual journey is more organic and circular in nature. Both perspectives provide pathways for expressing and experiencing our spiritual core. Our truest nature draws us toward a balance between the two. When one or the other is dominant, however, the imbalance of denying half our nature can potentiate far-reaching and long-lasting discord in many areas of life.

In the cosmology that has permeated most of Western philosophy and religion, the Divine is generally perceived as a transcendent creator and ruler of creation, yet separate from what *He* created. This cosmology promotes a view of spiritual growth that follows a linear and hierarchical path in which one moves away from things of the earth, which are considered lowest in the hierarchy, to move toward things of the spirit and the Divine, which are considered highest on the ladder. Because this cosmology has historically ranked women with nature at the bottom of the scale, women's experience of the sacred, as with so much of women's experience, has been devalued. Even when we have moved beyond believing this as truth, we are likely to carry this hierarchical ordering in some level of our psyches because of the pervasiveness of this attitude in Western civilization (Anderson & Hopkins, 1991).

The Feminine interprets "Be ye perfect as your heavenly Father is perfect"
to mean, "Be whole and complete, in both shadow and light, just as your

Mother, the Cosmos, is whole." (Report of the Committee
for the Spirituality of the Divine Feminine, Sufi Order of the West,
cited in Anderson & Hopkins, 1991)

Within non-Western spiritual traditions, and in the experiences of mystics within Western traditions, we find much less distinction between spirit and matter than we find in the hierarchical perspective. This same is true within women's experiences of spirituality and their spiritual journeys (Anderson & Hopkins, 1991; Borysenko, 1999; Burkhardt, 1994). Women's experience of spirituality (which aligns with the feminine nature of both women and men) reflects wholeness and interconnectedness that goes beyond the confines of a linear process. Some traditions consider women to be more innately aware of spirituality than men are. Perhaps women's biological cycles and connection with the life-giving process of creation provide opportunities for more intimate experience of the Sacred. We see this, for example, in many Native American traditions that honor a woman's menstrual or *moon time,* as a sacred time in which the woman is nurtured as she pays attention to her inner self, her dreams, and visions. The sacred focus of this time is not so much on personal growth, as on the good of the whole community and balance within the earth and heavens. In some traditions, major decisions were made by the women or through women's dreams and visions, honoring both women's special connection with the spirit world and their consideration of the impact of the decision on their children for several generations.

Anderson and Hopkins (1991) liken women's spirituality to a garden that can be entered by many gates. As a living entity with cycles and seasons, a garden sometimes needs much cultivation, but maintains a natural organic balance at other times. Women's spiritual journey values the process—the growing, shifting, and changing—where all elements can be included in and viewed as part of the whole. Being in the sacred garden involves both receptivity and choice. Receptivity, or grace, implies that though we can prepare for the direct experience of the sacred that can occur within the garden, how and when it happens is beyond our control. Choice is an act of conscious intention to both recognize and honor the sacred in every aspect of our lives, routine and mundane activities of living as well as the more centered and reflective times. The place where we find God is in the present moment, the here and now of our lives.

Spirituality for women is relational, intuitive, earthy, compassionate, sensuous, and mystical. Borysenko (1999) describes women's spiritual journey as walking a circle. In contrast to a linear and hierarchical path, a circle implies a process that is more intuitive, unplanned, and nonrational, leaving room for the unexpected—for changes and transformation to come through grace, our receptive openness to the Divine within us. She notes that a circle is defined by its center from which everything is equidistant, with no above or below, ahead or behind. Within this circle, a woman's center is her own heart, intuition, Inner Light, Spirit, the voice of God. It is here she seeks and hears the guidance for her journey. The metaphor of walking the circle implies that the spiritual journey is a process of continually orienting ourselves to the center of the circle, our sacred core,

> that Spirit that the Quakers call the Inner Light. The Buddhists call this *rigpa*, one's own true nature. Jews call it the Shekhina, "She who dwells within." The Christian mystic Meister Eckehart called it the Godseed. The Hindus call it the Atman. The Seneca tribe calls it the Orenda. The theological debate over whether God is immanent or transcendent doesn't make sense in a circular model. Everything is related and interdependent. In a nonlinear universe, either/or gets replaces by both/and. By grace, at any time during the journey, we can touch the center and know God. (Borysenko, p. 83).

Although the circle metaphor arises from women's experience of spirituality, the truths that it embodies apply to and can be part of men's spiritual experience as well.

 ## SELF-NURTURE: Attending to Self as Embodied Soul

Give yourself the gift of at least an hour, or better yet, a day in which you attend to yourself as embodied soul. Choose activities that nurture your spiritual self. You might spend time in nature, or reading, or in prayer, meditation, or worship. You might just want to be still. You might arrange to share the time with a special person, or have a massage, or care for your garden. Perhaps you will feel like dancing, singing, drumming, crying, or expressing what is going on in your inner self in other ways. Let your soul lead you to what you need in the present moment to connect with your spiritual core.

THE LANGUAGE OF SPIRITUALITY

Within Western societies the attitude that spirituality is private and separate from the secular aspects of life and the paucity of language for discussing and expressing matters of the spirit or soul contribute to the general discomfort we feel regarding matters of soul. The difficulty with the language of spirituality is evident in the nursing literature. (Burkhardt, 1989; Emblen, 1992; Fehring, Miller, & Shaw, 1997; Nolan & Crawford, 1997; Reed, 1992; Sussman, Nezami, & Mishra, 1997). The choice of a language for expressing spirit in Western cultures has generally been limited to that of science or that of religion derived from the Judeo-Christian tradition (Hall, 1997). Indeed, discussion of spirituality within nursing and other health-care literature often reflects Judeo-Christian values and perspectives regarding the Sacred, how we are to relate with others and the world, the place of suffering, forms and importance of prayer, and other aspects of the spiritual journey. With awareness that spirituality, as the essence of each person, transcends particular religious perspective, we need to expand or create both language and processes to allow room for each person's unique expression of spirituality.

Engebretson (1996) cautions that the Western cultural bias can lead to misinterpretation of spiritual expression and concerns. She notes that Eastern and nature religious traditions do not share assumptions of Western Judeo-Christian-Islamic traditions that include monotheism, transcendence, and dualism. Monotheism, the belief in one God that is above and beyond nature, contrasts with beliefs in the existence of many gods (polytheism), or the existence of the sacred in all living things (pantheism) found in Eastern and nature religions. The Western view of God as separate from humanity implies a sense of transcendence, meaning to exist above material existence. Focusing outward through ritual and prayer is a way people seek connection with a transcendent God. Eastern and nature traditions focus on the immanence of the Divine, experienced within each person. Meditation and spiritual exercises that draw one inward are common ways of connecting with the Divine in these traditions. Dualism, the separation of spirit and matter, a basic concept in Western traditions, contrasts with Eastern metaphysical traditions of monism in which reality is conceived as a unified whole. We see this in the African world view as well, which

> rejects the popular dichotomies between the sacred and the secular, the material and the spiritual. All life is religious, all life is sacred, all life is of a piece. The spiritual is real and permeates all existence so that the ancestral spirits, the living dead, are all around us, concerned to promote the well-being of those who are bound together with them in the bundle of life (Tutu, 1995, p. xvi).

In the West, the polarization of body and soul, science and spirituality reflects the institutionalization of dualism. These assumptions have a great impact on perceptions, definitions, and expectations of the spiritual experience within health care. Engebretson stresses the importance of recognizing these assumptions and cautions us about labeling spiritual issues as pathology, or about not recognizing them at all because they do not fit our familiar paradigm.

In today's world, people have many opportunities to interact with people from various cultures and spiritual traditions. We learn about traditions different from our own through books, media, workshops, personal interaction, and study with spiritual teachers. It is becoming more common to find a blurring of boundaries and blending of some Eastern traditions within Western religious practices. Some people express and experience their spirituality best in the distinctiveness of a particular religious tradition. Others address their spirituality by blending different religious and philosophical traditions. Still others experience their spirituality outside organized religious systems. Holistic practice recognizes and honors the unique ways that people express, experience, and nurture their spirit selves, both within, and outside of an organized religious context.

ELEMENTS OF SPIRITUALITY

Attempting to define spirituality is akin to trying to lasso the wind. We know the wind is there because we feel it and see its effect on things around us. However, it cannot be contained within imposed boundaries, conceptual or otherwise. The elusive and somewhat intangible nature of spirituality poses a particular challenge for those who feel more at home with phenomena that can be categorized, quantified, and measured. Understanding spirituality requires both intuitive and cognitive knowing. As we open ourselves to experience the inner reality of our spirituality, we become more familiar with both its tangible and less tangible attributes and manifestations. Through this, we discover that, rather than being hostile toward science, spiritual discourse illuminates and complements scientific debate (Nolan & Crawford, 1997).

Spirituality Described in Nursing Literature

The need for more conscious inclusion of spirituality in health care has prompted nurses to seek a fuller understanding of this most essential element of life and healing. Descriptions of spirituality have emerged from investigations of how the concept is used in the literature, and how it is understood by both healthy people and those experiencing illness. The following examples of spirituality described in Western nursing literature reflect the unfolding understanding and ongoing illumination of the concept for nursing. With a fuller understanding of the concept, nurses are better able to consciously and competently incorporate spirituality into care and healing practice.

Theoretical definitions of spirituality derived from syntheses of how the concept is used in the literature include "Spirituality is the unfolding of mystery through harmonious interconnectedness that springs from inner strength" (Burkhardt, 1989) and "Spirituality is defined as experiences and expressions of one's spirit in a unique and dynamic process reflecting faith in God or a supreme being; it is connectedness with oneself, others, nature, or God; and an integration of the dimensions of mind, body, and spirit" (Meraviglia, 1999).

Descriptions of spirituality that are synthesized from conceptual, clinical, and empirical knowledge in nursing include

Spirituality refers to the propensity to make meaning through a sense of relatedness to dimensions that transcend the self in such a way that empowers and does not devalue the individual. This relatedness may be experienced intrapersonally (as a connectedness with oneself), interpersonally (in the context of others and the natural environment), and transpersonally (referring to a sense of relatedness to the unseen God, or power greater than the self and ordinary resources). There is an expansion of boundaries inward, outward, and upward (Reed, 1992),

and "Spirituality is the essence of our being which permeates our living in relationship, infuses our unfolding awareness of who and what we are, our purpose in being, and our inner resources, and shapes our life journey (Burkhardt & Nagai-Jacobson, 2000).

Several grounded theory studies have explored spirituality from the perspective of participants. One study exploring understandings of spirituality among women in Appalachia describes spirituality as "the unifying force that shapes and gives meaning to the pattern of one's self becoming. This force is expressed in one's being, in one's knowing, and in one's doing, and is experienced in caring connections with Self, Others, Nature, and God or Higher Power" (Burkhardt, 1994). A similar study with men in West Virginia and Texas describes spirituality as "the essence of one's being permeating living in awareness and relationship" (Burkhardt & Nagai-Jacobson, 1995). From their grounded theory study of spiritual well-being in older adults, Hunglemann and colleagues (1996) describe spiritual well-being as "a sense of harmonious interconnectedness between self, others/nature, and Ultimate Other which exists throughout and beyond time and space. It is achieved through a dynamic and integrative growth process which leads to a realization of the ultimate purpose and meaning in life." Walton's (1999) exploration of spirituality of patients recovering from an acute myocardial infarction describes spirituality as "a life-giving force that comes from within which is nurtured by receiving presence from God, nature, friends, family, and

REFLECTION 1–3

- Recall that most research on spirituality reported in the nursing literature in the United States reflects a Judeo-Christian perspective. Consider whether similar studies would result in the same descriptions of spirituality if done in India, Japan, Ethiopia, Tanzania, or Sri Lanka.

- What elements or characteristics of spirituality do you feel are applicable across cultures and traditions?

community, and is based on developing faith, discovering meaning and purpose, and giving the gift of self."

In her phenomenological study of *Spiritual Well-Being in Appalachian Women,* Barker (1989) noted that the essential structure of spiritual well-being is encompassed in the metatheme of *Being Whole* and reflected through the interconnected and interlocking themes of Relationship and Self. Relationships with Deity/ Unifying Force, kin, others, and nature manifest in many ways and provide meaning and sustenance. A sense of Self as the place where spiritual well-being is embodied and reposes includes purpose in life, satisfaction, inner strength, responsibility, clear values, individual identity, and service.

LIVING OUR CONNECTEDNESS

Whatever the tradition or academic discipline, the many ways of describing spirituality, at some level or another, relate to our experience of living in the interconnected web of life. People grounded in Western traditions often initially speak of spirituality in terms of relationship with God or Divine Reality. In our research (Burkhardt, 1993; 1994; Burkhardt & Nagai-Jacobson, 1995) many participants began talking about spirituality with comments like "it's my total dependence on God," or "my number one priority is my relationship to God, so I pay a lot of attention to that." Other participants reflected a sense of an inner presence or being part of something greater than themselves although they did not use God-language. One participant related spirituality to "that nonmaterial reality that I think is part of every human being." Another stated that "spirituality is being connected to everything and knowing that it goes beyond every person to something much bigger than all of us together." In non-Western traditions, spirituality might be expressed as "walking in beauty" "following the red road" "seeking enlightenment."

Along with relationship with the Sacred Source, people reflect that relationships with others, nature, and oneself are core elements of spirituality (Burkhardt & Nagai-Jacobson, 2000). Relationship with self recognizes the integrality of our body-mind-spirit being. As an embodied soul, our spiritual core infuses and is expressed in our very being, in what we do, through our emotions, and through our intuitive and cognitive knowing. Thus, attending to any of these spheres provides an opportunity for connecting with and expressing the spiritual self. We know and experience ourselves as embodied souls within our relationship with others—both particular individuals and groups, and through our common bond with all of humanity. The joys and sorrows, love and hurt, harmony and discord, and giving and receiving of our relationships are potential doorways to deeper senses of ourselves as spiritual beings. People often experience a closeness with their spiritual selves and Sacred Source when they connect with nature, earth, environment, or universe. Our relationship with nature is a reflection our spirituality—our sense of place, belonging, and connectedness within the web of life. Each of these core elements of spirituality will be discussed more fully in later chapters.

 ## SELF-NURTURE: Finding Spiritual Sustenance

List five ways that you find spiritual sustenance. Consider how you can include two of these daily in your life for the next week.

Common characteristics of spirituality evident in the health-care literature suggest that spirituality is the life principle, the unifying and animating essence of our being that permeates our living in relationship, infuses our unfolding awareness of who and what we are, and shapes our life journey (Burkhardt, 1989; Burkhardt, 1994; Burkhardt & Nagai-Jacobson, 1995; Emblen, 1992; Mansen, 1993; Reed, 1992; Walton, 1996). Within our spiritual core, we discover life's meaning, our purpose in being, and our inner resources. Spirituality helps to ground our sense of place and how we fit in the world. Because it is practical and relevant to daily life, people experience spirituality in the mundane as well as in the profound, the secular as well as the sacred.

Spirituality is active and expressive. It is how we experience and live, in the present moment, our connectedness with our body-mind-spirit Self, with others, with nature or the cosmos, and with the Sacred Source, however we image or name this Source. *Spirituality is the search for right relationships more than it is the search for right answers.* Within the living of our connectedness, we experience all that life brings—the joy and sorrow, love and fear, discord and forgiveness, hope and despair, healing and suffering. Our spirituality shapes how we encounter mystery; discover meaning and purpose; offer and receive compassion, love, and forgiveness; and open our hearts to Love. Our spiritual core calls us into deeper relationship with ourselves and all of life so that we become more awake and aware and, ultimately re-member and re-connect with our wholeness, our holiness, and our healing.

REFERENCES

Anderson, S. R., & Hopkins, P. (1991). *The feminine face of God.* New York: Bantam Books.

Armstrong, K. (1993). *A history of God.* New York: Ballantine Books.

Barker, E. R. (1989). *Spiritual well-being in Appalachian women.* Unpublished doctoral dissertation, University of Texas, Austin, Texas.

Benson, H. (1997). *Timeless Healing: The power and biology of belief.* New York: Fireside Books.

Berry, T. (1998). Earth systems . . . human systems. In B. Webb (Ed.). *Fugitive Faith: Conversations on spiritual, environmental, and community renewal* (p. 31–43). Maryknoll, NY: Orbis Books.

Borysenko, J. (1999). *A woman's journey to God: Finding the feminine path.* New York: Riverhead Books.

Burkhardt, M. A. (1989). Spirituality: An analysis of the concept. *Holistic Nursing Practice, 3,* 69–77.

Burkhardt, M. A. (1993). Characteristics of spirituality in the lives of women in a rural Appalachian community. *Journal of Transcultural Nursing, 4*(2) 19–23.

Burkhardt, M. A. (1994). Becoming and connecting: Elements of spirituality for women. *Holistic Nursing Practice, 8,* 12–21.

Burkhardt, M. A., & Nagai-Jacobson, M. G. (1995, June). *Understandings of spirituality among men.* Presentation at the American Holistic Nurses Association and American Holistic Medical Association Conference *The Changing Face of Healing.* Phoenix, AZ.

Burkhardt, M. A., & Nagai-Jacobson, M. G. (2000). Spirituality and health. In B. M. Dossey, L. Keegan, & C. E. Guzzetta (Eds.). *Holistic nursing: A handbook for practice* (pp. 91–121). Gaithersburg, MD: Aspen.

Calabria, M. D., & Macrae, J. (1994). *Suggestions for thought by Florence Nightingale: Selections and commentaries.* Philadelphia: University of Pennsylvania Press.

de Mello, A. (1998). *Walking on water.* New York: Crossroad.

Dolan, J. R. (2000). *Communion meditations.* Anand, Gujarat, India: Gujarat Sahitya Prakash.

Dossey, L. (1989). *Recovering the soul.* New York: Bantam Books.

Dossey, B. M. (1998). Florence Nightingale: A 19th century mystic. *Journal of Holistic Nursing, 16*(2), 111–164.

Dossey, B. M. (2000). *Florence Nightingale: Mystic, visionary, healer.* Springhouse, PA: Springhouse Corporation.

Dossey, L. (1982). *Space, time & medicine.* Boston: New Science Library.

Doyle, B. (1983). *Meditations with Julian of Norwich.* Santa Fe, NM: Bear & Company.

Emblen, J. D. (1992). Religion and spirituality defined according to current use in nursing literature. *Journal of Professional Nursing, 8,* 41–47.

Emerson, R. W. (1983). *Essays & lectures.* J. Porte (Ed.). New York: Literary Classics of the United States.

Engebretson, J. (1996). Considerations in diagnosing the spiritual domain. *Nursing Diagnosis, 7,* 100–107.

Fehring, R. J., Miller, J. F., & Shaw, C. (1997). Spiritual well-being, religiosity, hope, depression, and other mood states in elderly people coping with cancer. *Oncology Nursing Forum, 4,* 663–671.

Fowler, J. W. (1981). *Stages of faith: The psychology of human development and the quest for meaning*. San Francisco: Harper & Row.

Fox, M. (1991). Creation spirituality: Liberating gifts for the peoples of the earth. San Francisco: Harper San Francisco.

Goddard, N. C. (1995). Spirituality as integrative energy: A philosophical analysis as requisite precursor to holistic nursing practice. *Journal of Advanced Nursing, 22,* 808–815.

Habito, R. L. F. (1993). *Healing breath: Zen spirituality for a wounded earth*. Maryknoll, New York: Orbis Books.

Hall, B. A. (1997). Spirituality in terminal illness. *Journal of Holistic Nursing, 15,* 82–96.

Hunglemann, J., Kenkel-Rossi, E., Klassen, L., & Stollenwerk, R. (1996). Focus on spiritual well-being: harmonious interconnectedness of mind-body-spirit—Use of the JAREL spiritual well-being scale. *Geriatric Nursing, 17*(6), 262–266.

Kollmar, D. (1998). Complete Self Attunement Workshop: Week 1 Intensive. Boca Raton, FL, January, 24–30.

Kollmar, D. (1999). Complete Self Attunement Workshop: Week 4 Intensive. Beckley, WV, November, 13–19.

Lesser, E. (1999). *The new American spirituality*. New York: Random House.

Macrae, J. (1995). Nightingale's spiritual philosophy and its significance for modern nursing. *Image, 27*(1), 8–10.

Mansen, J. T. (1993). The spiritual dimension of individuals: Concept development. *Nursing Diagnosis, 4,* 140–147.

Mbiti, J. S. (1975). *Introduction to African religion*. New York: Praeger Publishers.

Meraviglia, M. G. (1999). Critical analysis of spirituality and its empirical indicators. *Journal of Holistic Nursing, 17*(1), 18–26.

Moore, T. (1992). *Care of the soul*. New York: HarperCollins.

Nagai-Jacobson, M. G. & Burkhardt, M. A. (1989). Spirituality: Cornerstone of holistic nursing practice. *Holistic Nursing Practice, 3,* 18–26.

Nightingale, F. (1859/1992). *Notes on nursing: Commemorative edition*. Philadelphia: J. B. Lippincott.

Nolan, P., & Crawford, P. (1997). Towards a rhetoric of spirituality in mental health. *Journal of Advanced Nursing, 26,* 289–294.

Ornish, D. (1998). *Love & survival*. New York: Harper Perennial.

Picard, C. (1997). Embodied soul: The focus for nursing praxis. *Journal of Holistic Nursing, 15*(1), 41–53.

Reed, P. G. (1992). An emerging paradigm for the investigation of spirituality in nursing. *Research in Nursing & Health, 15,* 349–357.

Sussman, S., Nezami, E. & Mishra, S.(1997). On operationalizing spiritual experience for health promotion research and practice. *Alternative Therapies in Clinical Practice, 4,* 120–124.

Taylor, J. (1982). *Nurturing the creative impulse*. San Rafael, CA: Dream Tree Press.

Tutu, D. (1995). *An African prayer book*. New York: Doubleday.

Tsu, L. (1988). *Tao Te Ching.* London: Penguin Books.

Vardey, L. (Ed.). (1995). *God in all worlds: An anthology of contemporary spiritual writings.* New York: Pantheon Books.

Walton, J. (1996). Spiritual relationships: A concept analysis. *Journal of Holistic Nursing, 14,* 237–250.

Walton, J. (1999). Spirituality of patients recovering from an acute myocardial infarction. *Journal or Holistic Nursing, 17*(1), 34–53.

Watson, J. (1985). *Nursing: Human science and human care.* Norwalk, CT: Appleton-Century-Crofts.

Watson, J. (1999). *Postmodern nursing and beyond.* Edinburgh, Scotland: Churchill Livingston.Walton, J. (1996). Spiritual relationships: A concept analysis. Journal of Holistic Nursing, 14, 237-250.

CHAPTER 2

Healing and Spirituality

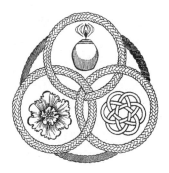

Jesus said to her, "Daughter it is your faith

that has made you whole. Now go in peace."

LUKE, 8:48

Healing and spirituality are intimately connected. Grounded in the understanding that spirituality is the essence of who we are as human beings, we believe that healing is essentially a spiritual process that attends to the wholeness of a person. The healing process occurs over time and is ongoing through our life journey. Healing is a way of living that flows from, reflects, and nourishes our spirituality.

Recent years have seen a re-awakened awareness of the relationship between healing and spirituality. The resurgence of a holistic view of persons among conventional health-care practitioners, coupled with exposure to views of sickness and healing within explanatory models from different cultures and traditions, have contributed to this awareness. Within a holistic perspective, we understand that every human experience is a whole person experience with body-mind-spirit components. We also recognize that the unitary person lives in continual interrelationship with Sacred Source, others, and all life forms on earth and within the universe. Contemporary science is learning anew what ancient and indigenous peoples have known—that all things are related. Individual healing occurs in relationship to the whole of life. Wholeness and healing imply a fluid, integral, and continual interaction within the spheres of the unitary self, and among relationships with family, friends, society, world community, and various levels of the natural and universal environment. Our choices regarding any sphere of our being or any of our relationships affects the balance and harmony of the whole. How we live and relate to others, how we care for ourselves as physical, emotional, mental, and spiritual beings, and how we relate to nature all influence our wholeness, healing, and holiness. As nurses, we recognize that the persons entrusting themselves to our care are more than the health problems that prompt their need for support. Each person is an unfolding story encompassing hopes and dreams, accomplishments and regrets, joys and sorrows, relationships, life experiences, processes of personal unfolding, insights, and different levels of awareness of their journeys to wholeness.

EXPERIENCING OUR WHOLENESS

Wholeness cannot be measured against a set of objective criteria, nor does it look or act any particular way. As nurses, we do not necessarily know what wholeness is or looks like for another. We often seek a wholeness beyond what is, rather than seeking to recognize and understand the wholeness that is present in our being as we are now. Our conscious minds divide, categorize, and seek to know all the details of the Whole. Our spirits, however, recognize the Whole in the interconnectedness of all life—the seamless garment of our being and experiences, where there is no separation. From the Buddhist tradition we learn that we become aware of our wholeness when we are awake—when we *see* what is happening in each moment, the natural order of things, how all things are interconnected, and how events unfold (Hagen, 1997). *Seeing* refers to *being with* what is happening in each moment, and is differentiated from what we *think* about what is going on. This includes being aware of our thoughts, preferences, mental calculations, and efforts to create or prevent certain actions or outcomes. Through the process of *seeing,* we recognize that our wholeness is that which sustains us, and is already in place.

Healing is a life long process of self-awareness, growth, and transformation that might become more evident when we experience illness or disease. Appreciating that healing reflects our journey to greater awareness of our wholeness enables us to recognize the organic relationship between healing and spirituality that is evident in their common grounding in wholeness. The work of healing, then, calls us to recognize the spiritual dimension of each person, including ourselves. As we attend to the wholeness of persons, we are aware that spirituality permeates every encounter, all that we are, and all that we do. The shared relationship between the caregiver and receiver acknowledging our common humanity and connectedness is both basic to healing and a manifestation of spirituality as well.

Healing and Holiness

Considering the interface of spirituality and healing calls us to clarify our understanding of terms related to these two concepts. In English, the words *heal, health, healing, whole,* and *holy* all derive from the same root: Old Saxon *hal (or haelen),* meaning *whole* (or *to become whole*), which is akin to the German *heilen,* and relates to the Greek *holos,* meaning *whole* or *entire.* The etymology of these words suggests that healing, wholeness, and holiness are closely related. Indeed, both healing and holiness draw us toward deeper awareness of and experience of our wholeness. Wholeness encompasses all of who we are—our body-mind-spirit being within our various environments and relationships and implies harmony within the unitary person.

Noting that synonyms for the word *harmony* include unity, peace, reconciliation, and connection, Quinn (1989) suggests that wholeness implies a fundamental sense of relatedness, a dynamic process of being in right relationship. This relationship contrasts with alienation and fragmentation in any area of our life. Whether we are alienated from our body, our inner self, the Sacred Source, our friends, family, environment, or society, we experience a breach in our wholeness and are dis-eased. True healing, addresses our various connections with a goal of reestablishing right relationship. An example of this perspective of healing is the Navajo belief that the natural state of all things in creation, including the human person, is that of harmony. To have a disease or illness indicates being out of harmony, and Navajo healing rituals focus on restoring harmony within the person and between the person, the spirit world, the community, and the environment. Even when a disease is "cured" by Western medicine, a traditional ceremony is necessary for healing, or the restoration of harmony, to occur. The goal of the healing ceremony, which includes the whole family and community, is restoration of a sense of connectedness within one's life, relationships, and environment.

Healing and Curing

Although the terms *healing* and *curing* are often used interchangeably, the distinction between these interrelated processes becomes apparent when they are examined within a holistic perspective of the unitary person (Burkhardt, 1985; Quinn, 1989). Although the word *cure* derives from the Latin *cura,* which means care of souls, in contemporary understanding curing refers to processes that attend to disordered physical or psychological parts of a person. Curing addresses disease, the broken or disrupted parts of a person, and restoration of the integrity of a specific component, usually physiological, of a person. Conventional medicine focuses on disease prevention and cure, generally equating cure with the elimination of the signs and symptoms of disease. Treatment and cure of disease is very important for our human existence, and modern medical advances in this area sometimes seem close to miraculous. Using antibiotics for an infection or surgically removing a diseased organ is considered a cure. Although the goal of curing is admirable, many diseases still have no cure. In the absence of a physical cure, practitioners often note, with deep regret, that their best efforts have failed and there is nothing more they can do. Contemporary medicine often loses sight of people's need for healing, whether or not a disease can be cured.

Healing, a process that is grounded in our wholeness, encompasses, yet goes beyond curing. Without implying "blame," healing acknowledges that disharmony in a whole person can manifest as disease or illness. Healing considers the personal response to and meaning of the apparent disease or illness, and seeks to understand the totality of the lived experience for the person. Physical, emotional, and spiritual concerns are all included as equally important considerations within the healing process. Healing addresses the various levels of our relationships as we move to greater awareness of our wholeness. Although healing can manifest as cure in one or more of the bio-psycho-emotional realms, it can occur in the absence of a cure. Paradoxically, a person can experience ultimate healing/wholeness through the nearing death experience (Singh, 1998). In his book *Tuesdays with Morrie*, Mitch Albom (1997) recounts the marvelous story of a man who experienced healing though no cure. A beloved university professor and very active person, Morrie Schwartz was diagnosed with the unforgiving and terminal illness amyotrophic lateral sclerosis (ALS). In taking in the impact of this "death sentence," Morrie chose to make the best of his life, to attend to his wholeness, "to live—or at least try to live—the way I want, with dignity, with courage, with humor, with compassion" (p. 21). Through the various phases of his physical deterioration, he reflected on the many blessings in life, both large and small, and helped others to experience these blessings. He encouraged visits from friends and students, enjoying the intellectual exchange and sharing the myriad of human experiences and concerns. Although not one to dwell in self-pity, he embraced his periodic feelings of anger, bitterness, and grieving related to his illness as part of the fullness of who he was. While having no hope for a physical cure, he could reflect on the many people walking around with a meaningless life because they are chasing the wrong things, and see that "the way you get meaning into your life is to devote yourself to loving others, devote yourself to your community around you, and devote yourself to creating something that gives you purpose and meaning" (p. 43). While watching his body "slowly wilt away," he could express his sense of being lucky to have all this time to say good-bye and his conviction that ultimately "Love wins. Love always wins" (p. 40). In the midst of dying, Morrie's healing became even more apparent.

Nursing and Healing

We learn from Florence Nightingale (1859/1992) that the focus of nursing is healing. She instructed nurses to put patients in the best condition for nature to act on them, to recognize that healing is a function of nature that is available to all of us. As a natural capacity of our being, healing is not given, provided or owned by the practitioner (Quinn, 1989). Although curing can be facilitated by impersonal means, and with minimal active participation by the one receiving cure, healing requires personal involvement in the process. Healing is not a technique or some-thing we do to another; rather, it is a process that is facilitated through caring rela-tionships that acknowledge our common humanity and connectedness. These relationships help to create the sacred space of healing. The paradox of healing is that, because all healing is essentially self-healing, we alone can do it, yet the rela-tional aspect of healing implies that we cannot do it alone. The examples noted ear-lier of healing within the Navajo culture and the story of Morrie Schwartz illustrate yet another truth regarding healing. Healing is not just for the individual, healing is for the whole community, for all one's relations. Healing within an individual cre-ates an energy that contributes to balance and harmony within all levels of our environment, both internal and external. Any focus on personal healing, leading to greater attunement with our wholeness, enhances planetary healing as well.

Before the advent of what we know as conventional Western medicine, spiritual-ity was considered an integral aspect of healing. As noted in Chapter 1, spirituality has been an essential part of nursing care from its beginning. With ever-expanding scientific knowledge and advances related to human health concerns, however, the belief that science can solve all problems has pushed the spiritual connection to health and healing into the background. The prevailing belief that solutions to health matters can be best addressed by science, and that any suggestion of other considerations in healing should be suspect, has helped to create the illusion of a chasm between scientific and spiritual perspectives. For many years, spirituality has been peripheral at best, in conventional Western health-care systems. However, there is a renewed interest in re-integrating this important element into contempo-rary practice—welcomed by some, viewed cautiously by others. The conventional medical paradigm teaches about disease and its treatment, with an ultimate goal of cure. Within this paradigm, there has been little sense of a need for the spiritual because of the trust that science would ultimately have the answers to human ills. However, there are still mysteries that science cannot explain. Some people live when science has predicted they will die. Some people develop health concerns or die for no reason that science can explain. Nor does science have clear understand-ing of why people with very similar clinical conditions and all the appropriate med-ical interventions can have quite different outcomes. Faced with these experiences, some scientists have begun exploring other factors that influence health and heal-ing, an exploration that leads us back to spirituality. Nursing has been at the fore-front of this exploration.

INFLUENCE OF CULTURE AND COSMOLOGY ON THE INTERFACE OF SPIRITUALITY AND HEALING

A large percentage of the world's population use health-care systems based on non- allopathic traditions of practice, or care for their health through self-care according to folk principles. Indeed, only about 10 to 30% of people worldwide receive health care primarily from conventional, biomedically oriented practitioners (Reed et al., 1994). Various cultures around the globe offer different explanatory models for understanding and dealing with health and illness, each having validity within its own context. Some models interface fairly easily with Western medicine, but others seem quite foreign to the western frame of reference. Many people who use allopathic approaches also ascribe to views from other explanatory models, and these views influence their response to explanations and therapies offered by the allopathic system. Because other explanatory models are often discounted within conventional Western medicine, people are less likely to discuss these views regarding cause and treatment of sickness with conventional practitioners. Consider, for example, a person receiving conventional medical treatment for an illness that he believes is the result of a hex. Unless appropriate interventions for dealing with the hex are initiated, the person might not respond to conventional therapies.

Examples of Different Explanatory Models

The biomedical model relates the cause of sickness to physiological factors such as microbes of many varieties, biochemical imbalances, and mechanical disruptions. Psychoemotional and environmental factors are considered, but spirituality is seldom acknowledged. Treatment focuses on eliminating offending microbes, fixing the imbalances, or repairing the disruption through pharmaceutical drugs, surgery and other therapies, and some lifestyle modifications.

Alberto Villoldo and Stanley Krippner (1987) describe the Candomblé and Umbanda traditions in Brazil, which derive from western African perspectives. Both of these traditions believe that humans have a spiritual as well as a physical body, that there are disincarnate spirits that are in constant contact with the physical world, and that humans can learn to channel beneficial spirits to assist in healing and evolution. Within these traditions, causes of disease include how one relates to others, the environment, God, and oneself, and healing requires that all these relationships be returned to harmony in addition to treating any organic cause. These traditions emphasize the importance of healing the spirit. Through entering an altered state of consciousness, the person can gain insight into the cause of illness and change patterns creating the sickness.

An explanatory model that has been a pervasive part of Western cultures before ancient Greece and Rome, and that is present in the Judeo-Christian tradition is that sickness is caused by the gods, or God. Healing therefore requires divine intervention brought about through prayer or other ritual. Two views pervasive in many cultures are that sickness occurs (1) when a person has broken a tribal law or taboo, which often affects the relationship with the whole community, or (2) through a hex or curse from another person. Healing is dependent on making amends for the transgression, or seeking intervention to remove or nullify the curse through the assistance of a medicine person or healer.

The tradition of the Pima Indians differentiates between afflictions that are futile to treat and those that are curable (Villoldo & Krippner, 1987). They believe that futile-to-treat problems, which include constipation, infant deformities, indigestion, and mental retardation, are permanent or will improve on their own. Curable problems include (1) "wandering sickness," which results from impurities that wander through the body (including germs) and is cured with herbs or medicines; and (2) "staying sickness," which results from improper behavior toward objects of power and requires the intervention of a shaman to restore the natural order.

Within the explanatory model of traditional Chinese medicine, theories of sickness relate to the concept of life force or vital energy. In this system, the body is organized as *Blood, Moisture,* and *Qi* (pronounced "chee") all manifestations of the same life force, which, together, represent all elements and processes of the soma and psyche, both visible and invisible (Beinfield & Korngold, 1991). All phenomena of the body result from the interaction among *Blood, Moisture,* and *Qi,* and sickness and healing address the relationships among the various factors affecting the generation, regulation, and accumulation of each. Disease occurs when there are patterns of disharmony; healing requires restoring and maintaining equilibrium and integrity among the dynamic and ever- changing relationships of the interconnected network that is the whole person. Beinfield and Korngold note that in the Chinese tradition, the heart enfolds the spirit and the blood, which communes with all regions of the body and houses the mind, and carries the spirit to all areas of the soma and psyche. In Chinese medicine, *spirit* refers to the totality of a person's life force, the outward expression of *Qi*, and includes the realm of the higher moral and spiritual faculties.

The Hawaiian Kahuna tradition holds that conflicts in mental and emotional energies, particularly fears and undue tension, cause illness. Healing involves breaking up tension-induced illness by stimulating energy flow or life energy through use of certain medicinal plants, types of colors and clothing, and healing foods (Villoldo & Krippner, 1987).

In our understanding of people as unitary beings, each individual's worldview is a blending of their culture and formal education. We learn cultural beliefs and values both formally, through directive education, and informally, through role-modeling. Informal learning often occurs by trial and error and is more unconscious. Through the way others react to what we say or do, we learn what is accepted and appropriate, and what is not. This more unconscious learning seems to become part of us even at the cellular level and is not as easily modified as is cognitive learning. Consider situations in which you react based on early upbringing, even though you might no longer intellectually hold your former beliefs and values. In health care, for example, the overuse or indiscriminate use of antibiotics despite information about increasing drug resistance of bacteria might be an example of learned behavior that contradicts current knowledge. Within a religious context, we might see older people who were raised in Catholic homes avoiding meat on Fridays regardless of their current faith affiliations. A more practical example is a mechanic who commented that even though cars today do not need to be warmed up by letting the engine run before driving the car, he has a hard time not warming up the car as he had seen his father do, and as he had also done for years. In the same way, people who are well schooled intellectually in the Western model can be affected by traditional cultural beliefs, whether or not they still cognitively hold the same values.

REFLECTION 2-2

In each explanatory model regarding sickness and healing described earlier consider the following:

- What are the beliefs about causes of sickness?
- How does spirituality relate to the understanding of sickness and healing?
- What is needed for healing to occur?
- Who holds the knowledge of healing, who needs to facilitate the healing process?

(continued)

• Describe your response (intellectually and emotionally) to these models.

Apply these same questions to your own worldview or explanatory model.

Culture, Cosmology, and Healing

Spirituality is an integral component of most explanatory models outside the Western worldview. This discussion will touch on the historical interface of healing and spirituality in several cultures, particularly those influencing the development of conventional Western medicine. We have more familiarity with the Judeo-Christian tradition that continues to have a predominant influence in Western societies, although increased cultural awareness and the wide interest in complementary and alternative modalities is prompting more openness to the healing benefits of other explanatory models.

The place of healing within any culture relates to its cosmology, that is, its beliefs about the nature of the universe, its origins, elements, and laws. Cosmology is an organizing way of viewing reality that incorporates both the physical plane and the transdimensional universe. A culture's cosmology is the context for ascribing meaning to, and determining relationships with, the various aspects of human experience. Each culture's cosmic story develops in response to the experiences, observations, insights, revelations, needs, interactions, and power relationships within the society. This story can shift and evolve over time with changing needs, new insights and knowledge, contact with other worldviews, and attempts by people within the culture to shift or maintain power and control. The worldview reflected in a culture's cosmic story influences roles and relationships among its members, between its members and other humans, and between its members and the natural and supernatural worlds. Beliefs about the Sacred, divine order and harmony, the source of health and cause of illness, the meaning of illness, suffering, life and death, and the presence and cause of good and evil all derive from the culture's cosmology. The cosmology also determines who can hold positions of honor and power, such as that of healer.

Within the cosmologies of most cultures across time, healing has been closely linked to understandings of the sacred and spiritual forces. For more than 100,000 years, and in many traditions today, the knowledge of healing has been held by the honored shamans or medicine people who attend to the general well-being of the community. Shamans are the revered healers in many cultures because they can commune with the supernatural world, the realm of the sacred. Shamans recognize the multilevel influences on disease and illness of our physical, mental, relational, emotional, and spiritual spheres and address all these needs in people's lives. Their communion with the powers and entities of the spiritual realm enables them to facilitate healing on these many levels.

Integral to shamanism is the awareness that all healing involves an experience of the spiritual, which can manifest in different ways, such as a sense of connection with the creative energies of all life or an encounter with the divine. In their book *Healing States,* Villoldo and Krippner (1987) describe healing beliefs and practices of shamanic traditions, shamans, and healers in North and South America. They note that shamanism is not an institutionalized religion but, rather, a tradition of knowledge about healing that transcends time and culture and manifests differently in various cultures. Shamans help to shape their society's cosmology by giving people a way of understanding their world and experiences. Shamanism refers to a consciousness that permeates life, incorporating attitudes and practices emphasizing loving concern and care for self, others, community, and Mother Earth. Shamanic traditions recognize the interaction between healing and personal lifestyle, relationships, and one's work. Within these traditions factors that contribute to illness include how one relates to the Divine, to others, to the Earth, and to oneself, as well as organic causes. Healing requires reestablishing harmony among all these relationships. These authors note that medicine women and men in North and South America believe that people rediscover their connectedness with nature and the divine through spiritual experience.

In tending to healing and the spiritual evolution of the community, shamans were the ones who located medicinal herbs, designed rituals, and created rites of passage. Villoldo and Krippner note that within different cultures a shaman might serve various functions such as artist, healer, priest, seer, storyteller, magician, and psychotherapist. These authors reflect that healing functions within a tribe resided primarily with the shaman in early hunting and gathering societies. As tribes became more sedentary, however, healing functions began to be divided between the shaman and others, leading to different groups of practitioners with specialized healing roles. Within the domain of the sacred (contrasted with the secular domain) four groups of practitioners emerged: the shaman, priest, diviner, and sorcerer or malevolent practitioner. These authors note that the number of specialized practitioners increased as a society's complexity increased, with different categories of healers holding different levels of stature.

Although all healers continue to be valued for what they offer, those who deal with the invisible realm often are considered of higher stature than are those who focus on the more mechanical aspects of healing. Achterberg (1990) describes two categories of healers in ancient Sumer, one that dealt with the invisible, magical, or spiritual realm related to disease, and the other that focused on the physical aspects of the problem. Among the Mazatec Indians of Mexico, three groups have special powers for healing (Villoldo & Krippner, 1987): The *brujos* and *brujas* (sorcerers) sell both cures and hexes, the *curanderos* and *curanderas* are herbal healers, and the *sabios* and *sabias* are the shamans or wise ones who have the greatest power for healing because it comes from Christ-Quetzalcoatl. The Navajo healing tradition provides another example of such a hierarchy of healers. Practitioners in this tradition include those who are consulted for diagnosis, those who are herbalists, and, most important, those who know the spiritual ceremonies that ultimately return the person to harmony within self, the family, community, and the natural world. Interestingly, within the Navajo perspective, Western practitioners belong to one of the first two categories of diagnostician or herbalist. Although contemporary society generally places higher value on these mechanical aspects of healing, traditional healing ways recognize that healing must address the spiritual.

In the ancient world, the esteemed roles of priestess, priest, and healer were often intertwined. Evidence from ancient Sumer, Persia, Chaldea, Babylon, and Egypt suggest that healing practices included physical interventions for disease such as use of herbs, other treatments, and surgery, as well as spiritual interventions such as prayer, dream interpretation, and other rituals. Both personal sickness and environmental disruptions and disasters were often attributed to spiritual beings—divine or demonic depending on the prevailing beliefs of the time. In her book, *Woman as Healer,* Achterberg (1990) notes that Western healing systems derived much from ancient Sumerian knowledge of body functions and disease. In Sumer, as in many ancient cultures, there was a connection between women healers and the religious beliefs. Women were respected healers in this culture because they could share the experience of the mysteries of birth, love, and healing embodied by the much-revered goddess, Inanna. Achterberg makes the following important observation regarding the influence of cosmology on the history of women as healers in the Western tradition:

Since the vocation of healer, particularly, is associated with the sacred, and the healing beliefs of any culture directly reflect the nature of the gods, only in those times when the reigning deity has had a feminine, bisexual, or androgynous nature have women been able to exercise the healing arts with freedom and power. (Achterberg, 1990, p. 3)

Women in many cultures have been the keepers of the healing arts. Perhaps this is because the work of healing, contrasted with that of curing, flows organically from our feminine nature that knows our wholeness. This perspective views the body-mind-spirit being as an intertwined and interpenetrating unity in which disruption to or healing of any one sphere affects the whole.

LEGACY OF WESTERN HEALING TRADITIONS

Knowledge, beliefs, and traditions from Sumer, Egypt, and India influenced the healing practices in Greece. In the cosmology of ancient Greece, illness was believed to be inflicted by the gods, and healing belonged to the gods as well, particularly to the god, Aesculapius. The temples of Aesculapius were the hospitals in ancient Greece, and the priests and other attendants of these temples were the healers. While staying at the temples, people would seek spiritual insight into their ailments through dreams and their interpretations, and have physical needs met through nourishing meals, being bathed, laying on of hands, receiving massages, and manipulating parts of the body. Healing in ancient Greece, including the teachings of Hippocrates, who was considered the founder of modern medicine, emphasized treating the whole person—body and soul.

Healing in the Hebrew Tradition

Healing in the Hebrew tradition was influenced by the many cultures with whom the Hebrew people lived and interacted, and by the belief in one God rather than many deities. As in other cultures, beliefs about the human person and sickness influenced the notion of healing in the Hebrew tradition. Within the Hebrew Scriptures, the person is viewed as a psychosomatic unity in which the bodily and spiritual dimensions are considered a single reality. The whole person is defined in terms of relationships—with others, self, the environment, and the covenantal relationship with their God. As with many tribal or close knit societies, one's individual identity is closely tied with that of the group, family, clan, and society (Kelsey, 1973; Seybold & Mueller, 1981). The notion of sickness in this tradition represented a rupture in relationship with God (the relationship that defined the Biblical person) and was considered a consequence of individual or communal sin. Marsh (1978) notes that the Biblical notion of sickness meant a loss of *rûah,* the spirit of life that God breathes into a person, enabling the person to be in relationship with God. In addition, sickness often carried with it a breach in relationship with society, an exclusion, and was viewed as belonging to the domain of death. The creation story in Genesis 3:7–24 provides an example of how sickness, more than something that happens to the body or mind, is an experience of a whole person within the context of multifaceted relationships. These passages describe several alienations (Spilly, 1981). An event takes place that causes a breach in relationship with God, thus destroying the harmony of Eden. Adam hides from God (alienation from God), blames Eve who blames the serpent (alienation from others), both notice their nakedness, are ashamed and cover themselves (alienation from true self), and are no longer safe with the animals and have to labor for survival (alienation from the environment).

The central belief set forth in the Hebrew Scriptures is that both sickness and healing are a manifestation of God's presence with God's people. This view is summarized in Deuteronomy 32:39, "Learn then that I, I alone am God, and there is no God besides me. It is I who bring both death and life, I who inflict wounds and heal them, and from my hand there is no rescue." We find throughout the Hebrew Scriptures the promise of health and prosperity for the covenant people if they are faithful to God (Amundsen & Ferngren, 1982). When illness occurs, restoration of fellowship with God is crucial for healing, and the chief means of restoring this relationship is through prayer. Secular practices of healing through physicians are rarely mentioned in the Hebrew Scriptures. In the early periods of Israel's history, physicians were often associated with magical and other cultural healing practices, and turning to a physician was viewed as a lack of trust in God. The change in this attitude over time is evident in the Book of Sirach (200–175 B.C.E.), which indicates that although God is still the primary healer, the physician and natural elements such as herbs are gifts from God and, thus, have a place in the healing process. References to healing in the Hebrew Scriptures reflect a holistic view of persons and the healing process that requires attention to relationship with God through prayer, with self through harmony within heart, mind, and body, and with others through right thoughts, actions, and attitudes. Healing within this worldview ultimately relates to the dynamics of covenant between God and Israel. Sickness is a consequence of turning from God, the source of life and blessing. The resulting rupture in relationship with the Giver of Life leads to alienation, which can only be healed when right relationship is restored. In love and fidelity of covenant, God offers healing, which occurs when God's love is accepted and the individual or nation returns to God.

Jesus and Healing

Healing in the Christian tradition is grounded in the life and ministry of Jesus. By the very fact that approximately 20% of the Gospels relate to Jesus' healing, we can see that healing played a prominent role in his ministry. His actions and teachings are evidence that he considered healing to be a sign of God's love and compassion for all people. Many of the Gospel healing narratives refer to Jesus having pity or compassion on the person(s). For example, Matthew 14:14 states that "when Jesus disembarked and saw the vast throng, his heart was moved with pity, and he healed their sick." In the society of Jesus' day, the sick person was still viewed as an outcast, which often meant being among the poor or marginalized. Jesus responded to this suffering by entering into relationship with the outcasts, seeing the uniqueness of each person, and restoring them to the community. He made it clear that his healing flowed from the power of God within him and was a sign of God's loving and saving presence. Healing for Jesus addressed not merely the illness, but the whole person in the context of illness and the relationships that define the person. Jesus addressed each person in his or her sickness and suffering as a unique individual, employing healing methods that met that person's needs. He healed through love, touch, word, forgiveness, presence, the use of natural elements, and faith, sometimes using one method alone and sometimes a combination of methods.

A WORD ABOUT TOUCH IN THE JUDEO-CHRISTIAN TRADITION

Humans have used touch in healing from their earliest existence. Healing through laying on of hands and touch was part of Jesus' own Jewish tradition and common within the healing traditions of the cultures to which he was exposed. In nearly half of the Gospel accounts of healing, Jesus uses touch or laying on of hands. The frequency of his use of touch suggests that this was his usual way of healing and offers us pause for reflection, especially in relation to contemporary research on the human need for touch and the use of touch in healing. In discussing Jesus' use of touch in healing, Seybold and Mueller (1981) note that there was a belief that there is a power within the miracle worker (Jesus) that flows out as a kind of aura. The transferal of this power to the sick person effects the healing, that is, where sickness is a deficiency of power, healing consists of an experience of newly acquired power, of becoming a new creation. Regarding laying on of hands, Diekman (1980) discusses the Israelite notion of the human person as a psychophysical unit in which the hand was viewed not just as an instrument but as an extension of one's self, one's personality, and one's power. Thus, touching another would be a sign of transferring something of oneself to the other. Current research on subtle energies and energy-based healing modalities supports this belief. *Healing from the Heart* by Graham, Litt, and Irwin (1998) and *Called into Healing* by Smith (2000) offer further discussion of the Judeo-Christian legacy of touch in healing.

Christianity and Healing

Jesus taught his followers about healing both the body and spirit, about wholeness, love, and forgiveness and sent them out to participate in and continue the ministry of healing. Modeling Jesus' ministry, healing was considered a natural activity of Christians and an integral part of life within the early Christian communities. As an expression of the creative power of God, given them as members of Christ, healing was a gift given to the whole community, not merely to a chosen few (Kelsey, 1973). Healing occurred within the community through prayer, laying on of hands, anointing with oil, faith, and fasting. Although the early Christian communities practiced and taught that healing was part of everyone's gifts and experience, a gradual shift away from healing as a way of life within Christian communities began to occur around the third century. Healing began to be associated primarily with special church services. Influenced by the prevalent Neoplatonist philosophy that saw body and spirit as separate, the church moved from the Biblical view of the person as an integrated whole. Accepting the notion that humans had a higher nature (soul, intellect, and will), and a lower nature (body, appetites, and emotions) the church's focus of healing began to emphasize care of soul. The church hierarchy again related sickness of the body with sin and promoted the notion that healing of sickness was dependent on confession of sins. Healing eventually became almost exclusively under the auspices of the Church, and by 800 C.E., the practice of primitive medicine in the Western world of the Latin Church was done primarily by monks and clerics (Cleary, 1982). Monasteries and convents became facilities for the care of the sick, poor, and persecuted. The lay healers (many of whom were women) were still available in communities; however, they were often looked upon with suspicion and accused of receiving their healing powers from forces other than God.

Although the practice of medicine by clergy decreased in the late Middle Ages, the church maintained a strong influence in secular medical practice even to the time of the scientific revolution in the 16th and 17th centuries. The philosophy that taught separation of body and soul prompted a split in the locus and focus of healing as well. Bodily healing belonged to science, but care of the soul and mind remained the realm of the church. The attitude that spirituality and healing are separate and that spirituality has no place in the world of science has been accepted by Western medicine for many years. People have responded to this false separation by seeking out spiritual healers and incorporating spiritual practices into their own healing.

HEALING AS A SPIRITUAL JOURNEY

As nurses who are called to be healers, we must recognize that the path of healing is a spiritual journey for both those in need of healing and those facilitating the process. The healer's path must incorporate care of the whole self, including attention to personal spirituality. Indeed, care of the spirit is a professional nursing responsibility and an intrinsic part of holistic nursing. How we care for and nurture ourselves as spiritual beings is an essential component of living in a healing way and influences our ability to effectively facilitate healing with another. The spiritual path is a life path that requires the ability and commitment to pause for reflecting and taking in what is happening within and around us, to take time for ourselves, for relationships, and for other things that animate us and to be mindful about how to nourish our spirits (Moore, 1992).

We must embody the interface of spirituality and healing. We integrate spirituality into our healing practice, not so much by what we do, but by who and how we are in every moment. Above all, we must come to know our own center and to live consciously from this inner place. As we become more facile with being in our own center, we are better able to attune or tune into ourselves in any moment, which then enables us to attune to others and whatever is in our environments. Such attunement grounds our ability to be a healing presence with another, sharing at the level of soul as well as of mind and body. With our presence, we create a sacred space in which every thought, word, or act makes evident the spiritual in the encounter. Living from our center enables us to recognize how spirituality manifests uniquely in each person and to be sensitive to particular ways of expressing spirituality that are supportive to those we encounter.

SELF-NURTURE: Supporting Spiritual Development

The healer's path must include attention to self-care, including personal spiritual growth. List five processes or activities that support your spiritual development, and regularly engage in at least three of them throughout the next week. You might wish to keep a journal of reflections on your experience.

FAITH, LOVE, AND RELATIONSHIPS

The most important thing in life is to learn how to give out love, and to let it come in. (Morrie Schwartz in Albom, 1997, p. 52)

Clinical observations and research suggest that love, faith, and relationships are especially important in the interface of spirituality and healing. They are manifestations of the deepest part of our being—our spirit or soul. These basic human needs relate each to the others, as you will see in this brief discussion, and throughout this book.

REFLECTION 1-3

Consider this statement: "The mandate to 'Love your neighbor as yourself' is not just a moral mandate. It's a physiological mandate. Caring is biological" (Lynch, cited by Ornish, 1998, p. 132).

- What do you think the author means by this statement?
- What do you believe or understand about the relationship between love and biology?
- How have you experienced the physiological effects of love and care in your own life?

(continued)

> • What does your spiritual tradition or life philosophy teach
>   about the interface of love and biology, of love and healing?

Love

The day will come when, after harnessing the ether, the winds, the tides,
gravitation, we shall harness for God the energies of love. And, on that day,
for the second time in the history of the world, man [humanity]
will have discovered fire. (Teilhard de Chardin, 1975, p. 87)

Love is a manifestation of our spirit. Love, not in the romantic sense, but in the sense of genuine care, compassion, and concern for the person's highest good, is a very powerful healer. Through his many years of working with cancer patients, Bernie Siegel (1986, 1989) has observed that many health problems relate to an inability to love ourselves and to feeling unloved by others. On the other hand, the ability to love ourselves and to love life lead to better quality of life, giving the body "live" messages. Siegel speaks of the importance of accepting ourselves as whole individuals, and the powerful effects on the body of unconditional love for self and others. Love, in this sense, implies accepting ourselves as we are in the present moment, including accepting our mortality. Being with ourselves and others in a loving way opens us to the energy of healing, of living our wholeness. Loving and living life fully brings healing even in the midst of dying. Dean Ornish (1998) suggests that our very survival as individuals, communities, and perhaps even as a species, depends on the healing power of love, intimacy, and relationships. His work with patients with heart disease has revealed that love and intimacy are intrinsically related to what keeps us well and what makes us sick, to what prompts happiness or sadness, healing or suffering. He believes that, although they may seem "soft," love and intimacy are actually the most powerful interventions he can offer to patients. The healing power of love manifests in the spiritual and emotional transformations that they often bring as well as in physical changes. Ornish notes that healing of the physical heart often follows the opening of the emotional and spiritual hearts. Research indicates that feelings of love and support can stimulate the immune system, predict the severity of coronary artery blockage, affect the development of ulcers, reduce the risk of angina pectoris, and promote longer term survival from serious illness and longer life in general. Bernie Siegel (1986) reminds us, however, that although love increases the likelihood of physical healing, it is *love,* not living forever, that is the goal. Loving makes life worth living regardless of how long we live.

Faith

In his book *Timeless Healing* (1997), Herbert Benson discusses the powerful influence of faith on healing. Faith refers to our various beliefs and expectancies about life, illness, spiritual matters, ourselves, and so on. Particularly important in health care are beliefs held by the patient, those held by the caregiver, and those generated by the relationship between the two. Benson suggests that our beliefs provide the grounding for an innate human capacity that he calls *remembered wellness.* The capacity for remembered wellness moves us toward healing. Through his years of research on the *relaxation response,* he has observed that, although the relaxation response process itself has positive health benefits, these effects are enhanced by a person's religious beliefs or life philosophy. He notes that affirmative beliefs of any kind, particularly belief in an eternal or life-transcending force, contributes to the effectiveness of bringing forth remembered wellness and that people whose focus draws on their spiritual convictions are more likely to use the process on a regular basis. He reports as well that people who, through eliciting the relaxation response, report a sense of presence of God or of an energy or power beyond themselves and who felt a closeness to this presence had better health results. Benson urges health practitioners to incorporate the power of faith into care with others by identifying beliefs and motivations important to each other, talking about and being willing to act on beliefs, and letting go and trusting the belief.

Research documents the influence of religious practice on healing (Koenig, 1999; Levin, 1996; Levin, Chatters, Ellison & Taylor, 1996; Levin, Larson, & Puchalski, 1997). The evidence suggests that many religious practices promote healthy lifestyles and behaviors that decrease risk for disease and enhance quality of life, healing, and general well-being. Religious participation provides a context for social support and a sense of connectedness that enhance physical health and emotional well-being. In his book *The Healing Power of Faith,* Koenig (1999) summarizes evidence from numerous studies of the impact on health of traditional religious faith and practice (primarily from the American Christian and Jewish perspectives). Among other things, he notes that, when compared with those who attend services less often or whose faith is not as strong, religious people tend to have healthier lifestyles, be hospitalized less often, cope better with stress, have better outcomes when they suffer from physical or emotional illness, have stronger immune systems, and generally live longer. Within these studies, *faith* refers to a confident belief in a supreme being, most frequently called God, who is loving and accessible, listens and responds to people, and desires good for humanity. Such faith provides people with a sense of meaning, satisfaction, and mastery in their lives.

Beliefs are powerful and can effect health in a negative way as well. People who believe they will get well are more likely to do so than are those who do not. Larry Dossey (1997) discusses how words, images, and beliefs can contribute to illness and even death. People who believe they have been hexed or cursed may become ill and even die unless the hex or curse is reversed. Such phenomena occur more often among people who believe the world is a dangerous or hostile place in which external forces may attack the individual who, having no inner resources to ward off the attack, must rely on outside help to combat the attack. Dossey suggests that medical diagnoses and prognoses, particularly those that imply a "death sentence" or that there is nothing that can be done, might carry with them an element of a curse. As health care practitioners, we need to be aware of the messages given in the language we use and to listen carefully for how our words are understood within the belief systems of our patients.

Relationships

> *The secret of the care of the patient is in caring for the patient.*
> *(Peabody, 1927/1984)*

Within a holistic framework, we understand that all things are connected. Our Spirit draws us to remember that implicit to our wholeness, and thus to our healing, is our connectedness with all life. Seeking healing, our spiritual being impels us toward union and communion within our body-mind-spirit self, with others, with God or Life Force, and with nature. Spirituality shapes and infuses our relationships, expresses and is experienced as we live our connectedness. We have seen that having a sense of belonging and being in right relationship with ourselves, others, nature, and God or Life Force contributes to our health and well-being. Actually, Ornish (1998) suggests that anything that promotes love and intimacy with self and others is healing, whereas things that foster separation, isolation, alienation, and fear contribute to disease and suffering. Being in loving and caring relationships has a tremendous affect on our health. This applies to relationships between patients and their health care practitioners. People want their practitioners to care about them. The imperative of caring (for self and others) that is basic to nursing practice can occur only within the context of relationship. Many facets of these relationships play a role in health and illness. What we experience as harmony or disharmony in any of these relationships varies. Every relationship and experience is a gift and an opportunity for discovering more of who we are, and for bringing us to a deeper sense of our wholeness, wherein lies our ultimate healing. We will discuss the interpenetration of spirituality and healing within each of these relationships more fully in upcoming chapters.

Prayer and Healing

Prayer is often the first thing that comes to mind when we speak of the interface of spirituality and healing. It is notable that Jesus' disciples asked not "teach us to heal" but "teach us to pray." Indeed, prayer has been an integral part of life and healing practices in all times and cultures. Most people, both those who are religious and those who are not, pray in one way or another. People pray in unique and varied ways, and most people believe that praying can heal illness. People generally would like their health-care providers to pray with and for them as well (Dossey, 1996). Prayer draws on and nourishes the healing energies of love, faith, and connectedness. Although we do not understand how prayer contributes to healing, people have always known that prayer can have a powerful effect on health and healing outcomes. Dossey's (1993; 1996; 1997) review of the scientific evidence of the influence of prayer on healing supports the benefits of prayer. Prayerful intentions that are directed in love and for the person's highest good have been shown to exert a positive influence on healing outcomes. Conversely, prayer has the potential to harm, terrify, and offend when the intention is contrary to the person's good, or what the person believes is needed. Matthews (2000) cites recent research on the healing effects of "soaking prayer" for persons with rheumatoid arthritis. In this study, prayer teams, prayed for and with patients for 12 hours, using a process that also included laying on of hands. Matthews notes that relationships and the power of presence and touch are all part of this type of healing prayer. Based on the evidence that prayer is an effective healing intervention, Dossey urges practitioners to compassionately and delicately incorporate prayer into routine patient care. Prayer draws on and flows from personal and communal beliefs, faith that there is a power from either beyond or within them that can bring about healing. The faith that prompts the prayer could be in God or Life Force, other spiritual beings, forces, or allies or might be a general trust in the healing power of Love. The relational aspect of prayer is evident in the care and concern for another or oneself that prompts the prayer, communal support, and sense of connection with divine or other spiritual beings. Further discussion of prayer and the spiritual journey is found in Chapter 6.

SPIRITUALITY AND PSYCHOLOGICAL HEALING

Addressing emotional or psychological concerns is another pathway to the spirit. The body-mind-spirit person is an integrated whole, so spiritual and psychological elements are interconnected. In fact, the term *psyche* means soul or spirit. Before the time of Freud, phenomena of the sentient realm that had no physical explanation were generally considered matters of the spirit and viewed in religious terms. As psychology has developed, however, matters of the soul have often been subsumed into psychological theory. Discussing the relationship between psychosocial and spiritual considerations, Puchalski and Romer (2000) point out that spiritual concerns can arise from questions commonly directed toward assessing the psychosocial domain such as "How are you coping with this illness?" and "What are the stresses in your life?" They note that assessing the spiritual domain requires us to move beyond how the person is coping and explore questions of meaning and purpose, relationship with God or the Divine, and issues of despair. For example, they observe that a person might be able to answer psychosocial questions by identifying family members who are supportive and professional helpers in areas of finances and resource management but still "at a very deep place inside himself or herself . . . is despairing. The person might feel that life has lost its purpose which might not come out on a psychosocial interview" (p. 130).

Historically, psychology has interpreted many spiritual experiences and manifestations as pathology. Although spiritual awakenings and deepenings might be accompanied by elements of psychological distress, it is inappropriate to label these spiritual issues as psychopathology. Interpretations of the life of Florence Nightingale offer an example of how behaviors, emotions, and reactions associated with individual experiences and expressions of the spiritual have been misinterpreted. Many of her behaviors and the health concerns she had after her return from the Crimea have been interpreted by some as psychological pathology, such as anxiety neurosis, malingering, depression, and stress burnout. Reviewing Nightingale's life from a broader perspective that recognized the presence of her deep spirituality, however, Barbara Dossey (1998a; 1998b; 1998c; 2000) has provided a fuller understanding of these behaviors.

Although the familiarity and comfort with the spiritual nature of different levels of consciousness found in Eastern and indigenous traditions has been limited in Western traditions, contemporary psychological models such as psychosynthesis, logotherapy, transpersonal, humanistic, and Jungian psychology offer pathways for incorporating the spiritual dimension into the healing process. The "dark night of the soul," which is part of the spiritual journey for many, could be a very important part of the process of moving to greater awareness and enlightenment. Spirituality can also be an important factor in healing emotional wounds and trauma. The Twelve Step program of Alcoholics Anonymous is an example of how spirituality is integral to such healing.

As nurses recognize the interplay between spiritual and psychological spheres, they can more effectively distinguish between spiritual cues, spiritual crises, and psychopathology and recognize opportunities to foster spiritual growth.

REFERENCES

Achterberg, J. (1990). *Woman as Healer.* Boston: Shambhala.

Albom, M. (1997). *Tuesdays with Morrie.* New York: Doubleday.

Amundsen, D. & Ferngren, G. (1982). Medicine and religion: Pre-Christian antiquity. In M. Marty & K. Vaux (Eds.). *Health/Medicine and the Faith Tradition,* (pp. 52–93). Philadelphia: Fortress Press.

Beinfield, H. & Korngold, E. (1991). *Between Heaven and Earth: A guide to Chinese medicine.* New York: Ballantine Books.

Benson, H. (1997). *Timeless healing: The power and biology of belief.* New York: Fireside Books.

Burkhardt, M. A. (1985). Nursing, health, and wholeness. *Journal of Holistic Nursing, 3*(1), 35–36.

Cleary, F. (1982). The church in health care: Reflections and projections. *Hospital Progress, 63,* 38–45.

Diekman, G. (1980). The laying on of hands in healing. *Liturgy, 25*(2), 11–14.

Dossey, B. M. (1998a). Florence Nightingale: A 19th century mystic. *Journal of Holistic Nursing, 16*(2), 111–164.

Dossey, B. M. (1998b). Florence Nightingale: Her Crimean fever chronic illness. *Journal of Holistic Nursing, 16*(2), 168–196.

Dossey, B. M. (1998c). Florence Nightingale: Her personality type. *Journal of Holistic Nursing, 16*(2), 202–222.

Dossey, B. M. (2000). *Florence Nightingale: Mystic, visionary, healer.* Springhouse, PA: Springhouse Corporation.

Dossey, L. (1993). *Healing words.* San Francisco: Harper San Francisco.

Dossey, L. (1996). *Prayer is good medicine.* San Francisco: Harper San Francisco.

Dossey, L. (1997). *Be careful what you pray for . . . You just might get it.* San Francisco: Harper San Francisco.

Graham, R., Litt, F., & Irwin, W. (1998). *Healing from the heart: A guide to Christian healing for individuals and groups.* Winfield, BC: Woodlake Books.

Hagen, S. (1997). *Buddhism Plain and Simple.* Boston, Charles E. Tuttle.

Kelsey, M. (1973). *Healing and Christianity: In ancient thought and modern times.* New York: Harper &Row.

Koenig, H. G. (1999). *The healing power of faith.* New York: Simon & Schuster.

Levin, J. S. (1996). How religion influences morbidity and health: Reflections on natural history, salutogenesis and host resistance. *Social Science and Medicine, 43,* 849–864.

Levin, J. S., Chatters, L. M., Ellison, C. G., & Taylor, R. J. (1996). Religious involvement, health outcomes, and public health practice. *Current Issues in Public Health, 2,* 220–225.

Levin, J. S., Larson, D. B., & Puchalski, C. M. (1997). Religion and spirituality in medicine: Research and education. *Journal of the American Medical Association, 278*(9), 792–793.

Marsh, J. (1978). A theology of anointing the sick. *Furrow, 29*(2), 89–101.

Matthews, D. A. (2000, October 12). *The faith factor.* Presentation at Ecumenical Institute, San Antonio, TX.

Moore, T. (1992). *Care of the soul.* New York: HarperCollins.

Nightingale, F. (1859/1992). *Notes on nursing: Commemorative edition.* Philadelphia: J. B. Lippincott.

Ornish, D. (1998). *Love & survival.* New York: Harper Perennial.

Peabody, F. W. (1927/1984). The care of the patient. *Journal of the American Medical Association, 252*(6), 813–818.

Puchalski, C. & Romer, A. L. (2000). Taking a spiritual history allows clinicians to understand patients more fully. *Journal of Palliative Medicine, 3*(1) 129–137.

Quinn, J. F. (1989). On healing, wholeness, and the haelan effect. *Nursing and Health Care, 10*(10), 553–556.

Reed et al. (1994). Alternative systems of medical practice. In National Institutes of Health, *Alternative medicine: Expanding medical horizons* (NIH Publication NO. 94–066). Washington, DC: Government Printing Office.

Seybold, K., & Mueller, U. (1981). *Sickness and healing.* (S. Stott, Trans.). Nashville, TN: Abingdon Press.

Siegel, B. S. (1986). *Love, medicine & miracles.* New York: Harper & Row.

Siegel, B. S. (1989). *Peace, love & healing.* New York: Harper Perennial.

Singh, K. W. (1998). *The Grace in dying.* San Francisco: Harper San Francisco.

Smith, L. L. (2000). *Called into healing: Reclaiming our Judeo-Christian legacy of healing touch.* Arvada, CO: HTSM Press.

Spilly, A. (1981). Alienation, reconciliation, unity: Dynamics in effective pastoral care. *Hospital Progress, 62,* 54–57, 66.

Teilhard de Chardin, P. (1975). *Toward the future.* (René Hague, Trans.). San Diego, CA: Harvest.

Villoldo, A., & Krippner, S. (1987). *Healing states: A journey into the world of spiritual healing and shamanism.* New York: Fireside Books.

CHAPTER 3

Mystery and Meaning

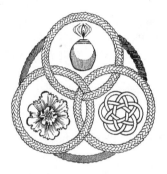

We shall not cease from exploration

And the end of all our exploring

Will be to arrive where we started

And know the place for the first time

T. S. ELLIOT—FOUR QUARTETS

Spirituality enables us to be with the mystery and meaning we encounter along our life's journey—to appreciate life as a mystery that we are called to live rather than as a problem we must solve. Where our mind seeks to understand the "why" of life experiences, our spirit draws us to know more fully the truth of our being as we live the experience. Throughout history, humans have devised varied explanations for the many events and experiences of living that do not seem to make sense. We want to know why there is suffering, why we are born, what happens when we die, why our family and life circumstances are as they are, why "this" is happening to me. Interestingly we do not ask "why" as frequently when we are joyful, feeling loved and loving, or feeling content with our lives. We wonder "what if" we were born at a different time, in a different family, followed another life path, could see the future. Our "why" and "what if" questions reflect an innate human need for having our lives and life experiences count for something—to have meaning and purpose in our lives.

MEANING AND PURPOSE

We never cease to stand like curious children before the great Mystery into which we are born. (Einstein, in Mayer & Holms, 1996, p. 37)

Understanding that meaning and purpose in life is a basic element of spirituality is well documented in the nursing literature (Barker, 1989; Burkhardt, 1989; 1994; Emblen, 1992; Haase, Britt, Coward, Leidy & Penn, 1992; Mansen, 1993; Meraviglia, 1999; Walton, 1999). Experiencing a lack of meaning and a sense of emptiness and unworthiness contributes to spiritual and emotional distress and can ultimately manifest as physical ailments as well. Viktor Frankl (1984) regards striving to find meaning as the primary motivation in life—that "something" for the sake of which to live. Although the ideals and values that provide a context for meaning may derive from a person's culture, family, society, religion, Frankl notes that meaning is personal and individual in that it must and can be fulfilled by each person alone. He believes that knowing there is meaning in life, having a sense of personal worthiness and purpose, can help a person survive the worst conditions. Willard (1998) writes that meaning is not a luxury but is essential to human life. He considers meaning to be " a kind of spiritual oxygen . . . that enables our souls to live . . . a 'going beyond,' a transcendence of whatever state we are in toward that which completes it" (p. 386). Having a general sense of meaning in life or being able to derive meaning from a particular experience such as an illness positively affects physical and emotional health, self-esteem, transpersonal and spiritual development, and sense of having the inner resources to deal with life's challenges.

Encountering mystery, uncertainty, and the unknown in our lives engenders two basic types of responses, neither of which is mutually exclusive because any experience can have elements of both. We might feel fear, anxiety, anger, and a tendency to recoil or at best approach mystery with trepidation. We could also respond with awe, wonder, gratitude, or a sense of adventure and embrace mystery with trust. Meaning unfolds as we are able to embrace both the fear and wonder of mystery.

Be patient with all that is unresolved in your heart, and try to love the questions themselves. Do not seek for the answers that cannot be given, for you wouldn't be

able to live with them, and the point is to live everything. Live the questions now,
and perhaps without knowing it, you will live along someday into the answers.
(Rilke, in Dass, 2000, pp. 151–152)

As nurses, we are called to address our own questions in the face of mystery, while recognizing that we cannot determine the meaning of an experience for another. We can, however, help people to draw on the inner resources and other supports that enable them to affirm or to discover meaning in their various life experiences. Although we need not have answers for their questions, we can be with them as they live their own questions. Spiritual caregiving calls us to be with another in openness and love, creating a safe and sacred space in which to explore the questions, delve into the mystery, and seek meaning. We start by assisting others to become more fully aware of and to honor their current feelings and reactions without judgment. We can acknowledge and explore that which gives meaning to their lives. Through reflections such as "You seem to really enjoy spending time with your grandchildren," "Your work at the homeless shelter seems to be very personally satisfying," "Your Bible study group seems very important to you," we help to name sources of meaning and open to further discussion of what is important in their lives. Reflecting our awareness of their fear or anxiety opens an avenue to explore factors contributing to these feelings. We can provide an opening with questions such as "You seem worried about your mother's x-ray." "From what you have been saying, it seems like you are wondering what your life has been all about." "What makes you feel that you deserve this illness?" Exploring where they feel alienated or disconnected from themselves, others, God or Sacred Source, or the universe helps in understanding sources of their suffering. Asking what helps them get through difficult times, what is important or meaningful in their lives, and how they nourish their spirits provides an opportunity for remembering resources that can be called on in this situation.

REFLECTION 3-1

- When and how have you experienced a sense of your life's meaning and purpose?
- Describe your sense of meaning and purpose today.
- What were the external or internal stimuli for these experiences?
- Describe how your values or sense of purpose have changed through your life. What has influenced these changes?

LIVING LIFE'S QUESTIONS

The Tao that can be told is not the eternal Tao. The name that can be named is not the eternal name. The nameless is the beginning of heaven and earth. The named is the mother of ten thousand things. Ever desireless, one can see the mystery. Ever desiring, one can see the manifestations. These two spring from the same source but differ in name; this appears as darkness. Darkness within darkness. The gate to all mystery. (Lao Tsu, 1972)

Life's deepest concerns and experiences are spiritual in nature. Because such concerns are not quantifiable, they are more authentically expressed as questions, tentative definitions, or as mystery—that truth which is beyond understanding and explanation (Burkhardt & Nagai-Jacobson, 2000). Our spirits call us to discover meaning as we live our questions and embrace life's inherent mystery. We discover meaning as we awaken to the experiences of our whole being. Meaning is something we feel and sense as a deep knowing in the stillness of our heart. In this sense meaning is not some thing that can be apprehended in a purely intellectual way, although we engage our cognitive self in comprehending meaning. Meaning, as David Steindl-Rast (1984) notes, is more like a light that illuminates our experience and allows us to see what is there. He reflects that the heartbeat of the spiritual journey is the quest of the human heart for meaning. We become aware of a restlessness in our hearts that can be satisfied, not by the many "things" of our world, but only by the "no thing" of meaning that we discover when our hearts rest in the Source of all meaning. This restlessness of the heart "leads from the misery of being alienated (often in the midst of pleasure) to the joy of being together with self, with all, with God (often in the midst of suffering) . . . To find meaning means finding how all belongs together and to find one's place in that universal belonging. And that means finding the heart" (Steindl-Rast, p. 37).

REFLECTION 3-2

- What words do you associate with the experience of mystery, that which is unexplainable?

- What in your life causes you to question or ponder? How do you seek support and insight as you live with these questions?

- How do you react when faced with the unknown, with uncertainty?

- Where do you find your support and strength?

ENCOUNTERING MYSTERY

The most beautiful thing that we can experience is the mysterious. It is the source of all true art and science. (Einstein, in Mayer & Holms, 1996, p. 38)

When we encounter that which is troubling or unexplainable, embracing the mystery often sustains us in the unknowing. What is beyond human understanding is considered mystery, and often beyond control. Fear, anxiety, and a need for explanation are common human responses to experiencing lack of control and being at the mercy of the unknown. The cosmology of a culture, religion, or spiritual tradition offers a way of relating to the mystery that is all around us. Cultural stories, myths, beliefs, and practices arise from these explanations. The stories change as understanding of how and why things happen deepens and becomes more clear. History shows us that the mystery of one era can become the known fact of another. Take, for example, explanations for the spread of disease before and after the discovery of microbes. Although we might discover explanations for some mysteries, many life experiences seem to defy explanation. We might understand what causes certain diseases or natural disasters, yet have no good answer for why they occur—at this time, to these people. We also continue to be faced with questions that philosophers, theologians, and common folk alike have pondered throughout the ages. Why are we here? How did our world, our universe come into being? What sustains us? Who or what is the Mystery beyond all of our understanding?

Ultimately, we all are dealing with these same questions at some level of our awareness. When faced with mystery, spirituality supports and encourages us as we question and seek to make sense of what is going on. The spirit-self calls us to enter ever deeper into Mystery with trust rather than fear, appreciating that moving further into the darkness enables us to come to know and appreciate the light. Because mystery simply is a part of our life journey, accepting and finding a comfort level with mystery is a part of our spiritual journey. Mystery may be understood as Truth that we cannot yet understand.

How people face the unknown is highly personal. The kinds of questions we ask, what gives us encouragement or solace, how we share or process our reactions, and the like vary among different people. Esber Tweel (2000) shares his story as an example of one person's journey into the unknown. In the midst of his roles as Episcopal priest and pastor, husband, father, counselor, and martial arts enthusiast, keeping in shape physically was important to Esber. So, it is not hard to imagine the deep concern and fear that he experienced when he started losing the use of his muscles for no apparent reason. One of the ways that Esber dealt with his experience of facing the unknown during the diagnostic phase of (and throughout) his illness was by keeping a journal and periodically sharing reflections on his process with his congregation. As you read this reflection about his encounter with the unknown, do your best to journey with him. Be aware of where and how questions of meaning arise, what engenders fear, where he finds solace, and how receiving a diagnosis was only one step in this journey with mystery.

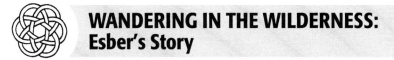

WANDERING IN THE WILDERNESS: Esber's Story

Several months ago when a tornado uprooted an oak tree and plopped it upon our building, a part of our substructure collapsed under its weight. One might say the muscle of our building was destroyed and a segment of our facility became vulnerable to the elements. It could not fulfill its mission—the task of shelter and comfort to our people. Within a couple of months, my substructure began to collapse, unbeknownst to me. A part of me that I felt was in good shape began to fail me, making me very vulnerable to the elements of living. When it began to happen, I fought against it with everything that I had, emotionally and physically. I did not want to give in to the breakdown that I was noticing. I had no idea of the storm that was raging within me. I remember awakening one night and telling my wife that I felt I was watching my body die, and I could not do anything about it. I felt powerless over my being; that which I had trusted, betrayed me. How was this happening? What was causing this? This became the wilderness wandering from within. During the time of the wilderness and the waiting for an answer as to what the name of the unclean spirit was that had invaded my body was agony. Your mind begins to play tricks on you. You think of the worst possible disease to the most minor one; but in the back of your mind you keep entertaining the black cloud which is the most traumatic one. You dance with it, it engulfs your mind, and at times you feel possessed by it. And finally there is the frantic rush to poke, to probe, to picture take, to blood suck, to analyze, to sticking of pins and needles, to electrical impulses on the muscles, to the biopsies; and from stem to stern you are scrutinized from the macro-world to the micro-world. It becomes "the invasion of the body snatchers!" Finally the long awaited word was verbalized—polymyositis. In first hearing it, I thought of some Chinese dinner plus squid! With this information, into the hospital you must go, where your identity is left at the door, where floppy gowns bare all, and where every secretion known to humankind is tested, bottled, and tubed. Injections are given, more pictures of your inner body are taken, more probing done. You become this biological and physiological phenomenon under microscopic eyes. Then comes the medication to shock your body back into a sense of stability, which puts you into a roller coaster spin—with its ups and downs, highs and lows, creating a shock wave internally which shakes every fiber in your system. Your body is in right field and your mind is in outfield. Bonhoeffer's words come to mind: "you may do with my body what you want and control every movement of it, but you can never control my spirit." This became the "calming of the storm." (Tweel, 2000)

FEAR AND STRESS

The fear and anxiety we feel when faced with the unknown or with uncertainty causes general tension and produces a systemic physiologic response within our whole being. The dis-ease engendered by our reaction to fear can manifest as a disruption in any sphere of our body-mind-spirit being. Fear, and the often accompanying anger, can arise from or prompt feelings of alienation or disconnection experienced in our relationships with ourselves, others, with nature, or with Sacred Source. These emotional responses cause feelings of further separation, which engender loneliness, questioning our belonging, wondering about our survival, and sensing the world as an unfriendly and unsafe place.

An editorial in the *Journal of Alternative and Complementary Medicine* (1999) discusses "diseases of meaning" as a major cause of suffering and death worldwide. This editorial echoes Margaret Newman's (1994) understanding of disease as a meaningful state that is ultimately a manifestation of health rather than an unavoidable alien entity aimed at afflicting or destroying the person. The editorial suggests that widespread disempowering paradigms, which are largely unconsciously held by individuals and societies, are at the root of diseases of meaning. Disease in these paradigms is viewed as failure or weakness rather than as an opportunity for growth, learning, and deepening awareness of who we are. Because our thoughts, feelings, and perceptions create biochemical changes, our perceived meaning regarding health and illness and how we live out these perceptions can be a determining factor in whether our health manifests as disease or as balance and harmony. The editorial suggests that we need to ask questions and develop processes to promote aspirational or inspirational health, derived from a shift in understanding and perceptions that address meaning in all life experiences, including that of illness.

REFLECTION 3–3

- Consider a situation in which you felt fear or anxiety when faced with mystery or uncertainty. How did this situation affect you physically, emotionally, spiritually?

(continued)

- How does your religious or spiritual tradition offer you support in dealing with stress, or anxiety, or the unknown?
- How does your religious or spiritual tradition contribute to feelings of stress or anxiety in any area of your life?

We know that our thoughts and emotions affect our total well-being and that stress contributes to illness within all spheres of our physical, mental, emotional, and spiritual selves. The same physiological response to a threat occurs whether the threat is real or imagined. The generalized stress response includes tightened muscles; increased heart rate; more rapid breathing with increased oxygen consumption; decreased blood flow to hands and feet, causing them to feel cold; increased blood pressure, brain wave activity, and sweating; closing down of the energy fields; and overall increased anxiety. Although these responses help us when faced with an emergency, when we chronically carry them in our being they can throw our systems off balance in many ways, including depressing the immune system.

Personal and cultural belief systems regarding the nature of the universe and of the Divine can contribute to healing or increase our stress when faced with uncertainty or the unknown. Believing the universe and the Divine to be ultimately friendly, loving, and supportive enables people to draw on this love and support and find meaning in the experience. In his book, *Man's Search for Meaning*, Viktor Frankl (1984) tells the story of a young woman in the concentration camp who, knowing she would die soon, reflected that she was grateful for her experience. She noted that before the travesty of the Nazi occupation she had been spoiled and not very interested in spiritual accomplishments. In her loneliness while sick in the camp she talked to a tree that she could see outside the window. She found great comfort and hope in the response that she heard through this conversation "I am here—I am here—I am life, eternal life" (p. 90). In contrast, viewing the universe as a dangerous place and the Divine as vengeful, punishing, or uninvolved can add to the experience of fear and anxiety in the face of mystery.

In the following reflection, Esber shares some thoughts regarding fears that arise when facing uncertainty. Consider what he has to say in relation to your own experiences of fear and in relation to what you have encountered with patients. How is his spiritual journey reflected in what he has to say?

WRESTLING WITH INNER DARKNESS: Esber's Continuing Journey

Evening comes and it's time to rest, but what does your brain do? It decides to wake up, even though you have been on drugs all day and you think something should knock you out. But these thoughts are stronger than any sedative. Your mind awakens to the goblins and the crawly things that hide behind the desk in secluded corners, behind the brain, which only come out when the sun goes to bed. The great dialogue and talk show appears on the stage of your mind, and suddenly questions appear before your eyeballs. "Where are you God?" "What happens if I die?" (I would be dead.) "What is death like?" "What would happen to my family and my children?" "Where would they live and what would they do?" "What would happen to the business?" "Will I be like this forever?" etc., etc. When this barrage of discouraging questions floods your brain from the cyberspace of your mind, your heart starts pounding, you start tossing and turning, and there is no possible way you can go back to sleep until you wrestle with your inner darkness. The questions and dialogue are not unusual. It's a way of the conscious mind emptying out its despair and suffering in order to give us a sense of cleansing and recognition. Even in the tomb of our minds, light does shine in the darkness. (Tweel, 2000)

SELF-NURTURE: Wrestling with your Fears

Esber offers these helpful hints for wrestling with our inner darkness, especially when it shows up at night. Try one or more of these when fear visits you.

- Go to the bathroom and relieve yourself, this is a physical act of relieving your mind and your body of what you don't want in it.

- The questions are there, allow yourself to pass through them, get out of bed and turn the light on.

- Let yourself know that these questions will be gone by the first ray of sunlight, you don't have to solve all of your problems entangled with your own fears.

- Find a place where you feel safe and secure in your own mind. Begin to imagine and physically see and hear the sounds that create an atmosphere of harmony and tranquility. It can be anywhere you want. It could be a fantasy or an isolated spot where you feel peace and safety.

- Read something away from your bed, it could be a poem, or a short verse that brings you back to focus.

- The best of all: sauté some onions with garlic, basil, and extra virgin olive oil. Make it a good sandwich, with a cold one. This will definitely keep you awake! (Tweel, 2000)

CONNECTING WITH INNER QUIET

Facilitating the process of being with mystery and discovering meaning, for ourselves or others requires a familiarity with, and ability to connect with, our inner quiet. Indeed, connecting with the inner self is essential for healing. Spiritual traditions throughout the ages have taught practices for pausing, calming, paying attention, and connecting with our inner selves. These practices provide a way of dealing with the stress response and accessing our innate potential for healing as they help us to trust in the uncertainty and open us to opportunities for experiencing love and support rather than fear. Connecting with our inner self and discovering our own inner resources, that which gives us strength, provide a lens through which we see meaning even in the midst of suffering. Within and through our inner self, we encounter the Sacred Source and have the opportunity to experience this Great Mystery, not as something to be feared, but as the very ground of our being. Using the metaphor of the ocean and the wave, the Mystery is like the ocean, and we are each waves of the ocean. In the same way that the wave is fully everything that is the ocean, so we are part of the Mystery and the Mystery fully abides in us. Our souls call us to remember that we are each an expression of this Great Mystery, and invite us into the inner stillness where we can access that which is beyond cognitive understanding. The goal of the spiritual journey is to enter more deeply into the Mystery, where we let go of our usual way of "knowing" in the cognitive sense and move instead to the knowing of our heart. When we open ourselves to Mystery, God, Sacred Source abiding in our hearts, we are transformed and relate to our various experiences in a different way. Entering into the mystery means letting go of our need to control and to know in the cognitive sense and trusting that we, as the wave, are fully part of the ocean. Recognizing our oneness with this Source of our being, our inner knowing is able to say "yes" to the mystery and be opened to discovering meaning in every circumstance, whether we judge the experience to be good or not. Regarding God's presence in all of life's circumstances, Elie Wiesel (1972) writes,

God is present even in evil, even in sin. He takes part in creation and chooses the side of man [humanity]. For whoever creates affirms that the creative act has meaning which transcends the act itself. And what is love if not a creative act, in which two beings fuse into a single consciousness scarred and healed a thousand times? Love's mystery resides in oneness and so does God's. "Whatever is above is also down below." Between the present concrete world and

the other, the one to come, there is a link as between source and reflection . . .
In man's [humanity's] universe everything is connected because nothing is
without meaning. (pp. 31–32)

Entering into the mystery helps us to see with different eyes, to recognize the
presence of the Sacred, of God in both joy and suffering, and to know that both
can be healing. The paradox of Mystery, that we see illustrated in various stories
of people shared throughout this book, is that the deepest suffering or "dark night
of the soul" can also be a source of great joy, even transformation.

 ## SELF-NURTURE: Accessing the Inner Quiet

There are many ways to access our inner quiet. Regular practice of
connecting with the inner self helps us to access this space more easily when we are faced with situations that may engender fear and anxiety or
prompt deep questions. We can access the still point within ourselves through
prayer of the heart and meditation. Pausing to pay attention to our breathing, to
carefully observe something in our surroundings, or to listen to sounds in our
environment are other ways of becoming still. Walking a familiar path; sitting
quietly in a favorite place; doing yoga, t'ai chi, or qigong; doing an activity that
relaxes us and requires little mental attention are other ways of connecting with
the inner self.

- Incorporate a regular practice of accessing your inner quiet into your daily life
  for 10–20 minutes once or twice a day. You might consider a practice such as
  the *Relaxation Response* (Benson, 1997), *Centering Prayer* (Keating, 1995), or
  some other process of meditation or prayer of the heart.

- Take a moment right now to attune to your breathing. Merely pay attention to
  your breathing without trying to change it. Follow its pattern. Feel the air moving through your nostrils and into your lungs as you inhale, and back again as
  you exhale. As you do this, pay attention to the space between your breaths.
  Spend a few minutes just being with you who is breathing. After a while notice
  how your physical self is feeling and what is going on with your emotional
  self—just observing, without judgment.

- When you are faced with mystery, are feeling anxious, or are dealing with deep
  questions, meet the mystery, anxiety, or questions in your inner quiet and just
  be with it. Allow yourself to feel the presence of the mystery, the anxiety, the
  questions, from the place of being grounded in your inner quiet. Pay attention
  to any insights or subtle shifts in your feelings without needing to have them
  change or to have answers.

THE MYSTERY OF SUFFERING

*The most helpful discovery of today has been that right in the midst
of my sorrows there is always room for joy. Joy and sorrow are sisters, they live
in the same house. (Macrina Wiederkehr in Rupp, 1997, p. 91)*

Suffering, one of the core issues and mysteries of our human existence, involves disconnectedness and lack of meaning (Cassell, 1992). People throughout the ages have struggled to understand the nature and meaning of suffering, particularly suffering that seems irrational. Cultural and religious traditions have been shaped in part through their attempts to make sense of suffering. Suffering may be a transformative experience that varies with each individual. Suffering relates to our attitude toward an experience and is different from pain, which is an experience that can prompt suffering. In other words, we can be in pain and suffering, or be in pain and not suffer (de Mello, 1998). The experience of pain is not always avoidable, whereas we can choose how we react to the pain. Reactions to suffering range from new depths of spiritual awareness to great despair, and many degrees or combinations of both experiences. This is illustrated in a story told by Anthony de Mello (1998, p. 71).

A certain master was asked by his disciple, "What has enlightenment brought you?" And he said, "Before enlightenment, I used to go around depressed; after enlightenment, I remain depressed!" But there is a great difference. Suffering means letting yourself be disturbed by depression. That is suffering. This much should be clear by now. Suffering means letting oneself be disturbed by pain, by depression, by anxiety.

Suffering that appears meaningless often engenders feelings of anger and frustration. Born of his own experiences of great suffering in the Nazi concentration camps, Frankl (1984) reflects that the ability to choose our attitudes in a given set of circumstances is the ultimate freedom that enables us to find the meaning in suffering. He writes,

If there is a meaning in life at all, then there must be a meaning in suffering. Suffering is an ineradicable part of life, even as fate and death. Without suffering and death human life cannot be complete. The way in which a man accepts his fate and all the suffering it entails, the way in which he takes up his cross, gives him ample opportunity—even under the most difficult circumstances—to add a deeper meaning to his life. (p. 88)

Suffering wears many faces, and we experience suffering in all of our physical, mental, emotional, and spiritual spheres. Suffering engendered by emotional, spiritual, or psychological pain is often more profound than that resulting from physical pain. We see this among victims of domestic violence who reflect "I would rather he hit me" than be subjected to emotional or verbal abuse. In his book *Ethics for the New Millennium,* the Dalai Lama (1999) observes that in the midst of the prosperity of modern society there is a prevalence of loneliness and alienation. Modern society's strong emphasis on autonomy and independence has caused people to lose sight of the underlying interconnectedness and interdependence of everything within the web of life. The lack of a sense of belonging or connectedness contributes to much of the psychological and emotional suffering that people experience. Such inner suffering in turn contributes to stress-related diseases.

Observing that meaningless suffering can lead to spiritual disintegration, Emblen and Pesut (2001) offer a model to guide care of people who are suffering. They note that helping people to find transcendent meaning in the suffering experience is an important attenuator of suffering. Attention to the five areas of assessment included in this model enable nurses to facilitate the realization of transcendent meaning in suffering by patients and families. In this model, assessment and intervention focus on the following: (1) authority and guidance—whatever people use to discover, express, and confirm their beliefs about illness and suffering, including who and what they draw on for guidance and direction; (2) experience and emotion—past experiences with suffering and current affective state, including experiences that support feeling good about who they are and that provide meaning; (3) community—relationships people draw on for support when suffering, including the type of support persons desire; (4) rituals and practices—reflective processes that help people cope with the suffering experience, including religious observances, prayer, meditation, journaling, physical exercise, and guided imagery; and (5) vocation and consequences—how the suffering is affecting duties and obligations, including identifying obligations that are particularly important and both current and future affect of the illness and suffering on the obligation.

The Dalai Lama (1999) notes that all people around the globe, whatever their circumstances, share a common desire to be happy and avoid suffering. The paradox is that the suffering from which we wish to be free is an inalienable part of our existence, and our experience of suffering connects us to others. He suggests that all the world's major religions provide directives regarding how to deal with suffering and achieve lasting happiness. Perceptions of what will bring happiness or cause suffering vary, but the inclination toward happiness and away from suffering is in our nature. Hope sustains us in our quest for happiness.

Hope

Hope is desire accompanied by expectation of fulfillment. The expectation of hope goes beyond merely believing or wishing and involves envisioning that the desired circumstances can become reality. In their research regarding hope, Morse and Doberneck (1995) identify seven abstract and universal conceptual components of hope that manifest in different patterns depending on the degree and context of the threat or predicament that is experienced. They describe hope as a multidimensional concept that includes: (1) a realistic initial assessment of the predicament or threat; (2) envisioning alternatives and setting goals; (3) bracing for negative outcomes; (4) realistic assessment of personal resources and external conditions or resources; (5) solicitation of mutually supportive relationships; (6) continuous evaluation for signs that reinforce the chosen goals; and (7) a determination to endure. These authors stress the importance of setting goals and developing a feasible plan for goal attainment that acknowledges risks and consequences of not attaining the goal, noting that people who do not know what to hope for are without hope. Because hoping is an active process, soliciting mutually supportive relationships help to sustain hope through the ongoing process of evaluating and modifying strategies across the time between goal setting to attainment.

Kaye (1996) suggests that the reality of hope takes on a different perspective with persons who are terminally ill. Although "becoming obsessed with hope for a cure in the face of advancing disease is inappropriate and becomes disheartening," there are realistic and appropriate hopes that give meaning to a person's days (p. 265). Examples of such hopes include being able to walk again, getting home for a time, feeling better tomorrow, being remembered, and having a stronger trust in God or Life Beyond the present experience. When we are caring for people who are dying, he encourages us to provide the best support we can as we realistically face the issues of the moment, restore as much control as possible to the patient and family, allow for their hope, and join our hope with theirs.

As an attitude of the heart, hope is a feeling, a passion for the possible that affects the whole person. Hope is future oriented, yet the anticipation of the goal or desire is in the present. In this sense, hope contains elements of both the already and not-yet. Steindl-Rast (1984) comments that the already and not-yet coincide in God and that hope is God's life within us that holds the present open for an ever new and fresh future. Hope can be a general sense that the future is somehow in safekeeping. When focused on more specific concerns, hope implies a goal or desire for a particular event or outcome. Where there is no hope, there is despair. How often as nurses have we seen a person's health status change when they "give up hope." On the other hand, the saying "hope springs eternal" reflects an energy of the spirit that continually prompts us to anticipate that tomorrow things will be better, or at least different! Hope helps us deal with fear and uncertainty, and enables us to envision positive outcomes. Hope is a significant factor in overcoming illness and in living through difficult situations. Frankl (1984) illustrates this with a poignant story of a friend in the concentration camp who had a dream in which he was told when the war would be over for him, when his camp would be liberated. As the date he heard in the dream approached and there was no indication that they would be freed on that promised day, this man suddenly became ill. The day his prophecy told him that his suffering would be over, he lost consciousness and died the next day, apparently of typhus. He had lost hope. Frankl reflects that the severe disappointment engendered by the lack of liberation lowered this man's resistance against typhus and caused him to lose his will to live.

In contrast to this type of experience, more recent research documents a positive correlation among hope, spiritual well-being, and religiosity (Fehring, Miller & Shaw 1997; Mickley, Soeken & Belcher, 1992). Intrinsic religiosity, the integrated and internalized expression of religious thought and practice in daily life, contrasts with involvement in religious practice more for the social support, security, or solace noted with extrinsic religiosity. These studies suggest that religiosity, particularly intrinsic religiosity, and sense of spiritual well-being enables people to find meaning in adversity and supports their self-concept. Hope is positively correlated with both intrinsic religiosity and spiritual well-being.

SELF-NURTURE: Compassion with Suffering

In his book, *Peace is Every Step,* Thich Nhat Hanh (1991) offers two meditations that assist in bringing compassion to one who is suffering by entering into their physical, mental, and emotional experiences of the suffering.

- Choose as the object of your meditation a person who is suffering. This suffering could be quite obvious, such as someone who is ill, has a physical or emotional problem, is grieving, is poor or oppressed, or it could be more subtle such as deep sorrow or past hurts. With your heart as well as your eyes, look deeply at the person and sense her or his suffering with your whole being. Pay attention to what you are feeling, and stay with the process until compassion arises in you and prompts more understanding and response to the suffering.

- Choose as the focus of your meditation a person who has caused you suffering, acknowledging that if they have caused suffering, they too are suffering. With your whole being, look deeply at the person and, without judgment, sense their suffering. In the process, sense what might have caused suffering for that person, and stay with the process until you feel compassion arising in you. When we appreciate another's suffering, we are less likely to harbor bitterness. On the contrary, compassion calls forth the desire to relieve suffering. With this process, we can be reconciled with the person even if he or she is not present because we have become reconciled within ourselves.

As nurses, we are confronted with suffering by the very nature of our work. Sometimes what we must do to help another move toward healing temporarily contributes to their suffering. Even our young patients recognize this, as we see in four-year-old Sheila, who would cry out when she was enduring spinal taps for monitoring leukemia, "you're hurting me, you're hurting me by accident!" Although our nature and vocation impel us to strive to alleviate suffering, at times we can do little more than be with the one who is suffering. Yet sharing another's suffering by being with that person is one of the primary ways we express care and compassion. Indeed, the word *compassion* means *to suffer with*. The Dalai Lama (1999) suggests that a level of concern for others is the unifying characteristic of spiritual qualities such as love, compassion, forgiveness, patience, tolerance, harmony, and sense of responsibility. Related to our concern for others is the basic human capacity for empathy, which, because it connotes our inability to bear the sight of another's suffering, is what "enables us to enter into, and to some extent participate, in others' pain" (p. 64). Our innate capacity for empathy is the source of compassion. The Tibetan concept of compassion, or *nying je,* denotes love, affection, warm-heartedness, gentleness, kindness, generosity of spirit, and a feeling of connection with others. Matthew Fox (1983) notes that within the Judeo-Christian traditions, compassion is perhaps the fullest divine attribute. The Judeo-Christian scriptures tell us that God extends compassion to all that God created (not only to humans). In Luke's gospel, Jesus says that we should be compassionate as our Creator is compassionate. Fox suggests that a consciousness of interdependence and equality of being among all of creation is essential to understanding compassion. Indeed, as both an emotional and cognitive response, compassion is grounded in the awareness of our interconnectedness.

Some suffering, such as that resulting from violence, war, and poverty, is created by humans, and thus avoidable. Suffering that is more difficult to avoid includes that associated with sickness, aging, death, natural disasters; having what we want taken from us; not obtaining what we would like even when we work hard for it; meeting with the unwanted; the uncertainty of meeting adversity; and lack of contentment (Dalai Lama, 1999). Whatever the source, we have a choice of how we respond to suffering. Our ability to connect with our inner resources influences our attitude toward the suffering, and this attitude affects how we experience suffering. One response to suffering that is avoidable is to work to eliminate the events and attitudes that cause the suffering. Some people embrace the mystery of their suffering and come to view it as a blessing through which they deepen in wisdom, joy, and inner strength, and gain a sense of inner peace. Viktor Frankl (1984), Morrie Swartz (Albom, 1997), Lisa Wayman, and Jean Watson (whose stories are included in this book) are examples of such people. Some people react to suffering with bitterness, anger, fear, and anxiety that only adds to their suffering because of the inner turmoil that these emotions cause. Some people look at suffering as a punishment or purification that they must endure to make amends for wrongs done. Some consider suffering to be an undeserved curse. And many people experience a combination of these responses as they encounter suffering.

Closely related to suffering are the concepts of spiritual distress and spiritual pain. The nursing diagnosis *distress of the human spirit* recognizes that, among the many kinds and degrees of suffering that nurses encounter, persons can experience spiritual pain as well as the physical and psychological pain that nurses may more readily recognize. Defining characteristics of *distress of the human spirit* offer insight into potential sources of spiritual pain such as anger against the deity; questions about the meaning of the suffering a person is experiencing; separation from religious, spiritual, or cultural ties; and changes in a person's beliefs or value system (Doenges & Moorhouse, 1998). Kaye (1996) identifies the following as possible components of spiritual pain: unfairness, unworthiness, hopelessness, guilt, isolation, vulnerability, abandonment, punishment, confusion, and meaninglessness. These sufferings are exacerbated by physical suffering, social isolation, practical worries, or unfinished emotional business. He reflects that the spiritual anguish that people often experience as they face death may relate to the past—such as painful memories or feelings of guilt—to the present—such as isolation or anger—or to the future—such as fear or hopelessness.

REFLECTION 3–4

Consider times when you have experienced suffering.

- What words describe your suffering?
- What was the source of your suffering?
- What enhanced or helped to relieve your suffering?
- How might you have lessened your suffering by responding differently to the experience?
- What supported you in the midst of your suffering?

As we have compassion for others, we must also be aware of and be with our own suffering. One understanding of burnout among health care professionals is that it represents not being able to find ways to tend the spirit as one suffers the suffering of another. Some people may not seek to immediately alleviate suffering. Personal response to suffering is influenced by sociocultural, religious, familial, and environmental factors. Thus, knowing about a person's personality, culture, religious traditions, and family background could assist the nurse in understanding the nature and meaning of suffering for that person. Nurses must also be aware of their own responses to and understanding of suffering in order to differentiate their perceptions from those of the patient. With this awareness, the nurse is able to be more fully present in an intentional, healing way with those who are suffering and to discern whether honoring another's suffering requires action, presence, absence, or a combination of these. Compassion, the ability to *be with* another who is suffering, is crucial, particularly when nurses confront suffering that cannot be alleviated and must simply be borne. The caring presence that is such an important part of being with those who suffer includes listening with one's whole being as another wonders aloud and expresses deep feelings regarding some of life's unanswered questions.

FORGIVENESS

> *Cultivating forgiveness daily softens our life . . .*
> *It makes room for life. (Levine, 1987, p 89)*

An inevitable part of our life journey is that we all make mistakes. We do things that we regret and for which we feel remorse, and we react to things that others do to us. Our actions or omissions can contribute to the suffering of others and to our own suffering. Wherever there is suffering there is, at some level, a disruption in our sense of connectedness with self, others, God, and the world around us. Estrangement occurs particularly when suffering results from an actual or perceived violation for which there is no acknowledgment or atonement. As intrinsic as suffering is to our human experience, so is the deep need and hunger for forgiveness, which is an important element in healing this disconnection. Festa and Tuck (2000) remind us that disease both within and between persons is a common consequence of interpersonal violation. They suggest that forgiveness can help prevent such diseases of interpersonal violation and contribute to healing when illness follows from the stress and emotional disruption related to these violations. Our beliefs about forgiveness, and our ability to offer and receive forgiveness, are influenced by our religious beliefs, cultural traditions, family upbringing, personal experiences, and how we understand the nature of God or Sacred Source. Consciousness of our interconnectedness is important grounding for understanding forgiveness. We must remember that forgiveness, though not the same as reconciliation, does open the door to the possibility of reconciliation. Whatever our beliefs, forgiveness and reconciliation ultimately flow from the place of our being that is aware that all things are related. Levine (1987) reflects that forgiveness is a way of letting go of armor that separates one heart from another and is also a way of connecting once again with our own hearts. He notes that in the deepest experience of forgiveness we discover that instead of an "other" to direct forgiveness toward, there is just a shared sense of the one heart and mind in which we all float. "Then, as in unconditional love, there is not forgiveness *for* another, but forgiveness *with* another" (p.91).

> *Forgiveness is one of the greatest gifts of spiritual life.*
> *(Kornfield, 1993, p. 284)*

Although we often think of forgiveness as something we offer to another, it ultimately has to do with healing ourselves as part of the interconnected web of life. Forgiveness is an antidote for the way we close ourselves off from other people because of the pain we have experienced as a result of our own short-comings or the reactions of others (Wieder, 2000). As an act of love, forgiveness is a way of extending compassion to ourselves and others, acknowledging that which separates and that which connects us. Rather than understanding forgiveness as something we grant to another or ourselves, nurse and artist, Lisa Wayman (personal communication, July, 2000) suggests that we are called to stand in compassion to witness forgiveness, either of me for myself, or another for her or himself. She reflects that

> in doing this kind of forgiveness I recognize that the seeds of another's wrong doing are present in myself. When I welcome another back to the whole, especially when I forgive a wrong done to me, I remove the barriers I have erected. Not only is the other now free to be in relationship with me, I, myself am unrestricted from the ineffable whole. Forgiveness is an act of love, and love is definitely the core of nursing.

Misconceptions about the nature of forgiveness contribute to difficulties we have with forgiving others, forgiving ourselves, and accepting forgiveness. In clarifying what forgiveness is and is not, Simon and Simon (1990) remind us that we must first understand that forgiveness is something that we do for ourselves, not others. Rather than a clear-cut one time decision, forgiveness is a by-product of an ongoing healing process. Levine (1987) suggests that learning to cultivate forgiveness in every moment opens the mind to the natural compassion of the heart. He encourages us to touch anything that we react to with resentment or condemnation with forgiveness instead, thus allowing the miracle of healing and balance to enter fully into our life in each moment. Forgiveness is a voluntary letting go of the right to retaliate, or hold anger and resentment in response to injury (Brush, McGee, Cavanagh & Woodward, 2001; Festa and Tuck, 2000). Contrary to commonly held beliefs, all these authors suggest that forgiveness is not forgetting, condoning, absolution, or a form of self-sacrifice; rather, it is a process of extending compassion to self or another. Forgiveness is an internal process, an act of the heart, that includes letting go of intense emotions attached to incidents from our past and acknowledging that we no longer wish to carry the load of grudges, resentments, hatred, and self-pity. Indeed, holding onto anger, bitterness, and resentment keeps us stuck in the past and less aware of and open to the opportunities for love and healing in the present moment. These emotions take a toll on our physical health as well as on our emotional and spiritual well-being. Seaward (1997) speaks of unresolved anger as a toxin or corrosive agent to the spirit that holds the spirit captive. He sees forgiveness as the antidote that releases the spirit to journey freely again. The process of forgiveness includes releasing the desire to punish people who hurt us, recognizing that whatever we do with the intent of punishing them only further disconnects us and does nothing to heal us. Along with letting go of resentments toward others, forgiveness calls us to recognize that any desire or need to berate or punish ourselves for past actions only alienates us from ourselves. Forgiveness enables us to re-connect with our true self and is ultimately self-empowering as it allows us to put the past in proper perspective and to live more fully in the present. Through forgiveness we free up energy once consumed by our anger, grudges, resentments, and focusing on unhealed wounds. We may then use this energy for opening to healing and moving on with our lives.

Forgiving ourselves is fundamental for spiritual growth and healing. Self-forgiveness is a process through which we acknowledge responsibility for our actions rather than focus on regret or guilt. Kollmar (1998) speaks of self-forgiveness as an energy, resource, and gift to ourselves that provides an opportunity to remove the energetic consequences from past thoughts and actions so that the cumulative energy of our past actions will not adversely affect the self. Basic to self-forgiveness is the notion of free will. Free will implies that we co-create our experiences through our own choices, and that the actual or energetic result of our thoughts and actions cannot be bypassed by God or the universe. Self-forgiveness opens us to receiving help from God or the universe as we acknowledge responsibility for our part in what we decided to create and as we are willing to let go of any energetic attachment to past actions and thoughts. For example, if we are feeling angry, the process of self-forgiveness helps us to accept responsibility for the tension that our anger creates, recognizing that this tension is affecting many areas of our lives, and promotes our letting go of whatever we are holding onto regarding the anger. This opens us to God's healing Light and allows the healing of the tension related to the anger to begin. In essence, self-forgiveness is the process by which we open ourselves to change in the areas we are responsible for creating, thus enabling us to open the door to receive God's grace and healing. As a way of illustrating the self-forgiveness process, Kollmar uses the following analogy: If you step on a thorn as you go for a walk, every step after that point is painful. The more you walk with the thorn in your foot, the more it hurts. As long as the thorn is in your foot, your body cannot heal, and instead must attend to the effects that the thorn's presence has on the whole body. Once you remove the thorn, however, your body can begin the healing process. Self-forgiveness, like pulling out the thorn, enables the natural self-healing energy that is a part of the universe to begin to have its effect and gives all of God's grace room to come to our aid.

SELF-NURTURE: Forgiveness Meditation

Forgiveness comes through an act of our will, a response of our heart, and grace that brings us to the place deep within our being where our experience of connectedness embraces our estrangement. Taking our needs for forgiveness into meditation is one way of cultivating forgiveness in our lives. Take your time with this process, giving yourself as much space as you need for each part of the process.

Begin the meditation by sitting comfortably and moving into your center. You can use any process that will help you to relax mind and body, such as paying attention to your breathing, progressive muscle relaxation, imagining yourself in a loving, safe place. After a few moments, bring your attention to your heart center and pay attention to what you are experiencing there, whether you feel your heart is open, or perhaps cluttered with many concerns. Pay attention to where your heart feels blocked or closed toward another or others because you have felt injured or violated . . . Allow yourself to feel the burden and pain that this estrangement is causing you, and the other person(s) . . . With compassion, acknowledge and be with that part of you that feels this pain, as you would be with a child who has been hurt . . . Allow yourself to feel how the resentment, anger, hurt, fear you have been carrying is contributing to this pain . . . With the same generosity and compassion, now open your heart toward the other, with the inner intent to release the burden of resentment, anger, hurt that you have been carrying . . . You may want to speak words such as "I forgive you," "I acknowledge that I, too, have hurt others through fear, hurt, ignorance," "I release us both from this burden" . . . You do not need to "feel" forgiving, merely have the willingness to enter into the process . . . You may just want to sit with the other in the Presence of Love, asking that Love open you to the healing needed in this relationship . . .

When you feel a sense of completion or readiness to move on, repeat this process focused on ways you have knowingly or unknowingly violated, abandoned, or betrayed *yourself* . . . With compassion, be with the part of you that feels the pain and burden . . . With the same compassion, be with the part of you that has contributed to this pain, embracing this part with acceptance and love, not judgment . . . You may want to voice your forgiveness, or just sit with yourself in the Presence of Love as noted earlier.

When you feel a sense of completion or readiness to move on, repeat this process focused on ways you have knowingly or unknowingly violated or betrayed *another or others* . . . Allow yourself as well, to feel the pain you have caused the other . . . Be aware as well of whatever fears, hurts, uncertainty, confusion may have prompted your behavior that caused the other pain . . . You may choose to speak words such as "I ask your forgiveness," or "I ask your compassion and willingness to release us both from this burden" . . . You may also wish to sit in the Presence of Love as noted earlier . . .

Repeat this meditation as a whole, or selected portions, whenever you are aware of issues of forgiveness in your life. You may at times feel a shift in yourself as you do this meditation, but you may feel no particular change. Forgiveness is a process that may take time. Always treat yourself with compassion, and honor your willingness to enter into this process. As you give time and energy to this process and continue to move into the deeper space of your heart and your soul, you open to the place of forgiveness within yourself that resides in the essence of Divine Love.

Forgiveness does not mean denying the hurt or the anger, rather, forgiveness must begin with acknowledging and processing our anger and hurt. Careful listening and observation for signs of anger, resentment, or hurt related to a patient's current condition or other relationships enables nurses to offer patients an opportunity to identify and explore these feelings and seek appropriate ways to process them. Reflecting "You seem angry about . . ." or "It sounds like you feel really hurt by . . ." gives the person permission to name the feeling and to talk about what is going on. Festa and Tuck (2000, pp. 82–83) remind us that patients might indicate that forgiveness is an issue by acknowledging the emotional disruption, grief, or personal distress in important relationships. Disruption in relationships can be evident as well in what is not said or done, such as the family member who never visits or who is not acknowledged in conversations about family and friends. These authors suggest that clinicians can provide an opening to exploration of these relationships by making an observation of the obvious such as, "you have said you are worrying a lot about how you will manage when you get home, what barriers exist in getting help from your adult children?" They also suggest more general questions through which clinicians can facilitate exploration of the need for forgiveness, such as "With whom would you like to be closer . . . What stands in the way or keeps you apart?" "If you had to call it, would you say you are moving closer together or further apart . . . What do you think accounts for that?" "If the relationship between you could be the way you wanted it to be, how would it be . . . What do you think could make it better?"

Events that cause anger and hurt also disrupt relationships, leaving us with a sense of loss. Seaward (1997) notes that when we acknowledge feelings of anger or hurt we often experience a time of grieving. He notes that people may experience feelings from anger to depression during this grieving process and may become stuck in feelings of victimization. Sometimes helping people to see that they are stuck is what is needed for them to choose a different way. Providing people a safe space in which they can talk about their experiences and see how holding on to the anger and resentment is affecting them can help them to see that they can choose a different response. Seaward suggests that the process of forgiveness moves from the phase of grieving toward detachment from emotions associated with the incident. Detachment implies an objectivity that provides a clearer sense of focus, which enables people to transform the emotional reactions, thus liberating them to move on with living. Listening for this phase of the process enables nurses to support people in releasing the hurt and reclaiming the power that they had given over to victimization. Nurses can help patients identify relationships in need of reconciliation and seek ways of beginning this process. Although a person's external circumstances might not change significantly, the change in inner attitude enables them to experience love and connectedness and to use their energy for life and healing. Throughout this process, as Festa and Tuck remind us, we must be aware that we do not know the optimal time for forgiveness to be offered or received, or even when a person might be expected to become aware of the need to seek forgiveness. Our focus regarding issues of and potentials for forgiveness relates to a primary goal of spiritual care-giving, which is to be alert for cues, and support processes that foster intrapersonal, interpersonal, and transpersonal healing and wholeness.

REFLECTION 3–5

- What are your feelings and beliefs about forgiveness?
- How have you experienced forgiveness in your life—both given and received, including self-forgiveness?
- Have you experienced hurts or are you holding grudges that you cannot seem to release? Consider how holding on to these feelings is affecting your life, health, and experience of connectedness. What would help you to begin to release these feelings?
- Consider a time when you experienced healing through forgiveness. What helped you in this process?

GRACE AND GRATITUDE

I do not at all understand the mystery of grace—only that it meets us where we are but does not leave us where it found us. (Lamott, 1999, p. 143)

Experiences of grace always contain an element of surprise, awe, or mystery—something unplanned and unexpected, yet just what we need in the moment. The Latin roots of *gratia* and *gratus* link the words *grace, grateful,* and *gratitude.*

Each of these words implies a sense of favor, thankfulness, and having a pleasing quality. Grace provides a framework for understanding those gifts of life that cause us to wonder and to feel that we are cared for in sometimes inexplicable ways. "Grace is uncontaminated conscious Light. It is Divinity" (Zukav, 1989, p.241). Grace opens our awareness to the experience of our wholeness, healing, and connectedness. That which is experienced as blessing is, at some level, an experience of grace. Experiences of grace are reminders that we are never alone and always have what we need.

REFLECTION 3–6

Where do you see grace in the following situations?

- He always seems to show up at the door right when I need him.

- I didn't know how I was going to get both food and medicine, then this check arrived.

- I wonder what made my spirits lift that morning, perhaps it was the rain after such a long drought.

- Just when I didn't think I could stand another bout of chemotherapy, my friend offered to go with me, and said, we'll take one day at a time.

- It just happened all of a sudden, this sense of peace came over me and I knew everything would be all right.

Grace enables us to know the something deeper in our lives that infuses our connectedness within the web of life. We may experience grace as a gift from God, Sacred Source, or from Life itself that enables, assists, and empowers us in the midst of difficult, and sometimes seemingly overwhelming circumstances. Through grace, we may experience more peace and acceptance or courage and endurance. Although our minds may suggest that unexplainable circumstances are coincidence, our hearts and souls recognize the gift of grace in the experience. Appreciating that we are all part of the One, the Mystery, we become more aware that within this wholeness there are no coincidences. Our experience of grace as a blessing that comes into our lives unearned, without merit, calls forth the response of gratitude.

If thanks is the only prayer you ever say that is enough. (Meister Eckhart)

Gratitude is a response of the spirit to the mystery of Love that flows through and sustains our life. Gratitude is the natural response to our awareness that life is a gift. Indeed, all in the universe is given to us, not something that we must earn. Grace enables us to see the gift, even in difficult and painful experiences. Gratefulness reflects our awareness of the gifts we are given, that all is gift, and nothing can be taken for granted. Steindl-Rast (1984) suggests that gratefulness is a measure of our aliveness, our ability to live life open to surprise in spite of the suffering and dying that living implies. Gratefulness brings more aliveness to our living. As we open more fully to the gratuitous universe, the sense of separation between giver and receiver begins to blur, and we know with greater clarity our interdependence one with the other. Steindl-Rast describes the circle of gratefulness in which the receiver of the gift offers an even greater gift of self by giving thanks, thus acknowledging the bond that unites giver and receiver.

Gratitude both opens us to the experience of joy and is an expression of joy. With grateful eyes and heart we feel ourselves as part of the flow and dance of all of life, and recognize the blessing both of every day occurrences and more notable experiences. Consider how you feel when you see a beautiful sunrise, smell the sweet scent of a flower, taste a favorite food, hear a child's joyful laughter, receive a call from a special friend, or meet the unexpected gaze of one who loves you. When we feel the touch of love and caring in any way in our lives, our hearts respond with gratitude. This response is prayer, that may not be spoken, or addressed to anyone or thing in particular. In giving thanks, we acknowledge the Sacred Source and Mystery of the gratuitous universe with some level of our being. For people in many Native American and other traditions, thanksgiving is a way of life. These traditions believe that all life is sacred, all thought is prayer, and that it is a privilege to be a human being and walk upon this earth. Viewing all as a gift, they do not take anything for granted, and constantly give thanks either in thoughts or words to and for all of creation.

LOVE–MYSTERY AND MEANING

The time will come when, after harnessing the winds, the tides, and gravitation,
we shall harness for God the energies of Love. And on that day,
for the second time in the history of the world, man will have discovered fire
(Teilhard de Chardin, 1975 pp. 86–87)

Love, the source of all life, is perhaps the greatest mystery of all. People across the centuries and in all traditions recognize the power of love to heal. Love is what sustains us. Indeed, as Larry Dossey (1996, p. 9) states, "the presence or absence of love can be associated with life-and-death consequences." Love has many facets, and, though described in many ways, no language can contain and express the whole. What we say here is but a mere glimpse of what has and could be written about love. Sacred texts and cultural traditions describe the energy of Divine or Universal Love as the animating principle, the life-giving force that holds the universe together in balance and harmony. Scientific inquiry reaches the same conclusion that love is "nothing less than the driving force of life and of the physical universe" (Jahn, 1996, p. 38). This same energy of love, residing deep within each of us is the source of our wholeness. Though sometimes quiescent, our internal energy of love is always available. Dossey (1996) writes that love unmasks our illusion of isolation, and provides evidence of who we are, filling us with a sense of being that is, in Underhill's (1961, p. 82) words, "great enough to be God, intimate enough to be me."

We do not become love; rather, love is who we are. Essential love is the experience of pure *being* that transcends the personal and separate of "I" and "You" revealing instead the oneness of "We" (Levine, 1987). Experiences of grace are reminders of love's abiding presence in our lives. Love prompts us to live from our hearts, our centers, where the ego is detached from outcomes. Indeed, love is the essential connection between heart and mind. Love is personal and universal, expressed and experienced as we give and receive care and compassion. Love flows from and infuses our interconnectedness. In discussing conceptualizations of love, Green and Shellenberger (1996) summarize the Greek classifications for the various ways we experience and express love. *Eros*, though originally implying love of the good, refers to what we understand as romantic love that involves sexual intimacy. The love of friendship, *philia*, implies support and commitment that goes beyond the relationship of an acquaintance. The bonds of family love, or *storge*, are stronger than friendship, cross generations, and promote unity within a group. *Agape* is altruistic or self-less love for others regardless of their circumstances or condition that involves giving to and caring for others without reward, sacrificing personal needs for those of others. *Koinonia*, love within a group that extends beyond family to the larger community, strives to maintain loving relationships through care and acceptance of others, and through forgiveness and reconciliation. Green & Shellenberger reviewed research that demonstrated the salutary effects of each of these forms of love on physical health. Based on their findings, these authors postulate three healing mechanisms of love:

- Psychophysiologic Process—in which health and healing are the result of internal homeostatic processes stimulated by positive interaction with other people, and cortical-limbic-hypothalamic mechanisms account for health and healing.

- Psychophysics Process—in which health and healing are the result of energy transmissions between people, and love is a radiant energy field accessible to living beings under certain conditions (e.g., loving intentionality, empathy, prayer, visualization, and altruistic action).

- Psychosocial/Behavioral Process—in which a social network of a loved one who encourages health behaviors promotes health by helping the person adopt and maintain these behaviors, and these behaviors, not love itself, are the ingredients of health, but they may be motivated by love (p.54).

The Judeo-Christian tradition holds that God is love, and those who abide in love, abide in God and God in them. As the essence of God, Love, in these traditions is the energy of life, a formidable power, and great healing energy. The healing energy shared through caring presence is ultimately the energy of love. Like our spirit, love is nonlocal and transcends place and time (Dossey, 1996). This enables the energy of love to be shared for healing at many levels, both when we are present with and distant from the one needing healing. Prayer for the good of another is an expression of and way of sharing love energy, as are energy healing processes such as Healing Touch, Therapeutic Touch, and Reiki. When awakened in us, love's energy manifests as both choice and emotion, and often underlies acts of courage and compassion that defy explanation. Indeed, Love both is the mystery and provides the meaning. Every act of forgiveness is an act of love. The trust and hope we experience when faced with mystery is grounded in love. Love supports us through and enables us to discover meaning in suffering. The light of love within us opens us ever more to awe, wonder, joy, and gratitude. Through Love, we discover more fully that Love is who we are.

REFERENCES

Albom, M, (1997). *Tuesdays with Morrie.* New York: Doubleday.

Barker, E. R. D. (1989). *Being whole: Spiritual well-being in Appalachian women: A phenomenological study.* Unpublished doctoral dissertation, University of Texas, Austin, 1989.

Benson, H. (1997). *Timeless healing: The power and biology of belief.* New York: Fireside Books.

Brush, B. L, McGee, E. M., Cavanagh, B., & Woodward, M. (2001). Forgiveness: A concept analysis. *Journal of holistic nursing, 19*(1), 27–41.

Burkhardt, M. A. (1989). Spirituality: An analysis of the concept. *Holistic Nursing Practice, 3,* 69–77.

Burkhardt, M. A. (1994). Becoming and connecting: Elements of spirituality for women. *Holistic Nursing Practice, 8,* 12–21.

Burkhardt, M. A., & Nagai-Jacobson, M. G. (2000). Spirituality and health. In B. M. Dossey, L. Keegan, & C. E. Guzzetta (Eds.). *Holistic Nursing: A Handbook for Practice* pp. 91–121. Gaithersburg, MD: Aspen.

Cassell, E. (1992). The nature of suffering: physical, psychological, social and spiritual aspects. In P. Stark & J. McGovern (Eds.), *The Hidden Dimension of Illness: Human Suffering* (pp. 1–10). New York: National League for Nursing.

Dalai Lama (1999). *Ethics for the new millennium.* New York: Riverhead Books.

Dass, R. (2000). *Still Here: Embracing aging, changing, and dying.* New York: Riverhead Books.

de Mello, A. (1998). *Walking on Water.* New York: Crossroad.

Doenges, M. E., & Moorhouse, M. F. (1998). *Nurse's pocket guide: diagnoses, interventions, and rationales* (6th ed.). Philadelphia: F. A. Davis.

Dossey, L. (1996). What's love got to do with it? *Alternative Therapies in Health and Medicine, 2*(3) 8–15.

Editorial. (1999). Diseases of meaning, Manifestations of health, and metaphor. *The Journal of Alternative and Complementary Medicine, 5*(6), 495–502.

Emblen, J. D. (1992). Religion and spirituality defined according to current use in nursing literature. *Journal of Professional Nursing, 8,* 41–47.

Emblen, J. & Pesut, B. (2001). Strengthening transcendent meaning: A model for the spiritual nursing care of patients experiencing suffering. *Journal of holistic nursing, 19*(1), 42–56.

Fehring, R. J., Miller, J. F., & Shaw, C. (1997). Spiritual well-being, religiosity, hope, depression, and other mood states in elderly people coping with cancer. *Oncology Nursing Forum, 4,* 663–671.

Festa, L. M., & Tuck, I. (2000). A review of forgiveness literature with implications for nursing practice. *Holistic Nursing Practice, 14*(4), 77–86.

Fox, M. (1983). *Original blessing.* Santa Fe, NM: Bear.

Frankl, V. (1984). *Man's search for meaning.* New York: Washington Square Press.

Green, J., & Shellenberger, R. (1996). The healing energy of love. *Alternative Therapies in Health and Medicine, 2*(3) 46–56.

Haase, J., Britt, T., Coward, D., Leidy, N. & Penn, P. (1992). Simultaneous concept analysis of spiritual perspective, hope, acceptance & self-transcendence. *Image: Journal of Nursing Scholarship, 24,* 141–147.

Hanh, T. N. (1991). *Peace is every step.* New York: Bantam Books.

Jahn, R. G. (1996). Information, consciousness, and health. *Alternative Therapies in Health and Medicine, 2*(3) 32–38.

Kaye, P. (1996). Spiritual pain. In *Symptom Control in Hospice & Palliative Care.* (Revised 1st Ed.). Essex, CT: Hospice Education Institute.

Keating, T. (1995). *Open mind open heart: The contemplative dimension of the gospel.* New York: Continuum.

Kollmar, D. (1998). *Manifestation.* Complete Self-Attunement Associates Workshop, Charleston, WV, August 30.

Kornfield, J. (1993). *A path with heart.* New York: Bantam Books.

Lamott, A. (1999). *Traveling mercies.* New York: Random House.

Lao Tsu. (1972). *Tao Te Ching* (Trans. Gia-Fu Feng & Jane English). New York: Vintage Books.

Levine, S. (1987). *Healing into life and death.* Garden City, NY: Anchor Press.

Mansen, T. J. (1993). The spiritual dimension of individuals: Concept development. *Nursing Diagnosis, 4,* 140–147.

Mayer, J., & Holms, J. P. (1996). *Bite-size Einstein.* New York: St. Martin's Press.

Meraviglia, M. G. (1999). Critical analysis of spirituality and its empirical indicators. *Journal of Holistic Nursing, 17*(1), 18–33.

Mickley, J. R., Soeken, K., & Belcher, A. (1992). Spiritual well-being, religiousness, and hope among women with breast cancer. *Image: Journal of Nursing Scholarship, 24,* 267–272.

Morse, J. M., & Doberneck, B. (1995). Delineating the concept of hope. *Image: Journal of Nursing Scholarship, 27*(4) 277–285.

Newman, M. A. (1994). *Health as expanding consciousness.* (2nd ed.). New York: National League for Nursing Press.

Rupp, J. (1997). *The cup of our life: A guide for spiritual growth.* Notre Dame, IN: Ave Maria Press.

Seaward, B. L. (1997). *Stand like mountain flow like water: Reflections on stress and human spirituality.* Deerfield Beach, FL: Health Communications.

Simon, S. B., & Simon, S. (1990). *Forgiveness: How to make peace with your past and get on with your life.* New York: Warner Books.

Steindl-Rast, D. (1984). *Gratefulness, the Heart of Prayer: An approach to life in its fullness.* New York: Paulist Press.

Teilhard de Chardin, P. (1975). *Toward the future.* (René Hague, Trans.). San Diego, CA: Harvest Book.

Tweel, E. N. (2000). *Unpublished personal journal of illness experience,* Charleston, WV.

Underhill, E. (1961). *Mysticism.* New York: Dutton.

Walton, J. (1999). Spirituality of patients recovering from an acute myocardial infarction. *Journal of Holistic Nursing, 17*(1), 34–53.

Wieder, K. (2000). *Meditation and Teshuvah: Exploring the Jewish Contemplative Tradition.* Centers of Contemplative Living, Gassaway, WV, September 8–10.

Wiesel, E. (1972). *Souls on Fire: Portraits and legends of Hasidic Masters.* New York: Touchstone Books.

Willard, D. (1998). *The divine conspiracy: Rediscovering our hidden life in God.* New York: HarperCollins.

Zukav, G. (1989). *The seat of the soul.* New York: Fireside Books.

Lisa Wayman's Story

Lisa Wayman, a nurse and an artist in Colorado Springs, Colorado, shares her experience of journeying with her son from the diagnosis of a malignant brain tumor to his death. She speaks of both the sorrow and the gift of this journey, her struggles, and her embracing of the Mystery, through which she has ultimately discovered meaning and is receiving healing.

I am a nurse, but the story I have to share is a personal story of suffering and joy. I have found suffering to be a transforming passage, and now find that I am more able to stand with my patients in their suffering since I have also suffered. I think often of Viktor Frankl's work, and how he echoed the Buddha when he said that all people suffer, the only real choice we have is how we are going to walk through it. I choose to share my story, not to make people feel sorry for me, or to make people cry, but so that other suffering may be looked at in a new way by the light of my suffering.

I am going to start my story by speaking of joy, which is, after all, just the opposite side of the coin. Years ago I had a meditation, which I go back to frequently. In this meditation I was walking along a canyon with steep, black rock sides. At the very bottom was just the glimmer of a little stream. Now, in my life I am very afraid of heights, but in this meditation I fearlessly jumped off the cliff. It was wonderful. I was free with the air rushing through my hair and across my body. As I got closer and closer to the bottom I realized that the water at the bottom was not a little stream, it was a large river, it had just been far away.

I dove into the water. It was not a hit or splash, just a changing of medium. I love to swim, and I started to swim toward the bottom. I didn't have to breathe, and the water flowed around me. The water was green, shot through with yellow light. As I swam, the light got stronger and stronger. Soon I could see the bottom of the river, bedrock which had been cut away, like diving into a quarry. The rock was glowing yellow, it was the source of all the light. I put out my hand and touched it, and when I did, I knew that I had touched the very bedrock of my soul, and that it was joy.

Over the following years I began to be able to see how that love light of joy reached from me to the people I loved. We were all connected with gold bonds of love. Eventually, like backing up the camera, I was able to see how the whole world was connected with a web of love. This connection with others, especially with my family and my friends, was the source of my joy. This love and connection also became the source of my greatest suffering.

My son, Joe, was diagnosed with a brain stem glioma September 7, 1996. He died February 21, 1998 at the age of 12. My love for him was the source of my greatest joy, and also my greatest suffering. I learned so much from this journey that I wish to share.

The first thing I learned was about denial. I had often looked at my patients and their families, (I am an ICU nurse), and wondered how they could tell me that nothing was wrong. Couldn't they see the same things I did? Did they think I said bad news just to say it? I really didn't understand the denial. Then I found myself in that place. I had, for the first, and hopefully last, time a curious split of person. My nurse self was standing outside myself. That part of me was looking at an MRI of a five centimeter tumor in the middle of my kid's head saying, "this is bad, this is going to be real bad." My mom self was close to my heart saying, "they do so much with childhood cancer now, it will be ok." I did not think that people were lying to me, or that this couldn't be happening. I just couldn't let the awful truth come into my heart. It took me about four hours until the two parts of me could get together, and I could deal with what was happening. That was valuable time though. I used it to collect all my courage, to take inventory, and to touch the joy in my heart again. Then I could get started on what was ahead.

What happened next was suffering. We did fairly well at controlling physical pain, it was mental suffering which was so hard. At first I could hardly breathe under the weight of just the idea of cancer. I started to pray, and I prayed with every breath, "please let my son get better, please let my son get better." Our friends started to pray, our family started to pray, people around the world prayed for Joe. "Please let him get better, please let him get better."

At this time I suffered a loss of the future. When we have children there are dreams that we take for granted. Simple things, like graduations, and girlfriends. I thought of possible daughter-in-laws and grandchildren. All of those simple things were now at risk. For Joe, the suffering was much more a loss of the now. Perhaps that is because children live so much more in the now. Joe lost his looks, his face became crooked from the tumor pressing on nerves of his face, he lost his hair from chemotherapy, he gained 100 pounds from the steroids. He eventually became wheelchair bound, and lost his independence. He did not usually look toward the future, he looked at today, what he could do now, and what he was missing through his illness.

Joe's primary way of dealing with loss was through humor. When his hair started to fall out from the chemotherapy it came out in big clumps. It was falling everywhere and driving him crazy. He asked me to shave his head. I did, and he cried. I told him, "well, if you are bald you will have to be something cool for Halloween." He pondered it for quite awhile, thought maybe he would be Uncle Fester. Then he came to me and said, "if I'm going to be bald, I should be Daddy." My kids have never see my husband, Charlie, with hair! So I bought some fake glue-on hair and made Joe a fringe and a beard. Joe and Charlie walked around together, both with glasses, discs in pockets, ID badges, and coffee cups. Big and little programmers. It was funny, and a great way of coping with loss of hair.

We learned how sacred every day is. We worked hard at maintaining a normal life. Joe went to school as long as he was able. He got in trouble if he picked on his sister Katie. He reveled in every day. We didn't have to wait for vacations or for that "someday"; we could now see today, this ordinary day as holy and special.

After only a few months it became apparent that Joe would die. I felt so bad to even think that. We hear so much now about how positive thinking can change outcomes. I think that the blessing I felt with every day, and the way I looked for gifts in all things, especially suffering, did change things. It allowed us to heal, it allowed us to live fully today. Did it make my son beat an illness with an almost nonexistent cure rate? No. Yet, I still felt guilty at times for thinking he would die. We all die, we all suffer. I have no miracle cures to boast of. I can only speak of the gifts of growth and healing.

When I started to realize that Joe would die (he had no remissions, no improvements), my prayer changed. I no longer prayed for Joe's life. I began to feel that I was not wise enough to say what the best outcome would be. I wanted it to be that he got better and became a most interesting man. I thought though that perhaps his job was to die well, and to teach and bless me by the way he lived. I started to pray, "Thy will be done." I started to let go. I didn't get to this point easily or quickly. I'd like to share a small story from this time to illustrate how I changed from thinking I knew what was best to an openness to any outcome.

In May of 1997, Joe was really ill. He was now totally wheelchair bound, a loss which he would mourn the rest of his life. He had decubitus ulcers in his inguinal folds from the weight gain and the sitting. He had micro fractures from the steroids. Then he started to vomit. He threw up all the time. We couldn't figure out why. He was long done with chemotherapy, radiation was over, but still, he vomited. We tried every drug we could think of to relieve this horrible nausea. No luck. Perhaps it was just the way his tumor was growing. I don't know. For Joe, this was terrible. All other things he had worked around and adjusted to. This, however, interrupted his whole life. He could no longer go to school, or boy scouts, or out with his friends. He couldn't even do crafts at home. All he could do was be sick.

By the weekend he was really ill. He couldn't hold down his medications, including his long-acting morphine, so his pain wasn't being addressed. He couldn't hold down his steroids, so he had a horrible headache. We decided to give him some intravenous (IV) fluid, and give him his medications IV also. He had a central line, so this was no problem. The medical supply people came out with a pump and tubing. The pharmacy sent fluid, steroids, and a morphine drip. The home health nurse called and asked me if I needed her to come out and start the IV. I told her no. It was Sunday night, and I had hung plenty of drips, was familiar with the pump. I could do it.

That is how I found myself standing in his room with 50 milligrams of morphine in my hand. I looked at him lying in his bed, so ill, and I thought, "if I ran this bag wide open, shut the door, and didn't come back until morning, he would be done suffering, and we wouldn't have to watch him suffer." I stood there for a very long time thinking that. Then I thought, "I have never, ever done this to a patient. I don't know what is best. I don't know when he should die." I hung the morphine at two milligrams an hour, which did well for him, kissed him good-night, and left the room. Thank God I didn't think I knew what was best. I let go and started giving up control. I didn't have to figure everything out, I didn't have to be in charge of everything.

After that, Joe stopped throwing up, and had the best summer of his life. He went to camp. Colorado has a camp named Wapiyapi, which takes kids with cancer and their siblings. Joe had a great time. He still couldn't stomach camp food, take him too near the dining hall at meal time, and he would throw up. So they fed him dry cereal and he was fine. The camp had camp Olympics, and they decided they needed something great for opening ceremonies. The councilors fixed up a zip line, attached climbing gear to Joe's wheelchair, and hoisted him up. He waved a flag on the way up, then, when he got to the top, they gave him a big squirt gun, and he sprayed all the kids on his way down. He had a great time! When he told me about that I said to him, "Joe, honey, you have always been afraid of heights, how did you do that?" he looked at me in the eye and said, "Mom, after you've had cancer, you aren't afraid of anything."

The other thing they did at camp was let him drive. That was not a planned camp activity. Some of the councilors had been sitting around, and they said, "If you were a 12-year-old boy, and you knew you were going to die, what would you most want to do?" Driving was what they came up with. Jamie had an old beat up truck, but it was standard, so Joe couldn't drive it. Austin had a new four wheel drive, which was automatic, so Joe drove that. I bet Austin regrets it now. During a meal time, when the other kids weren't around, they set up cones in a field and had Joe drive around them. He did pretty good, so they said, "put it in four, and go up that hill." So Joe put it in four, and putt-putted up the hill. He wasn't going to make it so they told him , "back it up, and gun it." So he did. He went flying up the hill, and just about the time he was airborne at the top one of the guys said, "isn't there a big log up there?" Sure enough, he landed with the log behind the front axle. When they stopped, Joe looked around like 'boy, am I in trouble now!' then he just started to laugh.

He had a summer full of events like that. Full of friends, movies, projects, ball games. For him it was worth it to be alive, even ill, if he got to live like that. I learned that when I was so afraid of future suffering, I couldn't live fully in the now. If I run from suffering, I also run from joy. I didn't want to miss one moment of his life, or of mine. Now when I can't seem to bring together two seemingly opposite ideas, like suffering and joy, I think of an example from Fritjof Capra's book *Tao of Physics*. He says that if we have two circles on a flat plane, they seem totally separate, even, perhaps, opposite. If, however, those two circles are seen as parts of a donut, a three dimensional figure, then they are not separate at all, but aspects of the whole (Capra, 1991, p. 151). Now when I cannot seem to bring two opposite ideas together I think "I am thinking on the wrong plane." Then I can bring them together.

Another thing I learned from that wonderful summer was the nonlinear aspect of terminal illness. I had previously thought that cancer would progress steadily downward until death. Perhaps I thought this because all of the patients I see in ICU with this kind of illness are at the end of their journey. Life has many more ups and downs and is full of more of the unexpected than I had thought.

One of the gifts of a terminal illness is the ability to say goodbye. In a way it is much easier than losing a child suddenly, but an 18-month kiss goodbye is very long. As Joe lost more and more function, he became more ready to go. He worked at saying goodbye. One way he did this was to complete a scrapbook called *My Stupid Illness*. It was a gift from Children's Legacy, founded by Katie Tartkoff. She takes black and white photos of terminally ill kids and their families. The scrapbook was a way for Joe to say what his life had meant to him. In it he said "my body is worse, but my spirit is better." Isn't that the point? We all die, but if your spirit is better when you go, you've done it right. I have to say though, that he was a terrible speller, and it really says "my body is worse, but my sprit is better."

I think that by the end of his illness, Joe was healed. He was not cured, his body deteriorated, and he died. He was, though, so much more himself. He was a child, but also was an actualized person. He did what he had come to do. He lived fully and joyfully.

The last really conscious act he did was to make Valentines. It was an effort of love, and he sent them out to many people. By the time Valentine's day came, Joe was unable to hold up his head. He couldn't use his scissors, or even the glue, but he wanted to make Valentines. So he sat in his chair at the table (a difficult task in itself by that time) and gave me directions. He wasn't speaking clearly, so it was hard for both of us. He would say, "big blue heart," so I would cut a big blue heart. He had me put the hearts so the points were together, and they made butterflies. It was a beautiful last gesture.

Now I will speak of Joe's death, not to make anyone sad, but because we die so poorly in this country, and he did not. When Joe could not do anything anymore, couldn't even swallow Jell-O, he was ready to go. The evening of February 20th we knew he wasn't doing well. Katie had been planning on going to a sleep over for the whole basketball team. We didn't want her to miss out on it, so we told her to say goodbye to Joe in case he went while she was gone. She went up to his room for a while, and when she came down, we asked her if she had said everything she wanted to. She said, "well, not quite." She had wanted to kiss him, but Joe disliked too many kisses. We told her to go ahead, after all, he couldn't hit her now, could he? So she went back up to his room and kissed him. He made such a face, like "eww, my sister kissing me"! It was pure Joe.

After she left, Charlie and I went to Joe's room. We held his hand and talked to him. We reminisced about the good times we had together. We told him how much we had enjoyed being his parents and how proud we were of him. I sang him to sleep when he was tired. Songs I had sung when he was small. He slept, and we left him. I was up several times in the night with him, as I usually was. He was unable to talk to me, but alert. I gave him a little ativan and sang to him again, comfort on the way.

At about six in the morning I sat bolt upright in bed and thought "there's something different on the baby monitor." I hardly slept those days, always with an ear out for his soft call. When I came fully awake, I realized that an agonal respiratory pattern had awakened me. I went into his room, and he was now comatose, with a slow respiratory rate of about six per minute. I went to get Charlie, since I knew he would go soon. Charlie came in, sat and held his hand for a while, then said to me "do you think I could go take a shower?" Poor Charlie, the waiting and the illness wore him so hard. I said sure, since I really didn't know when Joe would go. I sat and held Joe's hand. I had no more words. I had no more songs. I was just so tired. Finally I said to him, "I love you. You have done a good job. Go ahead, and I will see you when I get there." He took about two more breaths and he died. The room was so quiet without him breathing. I just sat for a minute in the quiet, missing him, but knowing it would be OK.

After that we partied. We had two funerals. He had gone to Catholic school, so we had a separate service for the school, since the church wasn't large enough for all the people who wanted to come. We had helium balloons, funny stories, pictures of Joe, and lots of food. We wanted him to go out in style. We wanted to celebrate that he had lived well. The quality of one's life is so much more important than its quantity. Of course we couldn't just let go in one day, but we started. I wrote this poem as a way to let go.

To Joe

I remember, little caterpillar,

When you came to me, so hungry for the world.

I joyfully opened my life to you,

And stuffed your ravenous heart full.

I fed you

Love,

Laughter,

Discipline,

Tears,

Jokes,

Starshine,

I watched you grow.

Soon, oh too soon for me,

You pulled the silken strands

Of your chrysalis close

And wrapped youself in

Love,

Friendship,

Suffering,

Humor,

Loss,

Courage,

I watched you change.

Your beautiful, strong body

Bloated and weak, unrecognizable,

But for the mischief in your eyes,

And the logic in your hands.

You grew

Stronger,

Lighter,

Deeper,

Closer.

I caressed you with strong hands.

Then you were something different;

A mystery glimpsed through the web,

Too lovely for the chains of the earth.

As you left you showered me

With sweet gifts.

A flash of color,

Light of knowing,

Blinding love.

Enduring joy.

I cried.

I cried with selfishness.

I yearned to hold you forever, To not release you to the

Unfathomable lover.

I'll remember you with

Joy,

Music,

Sadness,

Laughter,

Love,

'Til we meet in the singing JOY.

I am still me. I am still the person who dove to the light of joy. I have also been changed forever. My heart has been broken, and that is a good thing. Now the light of joy and love which used to seep up from my bed rock, gushes forth through my broken heart. This change in me has changed how I am with my patients. I know now that I cannot fix everything. It is still important to me to alleviate whatever physical suffering I can, but more important is that I am present with my patients. I stand with them in their suffering so that they may heal. I don't quite know how that standing in that place helps patients to heal themselves, but it can work as a catalyst. Healing can occur when dying.

I cry now at work. I never used to cry. ICU nurses are tough birds. Our daily work is dealing with some of the worst suffering imaginable. We don't cry, but I cry. I will talk to families about taking a patient off life support. I will help do it, and know that it is a good thing to not always run from death, but still, I shed a few tears. I do so because I know how hard it is to say goodbye, I know how precious life is and how hard it is to let go. I never get comments about how unprofessional I am, only about how much I care.

I don't talk about Joe to patients and their families. I don't think it is appropriate, and I want them to feel free to go through what they are going through without worrying about me and my suffering. I don't say his story in words, but I tell it with my hands. I know that it has changed who I am, and how I touch others, and that is enough legacy for me.

I now know what it is to stand in paradox. I can honestly say that losing my son was the worst thing that has ever happened to me. I miss him daily with a deep down heart longing. Some days my every cell cries for him. I cannot deny the pain and the suffering. At the same time I can say that losing Joe was the best thing that ever happened to me. I know more how to let go. I know more how not to be in control. I know more how every second of my life, and every cell of my being is sacred. I cannot do it all the time, but sometimes. When I stand in this place of paradox, when in the same time and the same place I hold suffering and joy, I find mystery, meaning, and healing.

REFERENCES

Capra, F. (1991). *The Tao of Physics* (3rd ed.). Boston: Shambhala.
Frankl, V. E. (1984). *Man's Search for Meaning.* New York: Simon & Schuster.
The Children's Legacy. (1991). *My Stupid Illness.* Denver, CO: The Hunt Alternatives Fund.

Healing Presence, Spiritual Presence

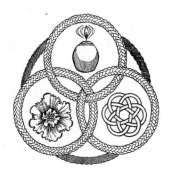

To bless is to put a bit of yourself into something.

It is to make holy,

to change something because of your presence.

MACRINA WEIDERKEHR IN RUPP, 1997, P. 135

Spiritual care begins with presence. The most fundamental and important way we integrate spirituality into nursing and health care is through our presence with those for whom we care. So often when we think of integrating spirituality into health care or nursing care, we consider how to incorporate prayer or meditation, sacred texts and rituals, religious beliefs and practices, and spiritual support persons into care planning. Although these are all important considerations, we often overlook the most readily available and essential resource for spiritual caregiving—ourselves. Incorporating spirituality into care with others is grounded in *who we are* and *how we are* with another. In essence, the presence of love we bring to any situation is the basic way we integrate spirituality into care. It is how we touch, and listen, and hear, and see, and sense, and speak, and sit with, and do all the tasks that are part of our care with another. Being a loving presence with another means that we are able to attune to our own spirit, our own heart center. We appreciate that we are all part of the Oneness of the Divine or Sacred Source, and within this oneness the experience of the other becomes, at some level, our experience too. When we encounter another at the level of spirit, we open to the sacredness of the present moment. This marks the place we are in as sacred, as holy ground. It is within this moment, and every new moment that the Divine is ever present, inviting us to open more to the fullness of who we are.

There are many ways of naming this presence, for example, loving presence, therapeutic presence, caring presence, transpersonal presence, transcendent presence, and intentional presence. Because the essential nature of these various understandings of presence flows from our spiritual core, we consider the essence of healing presence to be *spiritual* presence. Thus, unless otherwise noted, the term *presence* throughout this discussion refers to spiritual presence, which is the essence of healing presence.

UNDERSTANDING PRESENCE

Presence is the way that we are *with* another or others in the midst of all our interactions. How we are with another happens in a particular moment in time and is new as every moment is new. Presence reflects more of the non-instrumental aspects of our encounters and relationships with others that do not rely on words or tasks that the practitioner performs (Engebretson, 2000). According to Paterson and Zderad (1988), presence occurs within an intersubjective and transactional experience of a genuine dialogue with another, reflective of what Martin Buber (1958) describes as an "I-Thou" relationship. Paterson and Zderad describe presence as "a mode of being with the wholeness of one's unique individual being: a gift of self which can only be given freely, invoked or evoked" (p. 122). Presence in this understanding requires an openness, receptivity, and availability with the whole of oneself and involves reciprocity. Presence can be welcomed or rejected, but not seized or commanded. We reveal our openness and availability toward another in verbal, nonverbal, and energetic ways, our readiness to *be with*, and *be there* with our whole being. For Osterman and Schwartz-Barcott (1996), being with another spiritually, as well as physically and psychosocially, is the determining feature of transcendent presence. This contrasts with being physically present with another while you are focused on self or on a task, or even the experience of being physically and psychosocially present while interpersonally focused. The experience of transcendent presence includes a sense of peace, comfort, harmony, and oneness between nurse and patient.

One of my earliest memories of healing presence in nursing occurred when I was a novice in my first job as a "real nurse" in a large hospital for the treatment of and research about cancer. I experienced the whole hospital as a healing place, in spite of the immense pain and sometimes palpable suffering within its walls. I watched as patients were surrounded by the caring presence of not only the nursing staff but also of housekeeping staff who knew the patients by name, and dietary personnel who went the extra mile in providing nutrition to persons whose illness and treatment made eating difficult. One example of healing presence that I experienced occurred in my relationship with a young mother. A woman in her mid-thirties, she was dying and leaving behind two young children and a broken hearted husband. She was one of those persons who was special to the whole nursing staff, who touched us all by her courage and gentleness as she faced leaving behind her beloved family. One day, having given her some medication, I paused for a moment, and we held hands in silence. As I left the room one of her family members gave me a hug and said, "It was so good of you to take time to hold her hand." I could not speak at that time, but the knowing in my soul, even then, was "Oh no, you see, *she* was holding my hand." Indeed, my experience of that moment was of *her* healing presence for me. Even today when I think of healing presence I appreciate more and more that as caregivers we often stand in the healing presence of our patients on their spiritual journeys, privileged to be part of that journey

Space-Time: Physics, Mystics, and Presence

> *From atom to organism to person, the pattern that meets us*
> *in nature is that of connection and contact. In the world of living*
> *organisms, isolation is no where met. (Dossey, 1982, p.75)*

The oneness and relationship of all in the universe is a truth that shamans and mystics have known for eons and that scholars of modern physics and deep ecology are affirming. As we move beyond linear thinking, we appreciate more fully the web of life in which we are deeply intertwined and connected with all life. Mystics of many traditions reflect their experience that form and emptiness are two aspects of the same reality, form is emptiness, and emptiness is form. In the language of quantum physics, we hear that the same particles can appear as energy or matter. From physics, we learn that each atom is connected to all other atoms in the universe, exerting change on, and being affected by all these atoms. It is only through their relationship with all subatomic particles that we can comprehend any subatomic particles (Dossey, 1982). What we look at as parts can ultimately be understood only as an undivided, interrelated whole. We do not exist separate from the whole; rather, we share existence with this oneness or unity. Dossey (1982) discusses how quantum physics provides further insight into our implicit connectedness with all in the universe. He notes the work of John S. Bell, who postulated that given statistical predictions of quantum theory, an objective universe, that is, one that exists apart from our consciousness, is incompatible with laws of local causes. The implications of this theorem have been borne out through mathematics and experimentation demonstrating that "two particles, once in contact, separated even to the ends of the universe, change *instantaneously* when a change in one of them occurs!" (p. 100). Although separated in space these two particles remain in some way connected, suggesting an elemental oneness of the world. We live in a participatory universe in which we can never be detached observers. Nothing is totally outside, or other than ourselves; thus, even as an "observer," we are in relationship with, and at some level influencing, the observed.

Physics helps us to understand the intrinsic connection we have with others and that we can consciously evoke this connection in any situation. Neither what we perceive as matter, nor the space around it, are separate from each other. Consider the print on this page. Although it might appear separate from the space around it, in truth the print and the space are continuous. The space, however, allows us to see and understand the print because at the same time that it separates the letters and words, it also connects them. Applied to any encounter with a patient, we are always connecting because we are not separate from the space between us. Whatever energy we bring to an encounter, conscious or not, influences the interaction. Healing presence is a way of being with another with consciousness of our connectedness with self, with the patient, and with the healing energies of Universal Love, God, in this moment. Our intention to bring care and love into any situation brings a powerful presence that changes that situation.

EXPERIENCING SACRED OR DIVINE PRESENCE

The spiritual presence that we bring into our relationships with others flows from our connectedness with the Divine, the Sacred Source. We may be more conscious of this connection at some moments than we are at other times. People experience this connection in different ways, and our unique experiences may vary at different times in our lives. Our sense of the presence of the Sacred can be influenced by factors such as our spiritual or religious perspective, our culture, and our awareness of and commitment to our personal spiritual journey. Some people feel a very tangible sense of this presence; for others it may be more subtle. We might experience Sacred presence as a sense of peace, as joy and gladness, as gratitude, as insight, as a power or energy within us, or as that something that keeps us going when we feel we no longer can go on. The Divine may be felt as the presence of a friend, a guide, a parent, an intimate companion, as love, as universal energy, as beauty, or as light. We can experience Sacred presence through music, art, a day in the mountains, religious worship, sacred ceremony, teaching a child to read, or sitting with a sick friend. Mystics write and speak of how they encounter the Divine presence in both ordinary life experiences as well as in more numinous or visionary moments. For example, the Jewish mystical tradition teaches that God is equally in all things—in the compost as well as in the flower, in the light as well as in the dark, in joy and in sorrow and suffering, in health and illness. We need not seek God's presence in these circumstances, only be open to the presence that is already there.

REFLECTION 4–1

- How do you experience the presence of the Divine or Sacred in your life? Describe your experience at various places along your spiritual journey.
- What does Divine or Sacred presence feel like to you?
- Have you ever been surprised by a sense of the Sacred showing up unexpectedly in your life? What was this like?
- How does your sense of Divine or Sacred presence influence your presence with others?

Presence as Blessing

Presence is a way of bringing blessing to our relationships, to our world, to our life. Rupp (1997, p. 131) reminds us that, in the words of the Sufi poet and mystic Rumi, "wherever you place your foot, there rests a blessing." Rather than considering blessing an act that makes something holy, blessing is more truly our acknowledgment of the inherent sacredness that is already here. Our very presence, with awareness of the sacredness of all of creation, is a blessing. Because spiritual presence flows from the Divine or Sacred presence within us, we bless by our being. Rupp reflects that when we bless, we bring the touch of love, of goodness, of God-ness to others by both our presence and actions. She cites the example of Jesus, who did not offer or bestow many blessings; rather, "he *becomes* a blessing. His presence, his goodness, engenders life, strength, healing, courage, and vitality" (p. 135). As we bring spiritual presence into our encounters, we, too, become a blessing for those in our care. This blessing can come in very simple acts and moments of being with another, as seen with Annie and Mother J.: Annie, one of the members of the hospital dietary staff who brought meals to Mother J., was a source of joy and comfort to Mother J. during her hospitalization. Her presence always brightened up the room when she brought in Mother J.'s tray. One particular day she came in with the tray and then, in as gentle and natural a manner as any minister, she took Mother J.'s outstretched hand and prayed with her. Although there were several of us in the room, as far as Mother J. and Annie were concerned it was the two of them and the God to whom they prayed. I don't know what led Annie to pray with Mother that day (or then again, maybe I do), but I know that it was a blessing of healing in a situation that was beyond curing. In the hustle and bustle of a high-tech medical center, we were reminded of God's presence as a woman passing out meal trays took a moment to pray with a woman she called "my sister."

LOVING PRESENCE, HEALING PRESENCE

Love alone is capable of uniting living beings in such a way as to complete and fulfill them, for it alone takes them and joins them by what is deepest in themselves. (Teilhard de Chardin, 1959, p. 265)

Love is a very powerful healer; indeed all healing is grounded in love. Healing love goes beyond a feeling response, and sometimes might not even feel very loving. This love comes from the deep place of Spirit within us, and flows from our connection with God, the Life Force, Sacred Source. In describing healing love, Levine (1987) writes, "It is not the relationship of 'I' for 'other.' It is the sense of the inherent connection between the two that goes beyond duality to the oneness of being" (p. 67). Love is the ground of our being and, as such, is the essence of who we are. As described in 1 Corinthians 13 of the Christian Scriptures, this love is patient, kind, not jealous or snobbish, never rude or self-seeking, not prone to anger, does not brood over injuries, does not rejoice in what is wrong, rather rejoices in the truth and has no limits to its forbearance, trust, hope, and power to endure. When we relinquish all our preconceptions, judgments, ideas about what love is and is not, our sense of limitations of love, we become aware of this natural condition of our being that receives all things, all experiences, and all of who we are with equal openness and regard. The universal and always connected state of being that is love itself "is a condition not between beings, but within being. When I am in that place of love and you enter, then we are in love together . . . one does not have unconditional love for another. One is unconditional love" (Levine, 1987, p. 68). Love in this understanding is what enables us to be a sacred presence, healing presence with another. As we discover and attune to our essential nature of love, we connect with the vastness of being where we experience unity with and appreciation, love, and compassion toward all.

SELF-NURTURE: Being with and in Presence

Sit quietly in a place that, for you, is sacred space. This could be a place of spiritual ceremony, religious worship, somewhere in nature, an area of your home, or any place where you have a sense of the Sacred. Become aware of and sense the Presence of that which is more than you, or the more of you in this place. You might feel that you are with or in this Presence, or that it is with or in you. What is this like for you? Consider how you experience this Presence, whether it feels strong or subtle, active or quiet, personal or universal.

Choose a place that you consider a more secular or ordinary space and engage in this same process. Use this process to become aware of the Presence in your workplace or in a public place within your community.

INTENTIONALITY

Within the context of healing and nursing care, intention reflects both our purpose and motivation for care. At some level, intention is a conscious response to the question "how can I be here in the most healing way?"—both in the general way in which we practice and in particular situations with particular persons. Intention is a volitional act of love that flows from our spiritual core where we consciously align with creative essence and divine purpose (Dossey & Guzzetta, 2000; McKivergin, 2000). Intention involves being fully present in the moment and directing our inner awareness toward healing, wholeness, and the highest good, without needing to determine how healing will manifest. Healing intention is choosing to be an instrument of Universal Love, an instrument of God, of the Divine.

Being a healing presence with another requires that we are aware in the moment and that we choose to be in the moment in a loving way. Connecting with our essence of love, we make the choice to be this love with another. Within this choice is our intention to be with another with all the qualities of presence noted earlier. Intentionality in this understanding implies directing our awareness with purpose toward an object or outcome (Watson, 1999a). Intentionality reflects our beliefs and desires regarding healing. In choosing to be with another in a loving, healing way, I bring my awareness fully to this moment. I choose to be the energy of love in this encounter. I am conscious of making myself available to another, and I open myself to receive the other within the space of love in which there ultimately is no "other." Intentionality involves projecting a thought or idea, but is more than a cognitive process. Intentionality is rooted in our being, in our consciousness of being, and in our lived experience of our connectedness. Through intentionality we open ourselves to our greater connectedness with all life, acknowledging that the energy of life, of love, and the divine energy can and does flow within and through us and is available in this moment, in every moment. Intentionality is living in awareness of what is needed in this moment. It is heart awareness, soul awareness that includes, yet is deeper and more expansive than our cognitive knowing. Intentionality is a way of bringing consciousness to a situation, of opening to the greater knowing in any situation.

BEING PRESENT WITH ANOTHER

Presence is a person-to-person experience. Presence flows from being aware of my grounding in my own center. Within my center, I recognize that the Source of me is the Source of you. This is the place where we are one, yet distinct, the place where we experience our common humanity. Within this place, I can be with you without judgment, without needing you to change to fit my needs and expectations. From the place of my center I can receive who you are, I know that your fears, your hopes, your joys, and your longings are not so different from my own. This is the place where Mystery resides, where I can be with mystery and allow it to unfold—in me, in you, and in us together.

Presence is perhaps one of the clearest ways that Spirit, or the Sacred, manifests in and through us. Because this presence is a manifestation of Spirit, it is difficult to describe and understand from a purely cognitive perspective. We feel and experience presence, and in this way it is tangible, yet it is not measurable in an objective sense. When we speak of presence, we refer to the deeper essence of self that we share with another. This presence is a way of *being with* another, rather than having a primary focus on the tasks of *doing for or to* that person. Being with another implies being in the moment with all of who we are, attuned to the other in her or his uniqueness in the context of the lived experience of life at this time. This is a sacred process of relating heart to heart, soul to soul, whole being to whole being. These are *I-Thou* relationships, in which we recognize and meet God, the Sacred, in the other, contrast with *I-It* relationships in which we interact with others with the indifference or disdain that flows from not seeing their innate value (Buber, 1958). Boulding (1989) describes this relationship as listening to God in another person, being fully and totally there with another with all our physical senses and our intuitive senses as well. Presence is a way of being physically, emotionally, and energetically with another in a way that conveys our desire and willingness to hear, to know, to appreciate, and to receive who the other is and what the person is experiencing in this moment. The exchange of authentic meaningful awareness and essence that occurs when relating with another in this way promotes integration and balance in the healing relationship (McKivergin, 2000).

Let us clarify that when we speak of presence in terms of *being with* another, we do not mean to imply that we can only be present if we are sitting still with another, *doing* nothing! Rather, our goal is to be with others in this way in the midst of whatever we are doing with or for that person, whether we are sitting quietly or involved in much activity. Presence speaks to *how* we are with others and can change from moment to moment with no apparent change in what we are doing. At some levels, it is a shift in attitude or consciousness of where or how we are within ourselves and how we are choosing to be with the other. We shift to a different place from which we are listening, hearing, seeing, and being. For example, I, like most of us, have some patients that, for one reason or another, I find harder to be with than others. One such patient is a woman who has many chronic health problems and who seems little motivated to participate actively in her care. Because of my frustration and impatience with her (perhaps stemming from my inability to "make her better"), I often feel like I just want to get in and take care of her current complaint and move on to my next patient. It is easy to be in these encounters primarily from the place of my technical and clinical self, who knows how to obtain a good history, do a proper assessment, and decide on appropriate interventions based on what I learn through these processes. When my interactions come primarily from this place of my cognitive knowing, I often feel an uneasiness in myself and a strain or discordance between myself and the patient, even though what I am doing, saying, and suggesting are clinically appropriate. I have found, however, that when I am conscious of my attitude and make the inner shift to being with the patient from my deeper, truer, self, even in the midst of an encounter, that there is a difference in the whole interaction. What I am doing does not change, but how I am being with what I am doing is quite different because I move beyond personality and create more space for a soul-to-soul encounter. My presence flows from consciously being in my heart center, the place of inner listening, where I can listen, receive, and respond with my whole being. When in this space, I experience that my frustration and irritation seem less intense. I find that I am able to be more open to hearing her concerns within the context of her life as it is today, in this moment, rather than feeling that I'm just hearing the same old story again. I feel more compassion for and experience more of a shared humanity with her, which helps me to reconsider how I can be with her in a loving way without feeling that I need to, or even know how to, fix her life.

Let us shed more light on healing presence with some examples of when it was absent. Our friend, Nancy, shared an experience of a time when she was in the hospital, and, because of her overall situation, was crying quite intensely. She noted that two different nurses came into her room to attend to some task, did whatever they needed to do as quickly as possible, and left. Neither nurse acknowledged her presence or appeared to notice that she was crying, nor inquired about what was going on with her. Perhaps they were extremely busy, or feared they might need to "fix" whatever was going on with her, and felt inadequate. Sandra Melville (whose story is shared later in the book) describes a hospital experience in which healing presence was absent: "That night the IV was feeling funny, and I asked the nurse to check it. 'I don't know what you're worried about; you don't need the IV anyway.' (the nurse replied) . . . I started to cry . . . (later) another nurse came in to look at the IV. She flipped on the light, took in the tears leaking from my eyes and sniffed, 'I don't know what you're so upset about. You have nothing to cry about!'"

In contrast to these two experiences, Floyd describes a nurse whose presence was both loving and healing:

There was this nurse . . . I don't remember her name, but I can see her face. It was one of those nights when I just couldn't get settled down. I had too much going on between my ears. Boy, your thoughts can run away with you sometimes, especially when you don't know what's happening 'cause you've never been through this before. This cancer is an ugly thing. Well, it's the middle of the night and I put my light on . . . and this nurse came in, and she must have stayed with me for about an hour. She just sat down and asked me how I was doing . . . and we went from there. We'd talk about everything. I'd tell her some of my story, and she'd tell me some about her life. Then, every once in awhile, we'd get around to some of the things that were bothering me. I had about four or five things going on that were really eating my lunch, and over the course of the hour we talked about them all. She talked. I talked. I listened, she listened. I had questions. I'd never been through anything like this before. She has some answers, but she didn't mind saying when she didn't have an answer either. She could tell me what usually happened, make it easier for me to go into the unknown. Yes, I remember that nurse for sure. I think most nurses are like a part of heaven.

This nurse was with Floyd when he needed her, not when she had time for him on her schedule. She created a sacred space in which he could "go into the unknown," allowing him to set the pace of both moving away from and confronting the issues.

Holistic nursing calls us to cultivate this way of being with others in every interaction, fully attentive to the sacredness of every moment and of every person. Because presence transcends time and space, we can be present energetically with another in this way even when we are at a distance. Consider a time when you have felt a tangible sense of the love and support from a parent, friend, partner, or child even when you were separated by many miles. People often speak of feeling the presence of people who pray for them when they are ill or need support in other ways. Distant intentionality, nonlocal healing, and prayer are all ways of offering spiritual presence to others. (Dossey, 1999; Schlitz & Braud, 1997; Targ, 1997; Watson, 1999a).

- What helps you to *be* in the present moment? How is this different when you are alone compared with when you are in the midst of much activity?

- Recall an experience in which you felt you were truly present with another. How would you describe what presence looked like and felt like in this experience. What helped you be present with the other in this way?

- Recall an experience in which you felt you were unable to be authentically present with another. What factors limited your ability to be present in this situation? How did this experience feel to you?

SPIRITUAL PRESENCE

McKivergin and Daubenmire (1994) and McKivergin (2000) describe three levels of presence that can be evident in nursing or other encounters:

1. *Physical presence*: "being there" for another in physical service that involves body-to-body contact. Tasks of care and interventions such as examining, seeing, hearing, doing to and for, touching, and hugging are often carried out at this level of presence.

2. *Psychological presence*: "being with" another using self as an instrument for creating a therapeutic milieu addressing patient needs for comfort, help, and suppoørt. This level of presence involves mind-to-mind con-nection and can remain primarily focused in the cognitive realm. Com-munication skills including active listening, reflecting, nonjudgmental acceptance, and empathy, are necessary for this level of presence. Watson (1999a) notes that the therapeutic use of self and conscious intention to be available to another moves the nurse beyond the routine level of care toward a more authentic caring presence.

3. *Therapeutic presence*: is spirit-to-spirit, whole being to whole being connec-tion. This level involves "being with" and "being there" using all resources of spirit, body, mind, and emotions. Connection at this level is centered-self to centered-self, essence-of-love to essence-of-love, reflecting the spiritual dimension of presence. Being present at this level involves intentionality, openness, intuitive knowing, awareness of the interconnectedness of all life, and personal awareness of and attending to our own spirituality.

Jean Watson (1999a) translates the level of therapeutic presence into *transpersonal presence* because it is closely aligned with caring consciousness, intentionality, mindfulness, and transpersonal caring. By transpersonal she means

an intersubjective, human-to-human relationship, which encompasses two individuals in a given moment, but simultaneously transcends the two, connecting to other dimensions of being and a deeper/higher consciousness that accesses the universal field and planes of inner wisdom: the human spirit realm. At its core, transpersonal recognizes that the power of love, faith, compassion, caring, community and intention, consciousness and access to a deeper/higher energy source, i.e., one's God, is as important to healing as are our conventional treatment approaches, and is possibly even more powerful in the long run. At its root, transpersonal caring honors the unity of being, shifting levels of consciousness. It seeks to harmonize *being* for self and other in relation to one's deeper/higher self in the world (p. 115).

Therapeutic presence (McKivergin & Daubenmire) and *transpersonal* presence (Watson) are easily translated into spiritual presence as described by Savary and Berne (1988). They use the term *kything* to denote the concept of spiritual presence, a way of being with another that is beyond physical and mental presence, reflecting a spirit-to-spirit encounter that is experienced as communion. They note that, where our minds and physical senses tend to grasp elements and details of another, our spirits take in the essence or totality of the person. When we *kythe*, which is being spiritually present with another, we are in touch with that person's spirit or soul in a way that goes beyond being present to their physical, mental, or emotional spheres. Their term *kything* derives from an old Scottish word meaning to be manifest or to show oneself without disguise. In relation to spiritual presence, Savary and Berne extend the meaning to include making your spirit or true self manifest to another or to show your soul to another. Watson (1999b) echoes this in her reminder that because we are the instrument of caring presence, we have to be "up close and personal" in our way of being with others. The three essential steps to kything described by Savary and Berne (pp. 24–33) are a useful guide for learning or for further developing spiritual presence. These steps, which can sometimes seem to occur simultaneously, are:

- *Centering:* a holistic process of quietly and lovingly focusing attention on yourself—body, mind, spirit—until you begin to experience a sense of peace, inner calm, and relaxation, and become present to your whole self.

- *Focus on the other:* from your centered place, shift the focus of your attention to the other and use your whole being to truly *see* the person, until you feel yourself present to that person's spirit.

- *Establish connection or union:* communion happens as you establish spirit-to-spirit connection. This step can be facilitated by envisioning or

imaging a bond or connection between you and the other, and making a
choice to make what is imaged a reality.

SELF-NURTURE: *Kything* with Another

Review the process of *kything*. Using this process, ask a trusted
friend or companion to share in an experience of *kything* or spiritual
presence. Allow yourself to receive the presence of your partner as you are offering
yourself as presence to her or him. Be gentle and generous with yourself as you
move through this process, suspending any expectations or judgments, just being
open to the experience as it unfolds. You may want to share your experiences with
your partner, or express them in another way such as through poetry, prose, art,
movement, or music. Consider sharing this process with your partner several
times over a period of several days or weeks.

Transpersonal or spiritual presence acknowledges that the persons who come
together in a caring moment are in a process of being and becoming. What occurs
between the persons, and goes beyond either individual, can release inner power
and strength that promotes a sense of harmony. Spiritual presence potentiates the
self-healing process by facilitating access to our inner healer and opening access to
the healing potential of the universe. By entering into the experience of another
we find their hopes, fears, concerns, dilemmas in ourselves, and deepen our
awareness that we are all related. Essentially, we learn from others how to be
human in all dimensions of our experience of living as embodied souls. Watson
(1988; 1999a) notes that by deepening awareness of our common humanity we
are better able to stay connected with the human spirit and less likely to treat the
human person as an object that is separate from the spirit of the self and of the
wider universe. What Watson (1999a) describes as a caring-healing consciousness
is the source of healing presence, "a source and form of life energy, life spirit, and
vital energy which is connected to the energy of the universe, the universal energy
field" (p. 118). We recognize that this consciousness is unbounded, and
omnipresent, transcending time, space, and physicality (Dossey, 1991; 1999).

PRESENCE AS ENERGETIC CONNECTION

Presence is not a new concept in nursing, indeed descriptions of nursing presence as the nurse being with another with the whole of her or himself were evident in nursing literature in the early and mid-1960s (Doona, Chase, &

Haggerty, 1999; Godkin, 2001). Our understanding of the nature of presence has evolved as we have become more aware of the spiritual sphere, levels of consciousness, subtle energies, and ways of healing in various traditions. Nursing theories reflect that presence is a distinguishing feature of nursing care (Newman, 1994; Parse, 1992; Paterson & Zderad, 1988; Rogers, 1970; Watson, 1988; 1999a).

Nursing's development and practice of energy-based healing modalities has contributed to our appreciation that presence, as an energetic and spiritual connection, is a key factor in healing (Hover-Kramer, Mentgen & Scandtrett-Hibdon, 1996; Krieger, 1979; 1993). These modalities remind us that we do not stop at our skin. Energetically we are all constantly interacting with everyone and everything in our environment. The presence we are in any situation shifts and changes the energy of that environment, and these changes affect everyone in the environment, including ourselves!

REFLECTION 4–3

- Pause and describe your presence in this moment.
- Consider the energy or presence that you bring to your work (or any other) setting when you feel tired, worried, or unsure of yourself, compared with how you are when you feel happy, competent, at peace.
- Describe a time when another's presence decreased your comfort or increased your stress.
- Describe a time when another's presence brought you joy or peace.

Whether or not we are conscious of doing so, we energetically sense what is going on in our environment. Have you ever experienced feeling uneasy for no apparent reason when you were around a particular person or in a certain place? On the other hand, have you felt a peace and calm merely entering a spiritual sanctuary or being with a loving friend? Our energetic messages are often exchanged unconsciously. With intentional presence, however, we become more conscious of these exchanges. We choose how we wish to *be* in a situation, what kind of energy we wish to bring, to be in the situation. We also become aware of the energies that are not ours and choose how we wish to be with these exchanges as well. This choice grounds our intention, which sets the focus for the encounter. Our intention, which involves aligning our body-mind-spirit self with Universal

Energy, Love, God Energy, organizes and directs our energy in the present situation. Intention connects us with the spaciousness that is the more of who we are, both individually and together, connects us with the Source, and opens us to the love that we are.

QUALITIES OF NURSING PRESENCE

Presence is often hard to describe because it has so many faces and nuances. However, certain qualities or characteristics accompany the more subtle facets of presence. Hines (1992) describes six qualities of presence identified within nursing encounters: time with another, which includes a willingness to wait and stay with them; unconditional positive regard that affirms those in the interaction, is grounded in trust and respect, and provides safety; transactional being with another that includes verbal and nonverbal communication; valued encounter that involves an investment of self and action beyond the ordinary; connectedness or essence-linking that involves engagement with another who is recognized as making a difference in one's life; and sustaining memory, the enduring impact of the encounter.

When investigating factors related to nursing judgments, Doona, Chase, and Haggerty (1999) discovered that nurses had to talk about *being with* patients to discuss nursing judgments. These authors discovered that presence, viewed by some as the essence of nursing that distinguishes novice from expert, is inextricably related to nursing's focus on care with people. In the context of existential tension, the moment of nursing presence (which Watson would call an actual caring occasion) occurs when the nurse chooses to be available to a patient from the deeper self and the patient invites the nurse into her or his situation. This provides the opportunity and context for each to be present to the other. These authors identify six features of an experience of nursing presence:

1. *Uniqueness*: This presence encompasses a unique moment in time in which the nurse consciously chooses to encounter uncertainty in a situation, acknowledging the uniqueness of the patient and the uniqueness of the nurse.

2. *Connecting with the patient's experience*: The focus is on the person as a whole rather than on a particular task.

3. *Sensing*: This is openness to one's own inner sense and subjectivity as well as to cognitive information, and the ability to sift, weigh, and balance these multiple sources of data to determine what is really going on in the situation.

4. *Going beyond the scientific data*: This is awareness of patterns of response of a whole person that go beyond technical data and enable recognition of subtle changes and nuances in the situation.

5. *Knowing what will work*: Knowing the person as a unique being incorporates who the person is as well as the context of her or his experience.

6. *Knowing when to act*: In the tension of uncertain situations, this means going beyond objective data and trusting one's own sense and knowing of the right action and the right moment for action.

The findings of this study reflect that presence is as vital to nursing care as scientific and technical knowledge is and that presence grounds nursing judgments. Through their presence as they interacted with patients in various ways, including assessment and technical interventions, nurses were able to develop a better understanding of the whole situation, appreciate unfolding patterns, and see beyond the present to the possibilities inherent in the situation. As they continued to open to their own and their patient's experiences, they could envision possibilities for health in the situation and incorporated all this data in making clinical judgments. Godkin (2001) suggests that the ability to be a healing presence with patients relates to a nurse's level of competence and confidence in both clinical skills and professional interaction.

Spiritual presence is more frequently a part of nursing care than nurses recognize or acknowledge. Nurses might not name what they are doing as spiritual caregiving because they do not recognize it as such. I experienced this presence with nurses in a very busy outpatient surgery unit at a city hospital when I accompanied a close friend, whom I will call Maria, through a diagnostic procedure. The environment was one of much activity in a large room with many beds separated only by curtains. There was a continual turnover of patients who were in this space for both preparation and recovery. The nurses were very efficient as they attended to multiple patients. Despite the fast pace of the unit, I experienced each nurse who came into our space to be present with us in the moment as she completed necessary tasks. While taking the history, the nurse sat down and gave Maria her full attention. She expressed genuine interest in what Maria was saying and responded to her needs for explanation and comfort. For example, noting Maria adjusting herself in the bed, she got her an extra pillow. While competently performing technical tasks, the nurse oriented Maria to the procedure and provided an opportunity for Maria to express other questions and concerns. The nurse helped to allay Maria's anxiety through appropriate humor, encouraging Maria to use some deep breathing processes and supporting my presence with Maria. Although the nurse moved in and out of our space to care for other patients, while she was with us there was never a sense that she was rushed or that she needed to be someplace else. The presence of the nurse engendered a sense of trust. Although having someone accompany a patient as I was doing was not a common occurrence, I felt only generosity and welcoming from the nurses. Although these nurses might not identify what they were doing as spiritual caregiving, within all the technically competent care the nurses provided, Maria and I experienced their care for her whole being, body-mind-spirit. It was not something that they did in addition to other care, but how they were, and who they were in the care they were giving.

Caring presence guides nurses in the mystery of the moment, and ultimately contributes to and supports the patient's spirituality. This is evident in Joni Walton's (1999) exploration of spirituality of patients recovering from an acute myocardial infarction. Receiving presence was the core category identified in this grounded theory study. Participants experienced receiving presence from the divine, friends, family, community, creation, and health care workers. Through awareness of and willingness to receive this transcendent presence into their hearts, participants experienced comfort and peace, enhanced coping, and help in transitioning through phases of discovering meaning and purpose during their recovery. Walton notes that these caring connections between health care providers and participants helped to break the cycle of fear, anxiety, and chest pain. These connections provided a sense of hope, comfort, and trust in the treatment plan and ultimate healing of the heart. Presence supported participants in the vital spiritual processes of discovering meaning and purpose during their illness experience. Walton (personal communication, 1999) offers this reflection and personal practice of presence:

> Many patients are quick to recall experiences where they have not connected harmoniously with health care providers. I strongly believe that in order to move beyond the basic level of presence health care providers must use humanistic communications and behaviors. From the MI study I learned that all the participants wanted an encouraging, positive, caring nurse. I decided that I needed to incorporate some of their recommendations into my job in the open-heart surgery unit (usually only 1 or 2 days length of stay in ICU). When I transferred my patients to the floor I took several moments to tell them how proud I was of them and I congratulated them for all they had achieved in the past 24 hours. Then I gave them a hug. Each patient loved it. Many of them cried and would hardly let go of my neck. One day I was asked to transfer a patient out of the unit quickly so we could get an emergency AAA. I introduced myself to the elderly man and wheeled him to his new room. I decided that even though I just met him that I would tell him my routine transfer congratulations. I was surprised because he looked me in the eye gave me a hug and a kiss and said, "I love you so much." I looked at him and said, "I love you too." This was a profound experience for both of us and it happened in 3 minutes. I think that the atmosphere or environment that permeates the situation sets it up for a sacred moment.

This story reflects how easily presence can be integrated into our care with patients. It also illustrates that seemingly simple acts can communicate presence in a profound way. Within a brief moment in time, Joni trusted her own sense, connected with the patient's unique experience, opened her inner sense and engaged with the patient at the level of soul-to-soul, and communicated unconditional positive regard for the patient. She received and was received by the patient. Love was tangible in the encounter, which had deep meaning for both nurse and patient.

Certain qualities or features are evident in interactions in which we are present in a healing way with another (McKivergin, 2000). These interactions are marked by conscious giving of oneself without judgment in unconditional acceptance, understanding, patience, openness, honesty, love, and being available to another in a way that the other perceives as meaningful. Presence creates a sacred space in which to be with questions and wonderings, a space that allows for mystery without requiring that the situation be different. This requires an ability to be with another without needing to have the answers or to "fix it." Presence at this level acknowledges the gift and blessing of being able to participate with the other not by fixing or doing, but by being and sharing.

Joan Engebretson (2000) illustrates the power of presence with a poignant story of one of her nursing student's presence with a mother and newborn in a busy neonatal intensive care unit (NICU). The student had no role in the physical care of the infant, and was guided to "be with" the young mother who had just delivered a son at 23 weeks gestation. As the mother sat in a wheelchair next to her son's isolette, the student sat in a chair next to her, both in relative silence in the midst of the ceaseless noise of machines and conversations and activities of staff. As the baby's condition became less stable, the nurses invited the mother to touch her son, and eventually placed him in the mother's arms. The student continued to "be with" the mother, occasionally gently touching her shoulder, back, or arm, still with few or no words. Engebretson observed a noticeable change in the way the NICU staff approached the mother-baby-student trio through the course of the morning, noting that the staff "seemed to sense a special space in the unit extending about 3–5 feet around [the trio] . . . not intruding unless they had a specific need to do so. The mood in the entire unit also changed; there was a dramatically less hectic atmosphere in the unit . . . an aura of dignity was created throughout the unit" (p. 35). She recounted that the staff moved slightly slower, spoke more softly, and that their touch seemed kinder and gentler than it had been earlier. Throughout this time, she noted that the student seemed to be completely engaged with the mother and infant, engrossed in their interaction, and oblivious to the rest of the unit. Observing the mother's total absorption in the infant as his condition deteriorated, and most of the equipment was removed from him, Engebretson reflected that she felt "like time was suspended." She writes "by mid morning, the unit became considerably quieter and staff had gathered in a semi-circle 4–6 feet away from the trio. Nurses and doctors would move to attend to other infants and other tasks and return to stand in the circle . . . it felt like the staff had formed a human boundary to protect a space for what was about to happen" (p. 35). Throughout the next couple of hours, the student continued the silent vigil with the mother as the baby's condition deteriorated and his life slipped away. After the baby's death, the student accompanied the mother to a private room where the mother continued to hold the baby for awhile. After she transferred the mother back to her room, settled her in, and left her to sleep, the student, in reflecting on the experience with the instructor, noted that, although very sad, it had been a wonderful experience for her.

This story illustrates the very tangible impact that presence can have on the environment, as well as the blessing that it is for both those who offer and those who receive presence. Although it might be unrealistic to expect that we can spend the amount of focused time with patients as did this student, the energy of our presence in any situation can influence all that is going on interpersonally and within the greater environment. This story illuminates the value of silence and the ability to be with another in the mystery of the moment, without needing to have answers or to fix anything. We also see in this situation how the way in which nurses were present encouraged and supported the mother's presence with her son.

Supporting and encouraging presence of family and significant others is part of spiritual care giving. Family and others offer presence through physical contact such as stroking, hugging, holding; through photographs; by doing things for the patient such as bathing, cooking, dressing, bringing water, assisting with eating, running errands; and through overt signs of love such as verbal expressions of love and care, remembering special experiences together, touching, and being with (Wagner, 1999). We can both learn from family how to be present with patients, and help family to be comfortable in sharing presence with their loved ones as well.

CULTIVATING AND NURTURING PRESENCE

We are aware that being healing presence flows from our connection with our inner self and God or Sacred Source. It is a place of being that infuses our doing as we consciously choose to be in the moment in a loving way. It is a light and energy that permeates our own being yet flows through us and invites connection with others. From the vantage point of this presence, we recognize that spiritual questions and concerns manifest in many ways, often without specific reference to God, religion, or things traditionally considered to be of a spiritual nature. Being healing presence is an ability that we all have, a gift to be nurtured and cultivated.

We can be present for another only to the extent that we are present with ourselves. Thus, cultivating and nurturing presence must begin with deepening our ability to be present with ourselves, alert and aware of what is here, in the present. This is no easy task in our fast paced society where we seem to always be anticipating and planning the next thing we need to do, or wondering about something that has already occurred. Watson (1999b) recounted a story about an

Englishman, who, while traversing a region of Africa, was trying to make it to a particular destination by a certain time. After three days of pushing his African bushmen guides and porters faster than they would prefer to travel, they stopped and refused to go further. When he asked to know why, they told him they had been traveling so fast for so many days that they needed to stop and let their souls catch up. We too need to pause and make sure we are wholly in the moment—our souls, our minds, and our emotions with our bodies. We can begin by becoming aware of ourselves in the moment. What am I thinking? Are my thoughts related to the current moment or concerned about future or past experiences that take my awareness away from this moment. What am I experiencing physically and emotionally? How aware am I of my posture, the clothes touching my skin, areas of discomfort or tension? How aware am I of what I am feeling emotionally—sadness, joy, fear, worry, peace, love? How are my emotions showing up in my physical being, my relationships, and my spirit? What am I sensing energetically, and do I allow myself to trust these senses? We develop awareness by paying attention, by noting, without judgment or chastisement, when we are conscious in the current moment of what is happening within the various spheres of our physical-mental-emotional-spiritual-energetic being, and when we are not.

As we connect with the inner self and Sacred Source, we nurture presence. Spiritual traditions offer many approaches that assist us in seeking that quiet space within where we encounter mystery. Presence requires an ability to be still in the midst of activity—to experience our inner quiet even in the midst of a raging storm. Some people seem to have a natural ability to be in this space, but most of us need to cultivate this ability. We can begin by giving ourselves time each day to be inwardly still, to enter the quiet place within. From this quiet place, we experience our connection with Sacred Source or Universal Love, Life Energy.

SELF-NURTURE: Cultivating Presence

Spiritual practices of prayer of the heart or meditation enable us to attune to our inner self—to become familiar with our own sacred space and connection with Sacred Source. This space may sometimes feel dark and empty, yet is the space in which we come to know ourselves and experience our own sacredness and Love. The following are a few of the many ways you can nurture your ability to be present in the moment with yourself and others. Choose a practice that suits you that you can incorporate regularly into your life.

- Centering prayer (Keating, 1995) is an example of prayer of the heart, a form of contemplative prayer that opens our awareness, our whole being to the Ultimate Mystery, to God, beyond thoughts, emotions, words. The basic guidelines for centering prayer are

- Choose a sacred word (such as love, mercy, Lord, shalom, yes) or inner gaze (such as on a candle flame) that expresses your intention to be open to God's presence and action.
- Sit comfortably, with eyes closed, and gently and silently introduce the sacred word or inner gaze as the symbol of your intention to be open to God's presence and action within you.
- When you become aware of thoughts or other perceptions, images, reflections, return gently to the sacred word, viewing these thoughts as invitations to return to awareness of being in God's presence in the moment.
- At the end of the prayer period remain silent for a couple of minutes enabling the psyche time to readjust to external senses and fostering the ability to bring the atmosphere of silence into daily life.

Keating suggests incorporating this prayer into one's life for 20 minutes twice a day.

- Practicing the presence of God is an approach described by a 17th century monk, Brother Lawrence (1692/1958). For Brother Lawrence, the time of business was no different from the time of prayer for he recognized that at any moment and in any circumstance, the soul that seeks God may find God. This practice helps us to become more conscious of seeing God in all things and experiences in every moment. In the same way that Brother Lawrence found endless opportunities to experience the presence of God in his ordinary work in the kitchen, we too can experience God's presence in all the ordinary events and activities of our life—as we wash dishes, rake leaves, balance the checkbook, talk to a neighbor. This practice helps us see the holy in the ordinary.
- The simple practice of attuning to breathing can bring us to our centered space. Thich Nhat Hanh (2000, p. 82) offers several processes for developing mindfulness through becoming more aware of breathing. One process is counting the breath, which can be done sitting in a meditative posture or while walking.

    As you inhale, be mindful that "I am inhaling, one." When you exhale, be mindful that "I am exhaling, one." Remember to breathe from the stomach. When beginning the second inhalation, be mindful that "I am inhaling, two." And slowly exhaling, be mindful that "I am exhaling, two." Continue through 10. After you have reached 10, return to one. Whenever you lose count, return to one.

- Physical practices that include attention to breathing, such as t'ai chi, yoga, qigong, help us to be in the present moment. We are present with ourselves when listening and sensing into our body in the moment. You can do this right now as you are reading.

    Pause and slowly scan your physical self, paying attention to what you are sensing or feeling in each part of your body. Where are you experiencing tension or discomfort, or perhaps areas where you are aware of no feeling. Move your attention to one of these areas and just be with the sensation.

And be with yourself experiencing the sensation. Adjust your position and note any changes. Express gratitude and compassion to each area of your physical self. Turn your attention to your breathing, just noting how you are breathing without a need to change it. Staying aware of your body sensations, let your breathing inspirit your physical self even more, taking your whole being a little deeper into your spirit.

The same practices and process that enable us to be present with ourselves ground our ability to be present with others. Attuning to ourselves, or centering, is the grounding of all healing work. We see this in processes such as Therapeutic Touch, Healing Touch, and Reiki. Presence suggests an openness that embraces another, yet is able to differentiate between what I bring to the encounter, and what belongs to the other. Presence means that I listen to another with my whole being—body, mind, and spirit. I listen from the place of my own stillness, the place where we both can experience ourselves as whole. In this stillness is the dance of life.

BARRIERS TO PRESENCE

Although we are in continual interaction with those for whom we care, we are not always conscious of what we are bringing to the interaction in the present moment. We cannot be present if our focus is on something other than what is happening in the now. Presence can be uncomfortable because it requires an openness that exposes our own vulnerability (McKivergin, 2000). We may also be uncomfortable being with the mystery of another's journey, not having answers, or not feeling in control. Our discomfort can limit our ability to be present. When we are not grounded in our own inner self, our spiritual core, it is difficult to be with another at the deeper levels. The many distractions of professional tasks, responsibilities, insecurities, personal concerns and worries, and feelings of inadequacy impinge on our ability to be present. Fear about what might happen in an encounter, or about how others may perceive us can keep us from being truly present. Our own energy level affects how we are present with another, as does our general approach to nursing care. Self-awareness and self-care are key factors in identifying and preventing barriers to being healing presence for those in our care.

PRESENCE WITHIN THE DYING PROCESS

Conventional Western medicine still has difficulty dealing with the life reality of death. Practitioners often view death as a personal failure, and many people consider the outcome of death as a failure of the system. When scientific and technologic interventions to stave off death have been exhausted, many practitioners feel helpless, tell patients there is nothing more that can be done, and tend to withdraw. This time of life, however, offers nurses and other health care practitioners one of the clearest opportunities for providing spiritual care for patient and family. As a hospice nurse I was reminded of the poignancy of this time by a patient who said to me, "You know, you can be ready to die, but not eager. I still love the smell of breakfast cooking when I wake up in the morning." In such moments of shared journeying we know the mutuality of spiritual care and understand that our presence at this time is the primary healing intervention.

We are called to be present with a person and family who are deepening into their own awareness of self in the moment as they face all that dying and letting go means to everyone concerned. We share in the joy and humor of this time as well as in the pain and suffering. We saw both sides of this coin during the last few days of Mother J's dying process. One morning she opened her eyes as she woke and asked, "Why am I still breathing?" She had said her good-byes and was ready to go "home." On another occasion, Mother J's youngest daughter, Judi, spent the night with her at the hospital. Knowing that Mother loved music and singing, Judi began singing early in the morning. Judi says that Mother woke up thinking she had died and gone to heaven to the heavenly choir, and was quite disappointed to find that she was still in her hospital bed. Everyone got a laugh out of this.

Spiritual care during this time includes helping patients and family to be with their questions, uncertainties, and confusions as they deal with difficult choices, and with both expected and unexpected outcomes. Fostering and supporting important connections, facilitating healing of discordant relationships when this is needed, and facilitating the grieving process are part of this care. Joni Walton (personal communication, 1999) illustrates this with a personal experience of presence with a couple in the intensive care unit where she works.

> Yesterday I noticed a spouse hovering at the entrance of her husband's room with an expression of uncertainty. I immediately sensed that I needed to see if she needed me. I asked her "is everything ok?" She started crying and I put my arms around her and she cried for several minutes. Then she told me that the physician told her that her husband (who was sleeping) would only live several days unless he went on dialysis. She remembered him saying that he would not want dialysis. She said that she needed more time and was not ready to let him go (he had cancer). She said that she just could not make the decision and she did not feel strong enough to talk with him about it. I asked her if she would like me to talk to him and she nodded yes. I went into the room and pulled up a chair so that I could look him in the eye. His wife introduced me to Al. He opened his eyes and smiled at me. I could feel warmth and love shining through his eyes. I took his hand in mine and said, "Al, the doctor talked to your wife this morning and told her that your kid-

neys are failing and that you are dying. You may only live a few days without dialysis. Your wife is not ready for you to die and wants every day that she can to spend with you. If you choose to have dialysis you may live for up to 6 weeks. We don't know what the quality of those weeks will be. Connie will honor and support your decision." He smiled and said, "I will not have dialysis." Connie came to his bedside and put her arms around him and they cried. I let the side rails down, Connie laid next to him in bed with her arms around him. At that point I felt that this was a very sacred moment and I was an intruder. I slipped quietly out of the room. Now when Connie sees me she hugs me. Al will have a beautiful death surrounded by his loved ones. I felt that this experience that lasted about 10 minutes at the most was a deep and intimate level of presence.

In her book, *The Grace in Dying*, Kathleen Singh (1998) discusses how we are transformed spiritually as we die. She observes how her own attitude toward death changed as she allowed herself to enter more intimately into and participate more closely in the mystery of life and death with patients. Being able to be present with her patients in this way enabled her to observe how the dying process reconnects people with the source of their being. She reflects that the more we understand the path to the transpersonal realms that the world's wisdom traditions of every age outline, the better we understand the dying process. The transformative path of the spiritual journey is that same path we each traverse in the process of dying. An essential part of this journey is being present in the moment.

The heightened bodily awareness that accompanies terminal illness focuses the person's awareness in the present moment. Being present with the self fosters the process of what Singh describes as reintegration of the bodymind. Singh considers the transformation occurring through the dying process as the home of self-actualization, which carries with it a sense of existential meaning that equates with existing in the moment. She describes experiencing "heightened presence and awareness" and " a powerful sense of being" overflowing from people who are close to death, noting that "the sense of connection to the moment becomes very deep, very real" (pp. 135–136). The ability to be in the present seems to enhance a person's capacity to accept death.

Dying is essentially a spiritual process. Our presence with the one who is dying enables us to recognize and support persons as they move through the increasingly higher and deeper levels of consciousness that Singh calls the *Nearing Death Experience*. Because this process can occur anywhere from several weeks, days, hours, or minutes before death, the importance of nursing presence with patient and family throughout the dying process cannot be over emphasized. Transformational changes that occur during the dying process are subtle and experienced in the deep space within. The sacred space that healing presence provides supports the person through this very sacred experience. The subtleties of the process require nurses to connect with patients at levels beyond words, energetically, intuitively, soul-to-soul, the place of love where there are not two, but one. Being alert for subtle signals or qualities of the Nearing Death Experience enables the nurse to appreciate when the dying person enters into this important transforming experience. According to Singh (pp. 6–18), qualities indicative of the Nearing Death Experience include the following:

- *Quality of relaxation*: sensing the end of struggle, a letting go
- *Quality of withdrawal*: turning inward, back to one's center, detachment from worldly distractions and from all but one's closest loved ones
- *Quality of radiance*: a sense of brightening in the energy around the person, an inner illumination, brightness in the eyes
- *Quality of interiority*: spending more time in meaningful spaces of one's own interior where one experiences connection with both the within and the beyond
- *Quality of silence*: few words spoken, and when spoken are meaningful and deep, reflecting the language of love
- *Quality of the sacred*: sense of being on holy ground when with the other, sense of the intensity and presence of love
- *Quality of transcendence*: awareness moves between different levels of consciousness, beyond the identity of the personal self to a transpersonal consciousness
- *Quality of knowing*: sense of a larger vision and immediate knowing beyond that bound by space, time, and physical body
- *Quality of intensity*: sense of opening, enlarging, intensifying of the energy field and moving of energy through the energy centers
- *Quality of merging*: images of the Divine or Holy become more clear and the person might experience a blending with their image
- *Quality of experienced perfection*: sense that all is okay, their experience is appropriate, and they are absolutely safe

Singh reminds us that what we witness in the process of dying is grace all around us, often appearing in very subtle ways. The qualities of the Nearing Death Experience are all qualities of grace, which, for Singh, suggests that Spirit is their source, and indicates that *"in and of itself,* the dying process provides the human being with the experience of transcendence—which is the fundamental and purposeful dynamic of human life" (p. 14–15). Our essential nature, Singh posits, is to realize Spirit, as a fish is designed for swimming and a bird for flying, so is a human being designed for transcendence.

Being present through the waiting of the dying process can be difficult, for both patient and those who are companioning them in the process. In this time, we are called to be present with mystery and trust the grace of the process as we sit with our questions of why things unfold as they do. In my personal experience of being with Mother J. as she was dying, I found that the waiting was sometimes the hardest. Mother J. had decided to stop her chemotherapy and had finally been discharged home with hospice care. She was so ready to go home to be with her Lord. On a Sunday morning as she was in her bedroom with the sunlight streaming in, I sat beside her in silence. She was comfortable and the room was, for that time, a space of peace and quiet. We held hands in the easy silence, and then I said, "You know, Mother J., I feel like I'm waiting with you at the bus-stop for your ride home to come by." She squeezed my hand, smiled, and nodded. This was a gentle time of waiting on a lovely Sunday morning. As I was able to be present with her in this span of time, the waiting was peaceful. The wonderings about why death would not come, even though she was ready, dissipated, and somehow it seemed that, in this moment, things were, in fact, as they were supposed to be.

PRESENCE IN THE PRESENT

We need to remember that the present moment is all that is real, is all that we have. Our nursing care can only take place in the present, in the eternal "now" that is always a sacred moment. Watson (1999b) posits that the new cosmology for nursing's present calls us to ask the question "Where does spirit dwell in our world and in our work?" Then we must attend to the path that is deeper, more sacred. Following this path of the heart means being present with the sacred in the midst of the profane, the horrific, the unknown, the emptiness, the joy, and the ecstasy. This path leads us to ever deeper awareness of our own wholeness and interconnectedness with all of life, the Source of our spiritual presence, our healing presence with another, and with all others. Watson (1999b) reflects that the new cosmology for nursing holds the consciousness of this connectedness —that when we touch one, we touch all; when we heal one, we heal the whole; in caring for one, we are caring for many; when we honor self and our soul's journey, we honor other souls' journeys; by re-visioning ourselves and our own inner healing journey, we re-vision nursing and society; and in healing our own woundedness, we heal the profession.

REFERENCES

Boulding, E. (1989). *One small plot of heaven.* Wallingford, PA: Pendle Hill.

Brother Lawrence (1692/1958). *The practice of the presence of God: Being conversations and letters of Nicholas Herman of Lorraine.* Westwood, NJ: Fleming H. Revell.

Buber, M. (1958). *I and Thou* (2nd ed.). New York: Charles Scribner's Sons.

Doona, M. E., Chase, S. K., & Haggerty, L. A. (1999). Nursing presence. *Journal of Holistic Nursing, 17*(1), 54–70.

Dossey, B. M., & Guzzetta, C. E. (2000). Holistic nursing practice. In B. M. Dossey, L. Keegan, & C. E. Guzzetta (Eds.), *Holistic nursing: A handbook for practice* (pp. 5–34). Gaithersburg, MD: Aspen.

Dossey, L. (1982). *Space, time & medicine.* Boston: New Science Library.

Dossey, L. (1991). *Meaning & medicine.* New York: Bantam Books.

Dossey, L. (1999). Healing the nonlocal mind. *Alternative therapies in health and medicine, 5*(6), 85–93.

Engebretson, J. (2000). Caring presence: A case study. *International Journal for Human Caring, 4*(2), 33–39.

Godkin, J. (2001). Healing presence. *Journal of Holistic Nursing, 19*(1), 5–21.

Hanh, T. N. (2000). *The wisdom of Thich Nhat Hanh.* New York: One Spirit.

Hines, D. R. (1992). Presence: Discovering the artistry in relating. *Journal of Holistic Nursing, 10*(4), 294–305.

Hover-Kramer, D., Mentgen, J., & Scandrett-Hibdon, S. (1996). *Healing touch: A resource for health care professionals.* Albany, NY: Delmar.

Keating, T. (1995). *Open mind, open heart.* New York: Continuum.

Krieger, D. (1979). *The Therapeutic Touch: How to use your hands to help or to heal.* Englewood Cliffs, NJ: Prentice-Hall.

Krieger, D. (1993). *Accepting your power to heal.* Santa FE, NM: Bear.

Levine, S. (1987). *Healing into life and death.* Garden City, NY: Anchor Press.

McKivergin, M. J. (2000). The nurse as an instrument of healing. In B. M. Dossey, L. Keegan & C. E. Guzzetta (Eds.). *Holistic Nursing: A handbook for practice.* pp. 207–227. Gaithersburg, MD: Aspen.

McKivergin, M. J., & Daubenmire, M. J. (1994). The healing process of presence. *Journal of Holistic Nursing, 12*(1), 65–81.

Newman, M. A. (1994). *Health as expanding consciousness.* New York: National League for Nursing Press.

Osterman, P. & Schwartz-Barcott, D. (1996). Presence: Four ways of being. *Nursing Forum, 31*(2) 28.

Parse, R. R. (1992). Human becoming: Parse's theory of nursing. *Nursing Science Quarterly, 1*(5) 35–42.

Paterson, J. G., & Zderad, L. T. (1988). *Humanistic Nursing.* New York: National League for Nursing.

Rogers, M. (1970). *The theoretical basis for nursing.* Philadelphia: F. A. Davis.

Rupp, J. (1997). *The cup of our life: A guide for spiritual growth.* Notre Dame, IN: Ave Maria Press.

Savary, L. M., & Berne, P. H. (1988). *Kything: The art of spiritual presence.* New York: Paulist Press.

Schlitz, M. & Braud, W. (1997). Distant intentionality and healing: Assessing the evidence. *Alternative Therapies in Health and Medicine, 3* (6), 62-73.

Singh, K. D. (1998). *The grace in dying: How we are transformed spiritually as we die.* San Francisco: Harper San Francisco.

Targ, E. (1997). Evaluating distant healing: A research review. *Alternative Therapies in Health and Medicine, 3*(6), 74–78.

Teilhard de Chardin, P. (1959). *The phenomenon of man.* New York: Harper Torchbooks.

Wagner, A. L. (1999). Within the circle of death: Transpersonal poetic reflections on nurses' stories about the quality of the dying process. *International Journal for Human Caring, 3*(2), 21–30.

Walton, J. (1999). Spirituality of patients recovering from an acute myocardial infarction: A grounded theory study. *Journal of Holistic Nursing, 17*(1), 34–53.

Watson, J. (1988). *Nursing: Human science and human care.* New York: National League for Nursing.

Watson, J. (1999a). *Postmodern Nursing and Beyond.* Edinburgh, Scotland: Churchill Livingston.

Watson, J. (1999b). *A meta-reflection on nursing's present.* Presented at the 19th Annual American Holistic Nurses' Association Conference: Holistic Healing—Heritage to Vision, Scottsdale, AZ, June 16–20.

PART 2

Caring for the Nurse's Spirit

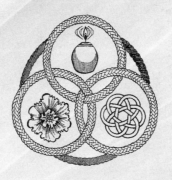

*R*ecognizing self as a spiritual being provides the basis for appreciating the spirituality of all persons. This section further explores the concept of spirituality as living our connections with God or Sacred Source, ourselves, others, and nature. Deepening our awareness of and nurturing ourselves as spiritual beings involves learning about and attending to all aspects of our relationships. Reflections and suggestions for self-nurture are offered to assist nurses and others in appreciating and nurturing themselves as whole persons and as embodied souls. The focus is on the uniqueness of each person's spirituality and soul journey or spiritual path. Processes that help us to care for ourselves, can be offered to our patients as well.

CHAPTER 5

Connecting with the Physical Self

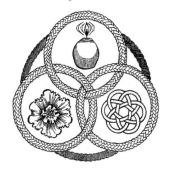

We are not spiritual beings trapped in a carnal experience.

Spirit is dancing in our molecular structure

and flowing in our bloodstream.

Physical form is the way we experience spiritual reality on earth.

ELIZABETH LESSER, 1999, P. 242

Attending to our physical selves is an important part of nurturing ourselves as spiritual beings. We are embodied spirits; that is, we are essentially spirit beings who have entered physical form, rather than physical beings that have a soul or spirit. As has been noted in previous chapters, the body, mind, and spirit are interconnected manifestations of our wholeness. We come to know the world, and we experience and express who we are, including our spirituality, through our physical selves. All our connections are mediated through the lens of our physical being. Although we live in our bodies, we are often aware of only a small percentage of what is going on in our physical selves. Unless we have pain or some other discomfort, feel hungry or tired, experience caring touch or other physical pleasure, or are concerned about how we look, we often are fairly unaware of our bodies.

Connecting with the physical self involves becoming more aware of and attentive to our bodies, which provides an avenue for deeper connection with our spirits as well. This chapter offers reflections on spirituality and the body sense, on breathing, touch, and movement as vehicles for spirit, on nourishing and caring for the physical self, on welcoming the sensual self, and on trusting our body wisdom.

REFLECTION 5–1

- How do you nurture and express your spirit through your physical body?

THE BODY SPIRITUAL

Perspectives vary in different spiritual traditions regarding the relationship between physical experience and spiritual practice. For example, some Christian sects consider the body, especially sexual expression, a barrier to the spiritual. In contrast is the Jewish tradition that sexual intercourse, especially on the Sabbath, is a *mitzvah* or blessing. Viewing the body as a vehicle for accessing our inner resources contrasts with traditions that suggest we must deny, transcend, or tame the body to gain access to the spiritual realm. Lesser (1999) reminds us that nothing in physical creation is inherently more sacred than anything else and that the energy of consciousness is as precious in the form of skin, organs, or blood as when it manifests as thought or emotion. She considers it tragic that the body was falsely accused for the sins of humankind, and thus rooted out of Western religious tradition, noting that, as materialized spirit, our bodies are as sacred and miraculous as any part of God's creation.

Both religious and cultural training influence attitudes about the body. Western religious systems have traditionally offered a dualistic perspective of life that separates things of earth from those of heaven, including a split between body and soul. Such dissociation of the body from the spirit engenders a general sense of devaluing the body as unholy and even unclean. Lesser (1999) postulates another influence on the separation of the body from spirituality in Western culture.

The advance of industrialism in the Western world also spawned negative attitudes toward the human body, and toward our shared body—the earth. Industry, large-scale agriculture, and urban living took away an immediate, physical connection to the natural world, to animals, and to a meaningful relationship between the fruits of physical toil and the fruits of the earth. As the tools to control nature became more and more effective, and as men and women became less identified with the land and animals, we lost a vital connection to our own bodies. A lack of knowledge and respect for the wilderness marches hand in hand with the disdain for the wild, animal nature of the body . . . the more separate one feels from the physical body, the easier it is to control and abuse the natural world, which leads in turn to a further distancing from a caring, loving relationship to the body. (p. 243)

All things are connected in the web of life. Attending to the physical self nurtures spirit as well and promotes more love and care for all of life.

In caring for others and in accepting care from others we experience
the spiritual community which can only take place in this world,
in the flesh. (Krysl, 1989, p. 1)

Our spiritual experience is mediated through the body sense. Some traditions give little direction about including the body in spiritual practice, but others are quite specific. Spiritual and religious rituals in many traditions require certain postures (e.g., standing, sitting, kneeling, prostrating) or movement (e.g., dancing, spinning, walking, swaying). Bathing, fasting, or other ritual purification of the body are included in many spiritual traditions as processes that facilitate spiritual openness. One example is the Native American purification or sweat lodge, a spiritual ceremony in which prayers are offered for particular needs and healing (Mails, 1988). Participation in a purification lodge may be done in preparation for another ceremony or for the spiritual, physical, and emotional benefits of the lodge itself. Spiritual ceremonies in some traditions involve adorning the body with color, design, jewels, herbs, or special garments. The physical deprivation or pain that is part of some spiritual practices leads to deeper spiritual connection. Fasting and ceremonies such as the Lakota Sun Dance are two examples. In African traditions, communal acts of worship are often occasions for singing, myriad forms of dancing, drumming, and clapping that engage the physical self as an instrument of worship (Mbiti, 1975).

The Body in Spiritual Practice: Scott's Story

(Scott Thompson is a psychotherapist, nonpracticing attorney, and Zen enthusiast.) I went to the Zen monastery when I was twenty-eight, in the cool, bright light of October, amid flickering yellow leaves. The life was tight and disciplined. The monks taught you how to eat, sleep, sit, use the toilet, work and chant, and all these activities were framed with instructions on exactly how to position the body. They emphasized *meditation*—sitting with a straight back on a black cushion stuffed with kapok, the legs folded into some version of the lotus posture. They eventually taught people to meditate in chairs, still sitting on a firm, flat cushion, with the back straight—reasoning that, after all, it's the Japanese—not us—who are accustomed to thriving on floors. We sat in meditation thirty to forty minutes in the morning and twice more in the evening. The work, five to six hours every day, was all manual labor—cleaning, sweeping, straightening old nails, tending to goats, digging trenches. They enforced stone silence the whole day except for half an hour of light social conversation during evening tea.

Zen teaches, among other things, that body and mind are *one,* always interrelated, each expressing the other. In his book, *Zen Mind, Beginner's Mind,* Suzuki said, "The most important things in our practice are our physical posture and our way of breathing. We are not so concerned about a deep understanding of Buddhism." I was a Buddhist for the next fourteen years, and have continued the meditation practice for over twenty years. Now the peace from it is so deep I would rather miss eating (well, almost).

Ten years ago I "got saved"—no kidding—which was an overwhelming experience—also puzzling. I loved learning about grace and truth and studying that good book, but to save my life I couldn't find any instructions on precisely what to *do* with my body in Christianity, including sitting in prayer. The generalized stuff—"pray on your knees"—was of no help, because the multitudes of subsidiary questions go unanswered: should the knees be on a cushion and if so made of what material? How *long* should one pray—twenty minutes, forty minutes, an hour? Twice daily or is once enough? What about the distribution of the weight and the angle of the back, and also are there stretching exercises to help one pray with greater comfort and strength and stability? Is prayer on the knees good for the back and digestion and if so what changes are typical? Finding no answers, I kept sitting Zen, now with a Christian heart.

The dearth of such information in Christianity seems weird to me, and suggests that the ancient Judeo-Christian foundation upon which this glittering, grandiose culture of ours is built has a crack or two of seismic dimensions. The fault line is in fact *separation of mind and body,* precisely the breach the Zen tradition works so assiduously to heal. The great Western philosopher Descartes said, "I think, therefore I am," which suggests that thinking, in and of itself, is somehow more special (or spiritual) than using the toilet or peeling potatoes.

Carefully examine American professional "education" of nurses, doctors, lawyers and MBA's and you will find this *disconnection* at the very heart of the training. When I was in law school, years before going to the monastery, we were pressured by every means imaginable to work until our bodies became as oblivious to stress as pillars of concrete. I eventually allowed myself, after putting up the best fight I could muster at the time (beer and bridge) to be pulled into this epistemology of overwork. What getting sucked in got me was esophageal reflux disease, for which I take medication to this day. By subjecting their numb bodies to abusive workloads, young professionals keep businesses, law firms and hospitals afloat, and the older professionals who hire them awash in plentiful incomes. It might be worth asking yourself: *who benefits?*

Zen meditation practice seems austere, and getting the hang of it does take awhile. The actual difficulty is that entrenched concepts and habitual behaviors are relentlessly challenged by the meditation. But the body loves it—let me explain. I sit twice a day, morning and evening, and knock off on Friday night. Morning meditation, as a rule, is an epiphany. Evening meditation is quite variable, in response, I believe, to work stress and other conundrums. On many nights, thinking I am drained, I actually find the meditation bright yet, paradoxically, quite relaxed. On other evenings I discover, to my surprise, that I quickly have to fight off exhaustion and go to bed immediately after I'm done. On still other nights, thinking I am all right, I find that my body twitches constantly in an effort to throw off a massive block of tension, and the thirty minute meditation seems to last hours. When *that* happens, it's time to have a careful look at what came down during the day and make some changes, *because the body is damn unhappy.* I am repeatedly struck by how easily, in the course of even a single day, the mind can disconnect itself. Perhaps this is a special vulnerability of our species. So if you want a happy, grateful body, learn to sit still. If you don't believe this, do your own research. Find out who lives longer—Zen masters or doctors.

SPIRITUALITY AND THE BODY SENSE

The body is the instrument through which we experience our existence and access the wisdom of God. In the body we have our comedy and our tragedy, our joys and sorrows (Krysl, 1989). de Mello (1978) reminds us that many people live too much in their heads, more conscious of thinking and fantasizing than of the activity of their senses. Indeed, the body is the vehicle through which our spirit or soul exists in time and space. When we are "cut off from the knowing that is proper to our bodies, we lose that integral awareness through which we can resonate as living cells within a Larger Cosmic Organism" (Campbell & McMahon, 1985, p 13).

The wondrous instrument of the body is always in the present moment (de Mello, 1978; Kollmar, 1998). This is in sharp contrast to the mind and emotions, which can live in the past, in the future, or in fantasy (and rarely in the moment). This aspect of the body, of living in the *now,* is more profound than it may appear at first glance. When we pay attention, the body can guide us to the rich inner resources of ourselves that are only available in the current moment (Gwynn, 2000). "Your soul talks through your body, which gives you a here-and-now experience of your truth. If you want to know your truth on any subject, look to your feelings. Checking in with your body is the fastest way of doing this" (Walsch, 1999, p.74). Gwynn (2000) suggests that the body might be the most mystical aspect of ourselves in that it can have a direct experience of spirit. The body is closely connected to the inner child, particularly the magical-mystical-spiritual child. Sensing into the body enables us to recognize that our body is resting in our spirit. The body, and more particularly, what is called the *body sense* or *felt sense,* is a doorway to the soul (Campbell & McMahon, 1985; Gendlin, 1982; Gwynn, 2000; Kollmar, 1998).

We listen to and become aware of what is going on in our bodies in several ways. We can be aware of things such as our posture, our breathing, our sense of fatigue or alertness, or our experience of the temperature in the room. We can attend to where we are feeling discomfort or tension in various areas of the body, as is done with progressive muscle relaxation exercises. Attuning to the *body sense* or *felt sense* may begin with attending to our posture or feelings of discomfort, but moves us to more subtle physical awareness. We attune to the body sense by listening into the body as a whole—the feeling of the body in the space that it occupies in this moment (Kollmar, 1998). It is as if we are listening with the whole body to whatever we are experiencing. Being present to the body in this way is neither an emotion nor a mental exercise of imaging the body. The felt sense is physical—paying attention to what we are feeling in the body from the body's perspective, just being present to the experience without labeling or analyzing it. This is a very different experience than listening from the mind's perspective. Although the felt sense has emotional and factual components, it is larger and more complex than any single emotion (Gendlin, 1982).

Although the body sense is a physical sensation, not an emotion, it can accompany emotional experiences. Consider a time when you were anticipating the visit of someone special and you felt a sense of excitement throughout your whole being. The excitement was an emotion, yet had a pervasive physical sensation—a felt sense. Another example is the experience of being in a bath or shower in which you begin by feeling the warm water touching your skin. As the warmth seems to penetrate your muscles, and you begin to feel your whole body relaxing, you may also begin to feel a deep sense of relaxation that is physical, yet pervades your whole being. You may even have the sense of becoming one with the water. It is as if you are listening with and aware of your body as a whole, a sensation that is physical yet coming from a deeper place within. This, too, is a felt sense. Because we are not familiar with this part of ourselves, the felt sense may at times seem so subtle that we wonder if we are imagining it. As we learn to attune to the body sense, however, we discover that it is a bridge to the deeper levels of ourselves, where we become conscious of being conscious, and know ourselves as whole.

Developing the "felt sense" that comes through an unmediated (by the mind) experience of the body allows the part of us that is greater than the mind to give us its wisdom. Attuning to the body sense involves a process of allowing and receiving whatever life is offering without judging or trying to change what is there. For instance, if you are feeling sad, just be with the feeling of sadness and how it is showing up in the body rather than try to analyze it or make it be different. This process is participatory, not passive. It goes beyond merely observing what is occurring within ourselves to participating in it consciously and energetically, again without judging or trying to change it. It is listening to life with openness and expectancy but without particular expectation.

Being present with our current experience allows us to tap into our body's natural wisdom, and the deeper wisdom beyond that. It allows us to access the inner space of ourselves where we can receive knowledge as a whole, a way of knowing that is aligned with spirit. The mind, in contrast, cannot *know* in this way, but arrives at knowing in pieces through analysis, interpretation, and outline. In addition, the mind must reference whatever it experiences to what it already knows, its memory and previous understanding. There is no room for something truly and entirely new to show up. By being completely present to our body sense in the moment, and allowing ourselves to deepen further into that experience, we make the room for what is completely new.

Often, especially at first, there is discomfort in really being present to the body. Because the body is present to all that occurs within us at all levels in every moment (even if our minds or emotions do not want to be present to what is occurring), it can become a storehouse for leftover, unprocessed, energetic attitudes, conditioning, and unresolved issues (Kollmar, 1998). It is not natural or healthy for the body to be such a storehouse. The body may set up a field of resistance because it is holding that which does not belong to the body. We might experience this bracing as discomfort, pain, tightness, numbness, or sense of "nothingness" (like an energetic fog) when we turn our attention to particular parts of the body. Willingness to be with the body as it is in the moment is a way of bringing love and healing to our whole being. Once the body feels our willingness to be with it, to listen to it, openly and uncritically, it begins to discharge that which does not belong to it. As it increasingly becomes more trusting and comfortable with us, the energetic dynamics of the body change, creating more space for spirit or the divine to come through.

In our healing practices, as in any situation, an important question to ask is "Am I embodied? Am I in my body? " Consciously being *in* our bodies in whatever we are doing enables us to be aware of experiences *from* the body's perspective, that is, to be with the whole felt sense of the experience. Being aware *from* the body offers a way of approaching life that includes more of who we are rather than relating to life primarily from a pattern that includes only part of us.

As we learn to relate to life with expectancy without particular expectation, we become more comfortable with the place of "not knowing" where we can be vulnerable to ourselves and the experience of the moment with each person. As noted earlier, this gives access to dimensions beyond the body allowing room for something completely unexpected to open and come through. Being with the body sense enables mental, emotional, and physical healing even without cognitive understanding of the process.

 ## SELF-NURTURE: Body Awareness Meditation

Close your eyes and be with your breathing—inhale slowly and deeply, and exhale fully. Feel your body in its present position and make peace with yourself. Be aware of the space of your breath as you continue to be with your breathing. Bring awareness to your spiritual heart, which is a doorway to your divinity, the part of yourself that is whole and complete. Feel the space of your spiritual heart as you continue to breath and settle into the feeling of your body in this space at this time. At your heart center, ask that your inner power of relaxation emerge from your inner center of divinity and wholeness. Feel the feeling of your power of relaxation coming forth from your infinite source and spreading through the body to all areas that are braced, defensive, tight, anxious. Allow relaxation to spread; no need to think about relaxation, it is an energy to feel. Bring your awareness to the top of your head. From here, slowly bring your awareness down through the body—feeling each part of the body. When you find you are caught up in the idea of your body, let go of the thought of your body and come back to the feeling of your body. Feel your crown and all the muscles of your scalp. Then move your awareness to your forehead, feeling relaxation coming here. Continue to feel down through your face and the back of your head, feeling the muscles receiving relaxation. You do not need to visualize your body, or to imagine it; your body is there to feel. Settle into the feeling of your body, letting the muscles disengage as your body feels your attention. Feel the relaxation coming down through your neck and throat, then into your shoulders. Move your awareness to your right shoulder, then slowly down through your arm to your right hand. Feel the muscles and tendons releasing any gripping, letting your body respond to your loving awareness. Then bring your awareness to your left shoulder, slowly exploring the feeling down your left arm into your left hand. If any part of your body is difficult to feel, be patiently present, continuing to explore the feeling in your body without thought. Move your awareness down through your chest noting sensations there, and feel the feelings of your upper back. Be aware of your stomach, feeling the feeling of your stomach responding to your relaxation. As you continue to explore your body, feeling each area, feel the peace and relaxation that comes from being with and feeling your body. Continue down through your abdomen and lower back. No need to struggle against the feeling of tension. Just acknowledge where it is difficult to feel and where your body is bracing and your body will begin to take on relaxation. As your body begins to relax, your feeling body, your energy body will begin to respond, and you may begin to sense a vibration and energy in addition to the feeling of the blood and the nerves. Bring your awareness to your pelvic area and buttocks, then into your legs, feeling these areas of your body responding to your attention. Come all the way down through your legs past the knees and through your feet. Feel the feeling of your whole body. Noticing your whole body, feel the feeling of your body relaxing, and accepting the affection from feeling the body. As you continue to breathe and to make peace with having a body, acknowledge the body as a great barometer for your life that lets you know exactly how you are being affected by everything that happens moment to moment in your life. Feel how your body is always living with your life in each moment, constantly informing you of what is so and what is real. The more familiar you become with your body, the more familiar you are with your divinity. (Adapted from Kollmar, 1990).

THE TOUCH CONNECTION

We locate ourselves in space and time through touch. Touch is our earliest (and perhaps final) way of connecting with the physical self. A basic human need, touch is essential for our overall health, development, and well-being. It is similar to our need for water, without which we cannot survive for long. Like water, however, certain kinds of touch can also be harmful. Infants come to know the world first through touch, and even before birth the developing fetus is surrounded and caressed by fluid and the womb. In research published more than 30 years ago, Vidal Clay (1968) noted evidence that, in the first four months of life, tactile communication is biologically essential to humans, and that "throughout the life cycle it is physically and psychologically useful in returning the individual to normal functioning after experiencing stress and is the main avenue through which the human need for intimacy and acceptance is satisfied" (p. 204).

When we appreciate that the skin through which touch is mediated is the largest organ of the body, the importance of touch becomes self-evident. Our skin covers about 19 square feet, accounts for 18% of our body weight, and contains more than 5 million touch receptors. Stimulating the skin communicates messages to various parts of the body via the brain and nervous system. Celebrating and experiencing the wonder of our physical being is a way of honoring our wholeness. Marilyn Krysl's poem *Skin* reflects this celebration.

SKIN

Because skin is the first organ
to form in the womb, and first things
are of first importance
Because skin is the largest
organ—an adult's skin
weighs six pounds
and stretched out
covers eighteen square feet
Because there is more of it to attend to
than anything else
Because the skin's resilience
can only be experienced
Because it feels superior by far
to silk or challis
and in addition is lovely
to look at, nothing by Cardin
comes close to it
Because it's the organ with which we experience wind,
which most loves water,
Because it's the organ through which we begin
to discover each other
because, because, because, because,
and for all these good reasons
hurry out and touch someone now!
Delay in this matter
is not
a good idea,
you have delayed too long
already, your suffering brothers and sisters
are waiting, you can hardly expect them to wait
much longer, and remember
when you touch another
person,
the skin
gives off a chemical
which makes them
and you
feel better
more alert
more cheerful
more willing to take chances

more open to new experiences
more generally obstreperously intent on securing
the greatest good for everybody
and more likely to say NO to the MX
and YES to the levy for the public schools
After all, it's
the organ
through which we take in
the light we give out

(*MIDWIFE and Other Poems on Caring,* Marilyn Krysl, New York: National League for Nursing, 1989, Jones and Bartlett Publishers, Sudbury, MA. www.jbpub.com. Reprinted with permission.)

REFLECTION 5–2

- When do you feel most like you need to be touched? When would you rather not be touched?

- Does touch ever enliven your being and help you feel connected to something greater than yourself?—perhaps the feeling of the wind on your face, the comforting hug of a friend, the cool water of a lake on a hot day.

- When have you experienced a sense of spiritual connectedness that felt physically tangible?

- Has the experience of unwelcome or hurtful touches contributed to a sense of disconnection from your body or the need for emotional or relational healing?

- Describe a time when you used touch to relate to another.

Have you ever noticed how the language of touch permeates our lives? For example, when you hear the word "feeling," does it bring to mind an emotional response, something that is experienced within your being, or do you think of feeling in the tactile sense? Truly, it is both. Emotional feelings and tactile feelings are very much interconnected. Feelings, according to Walsch (1996), are the language of the soul. What we experience emotionally manifests in our physical, energetic, and spiritual beings in one way or another. We often choose the language of touch to express that which is meaningful in our lives. We speak of being "touched" by kindness, "feeling" uplifted or downcast, being "knocked off" our horse, "embraced" by light, "held up" by prayer, "tickled" by a remembrance, or "cradled" by friendship. Through the experience of touch, we connect with our spiritual and emotional beings as well as our physical bodies.

Touch has been integrally associated with healing in most cultures throughout history. Ancient traditions teach us that healing is essentially a spiritual process that attends to the wholeness of a person. In these traditions, the healer and spiritual leader, priestess, or shaman are the same, and healing rituals are spiritual ceremony. Recall that the English words *healing, whole,* and *holy* all derive from the same roots: Old Saxon *hal* and Greek *holos.* Before the dominance of biomedicine, touch was a key component of healing processes. Many healing traditions and spiritual rituals employ touch through anointing the body with oil, herbs, sacred corn meal, or other substances; through ritual cleansing or purification; through laying on of hands for both diagnosis and healing; and through use of ancient healing modalities, such as acupressure, acupuncture, and qigong, that promote balance and harmony in the life energy or *chi* of a person.

SELF-NURTURE: Daily Anointing

This practice of daily anointing from the ancient Basque mystical tradition is adapted from Judy Ostrow's (1999) presentation "Ancient Ways—Modern Methods: Accessing Inner Guidance Through Cross-Cultural Healing Practices." It can be done using sacred or healing water or oil, or by merely touching your fingers or hands to each place. Each morning upon rising anoint in turn your eyes, ears, lips, heart, hands, and feet as you say, I anoint

- My eyes for clear seeing
- My ears for deep listening
- My lips to speak the truth without blame or judgment
- My heart to be open, clear, strong, and full
- My hands to reach for what has heart and meaning
- My feet to walk in a grounded and self-responsible way

The therapeutic use of hands in healing appears to be a universal human act and an ancient example of our ability to connect with and help each other as humans (Krieger, 1979). The use of touch in healing flows through religious and cultural traditions from ancient times to the present. Ancient Indian Vedas, Polynesian Lomi, and Native American traditions all describe healing massage, and, 5,000 years ago the Chinese recorded a system of touch based on acupressure points and energy circuits (Shames & Keegan, 2000). In the Christian Scriptures, the frequency of Jesus' use of touch in healing, particularly in response to physical ailments, is significant. The terms *touch* or *laying on of hands* are used in 18 instances of healing or raising from the dead in the Gospel of Mark, in 12 such incidents in Matthew's Gospel, and in 10 healing encounters in Luke's Gospel (Diekman, 1980). As noted in Chapter 2, regarding biblical accounts of Jesus' use of touch in healing, scholars point out that there was a belief that a power within the miracle worker (Jesus) flows out as a kind of aura. The transfer of this power to the sick person effects the healing. Where sickness is viewed as a deficiency of power, healing consists in an experience of newly acquired power, of becoming a new creation (Seybold & Mueller, 1981). This understanding relates to the Israelite notion of the human person as a psychophysical unit in which the hand is viewed not just as an instrument, but as an extension of one's self, one's personality, and one's power. Thus, touching another would be a sign of transferring something of oneself to the other.

REFLECTION 5–2

- How do you nurture and connect with your physical self through touch? How often do you experience self-nurture in this way?

- How comfortable are you with receiving touch from another? With touching others?

- In what ways do you experience a connection with your deeper self through touch?

- Recall your first memories of touch.

- Think of a time you have intentionally used touch to comfort another.

There are many ways to connect with the physical self through touch. Healing processes such as massage, Therapeutic Touch (Krieger, 1979; 1993), Healing Touch (Hover-Kramer, Mentgen, & Scandrett-Hibdon, 2002), and other energy-based and body therapies help us attune to the body and promote relaxation, healing, a sense of well-being, and overall self-awareness. These therapies open our awareness to where we hold tension or feel at ease and enable us to become more familiar with how the body tells our biography. Touch is a common way of connecting within our every day lives—a simple hug, holding another's hand, bathing, folding clothes, and sexual intimacy are but a few examples. We receive and give love, care, and support through various kinds of touch. When we are hurting, our whole being cries out to be touched, and touch helps heal what we hold in our bodies related to physical, spiritual, and emotional distress and trauma. As we express love and care for our whole self through touch, we experience a deeper connection with our body-mind-spirit unity.

REFLECTION 5–3

- How well do you know your body and how it works? Do you have a sense of how your muscles attach to your bones, what your internal organs look like and what they do, and how food is digested and assimilated into your body?

- What physical features or characteristics of yourself do you like or wish you could change?

- Are there parts of your body that you are hesitant to touch or that you feel are shameful or should be hidden?

- In what ways are you conscious of using your body to communicate with others?

NOURISHING AND CARING FOR THE PHYSICAL SELF

We are prompted to care for what we love. Lesser (1999) notes that without a basic respect, and even reverence for our bodies, we will not be instinctually drawn to nurture them. She reminds us that, to bring healing to and incorporate the body into a spiritual understanding of ourselves, we need to fall in love with, and get to know our bodies as they are now—not as we might wish them to be. Knowing, loving, and accepting the body is basic to being able to energize and heal it. As we embrace our bodies with loving attention and acceptance, we become more aware of what the body needs for healing and staying healthy. We also become more adept at drawing on and trusting the body's innate wisdom.

Our nourishment is affected by what we take into our bodies through all of our senses—the air we breathe, substances we inhale, what we absorb through our skin, light and energy that comes to us through our eyes and skin, the sounds we hear, as well as the food and other substances we ingest. How we care for and nourish our bodies affects our physical, mental, and spiritual capacities and well-being. Caring for the physical self requires awareness of what is nourishing for us, with attention to balance—of energy needs and caloric intake, of rest and activity, of necessary nutrients, of noise and quiet, and the like. Nutrition, exercise, sleep, rest/relaxation, and health challenging habits are important considerations in caring for the physical self. Because each of us is unique, what we need and how we express loving care for ourselves in each of these areas is different. Various traditions, resources, and fads offer different guidelines and practices for promoting healing and healthful living. Discerning the merit of different options and whether they are right for you often presents a challenge. Listening carefully to your own body's wisdom helps you make healthful choices at various points of your journey, as you recognize that what your body needs also changes along the way.

Nutrition

> *I try to see eating more and more as an occasion to refresh the soul*
> *as well as to replenish my body. Whether I eat a communion wafer or*
> *a crab cake, a fish sandwich on the run or a can of beans over a campfire,*
> *food itself mediates God's life-giving care. (Jones, 1999, p. 77)*

Nourishing our bodies can be a reminder of our connectedness with the earth, with God, and with others. In many traditions people pause before eating to acknowledge the gift of what they are about to receive in the form of food for their bodies. People who live close to the earth teach us that the relationship we have with the earth and her gifts of food plays a role in how we are nourished. Indigenous cultures often include prayer and ceremony around planting, harvesting, hunting, and preparation of food in recognition of the interconnectedness of all of life—that these life forms, which are a gift of Creator, give their lives that we may live. Raising our own food is no longer a common occurrence for many of us. However, through the way we prepare and eat our food, we can still bring a conscious recognition of our connection with the Life Source and life forms that nourish us, and the people involved in bringing the food to us.

Nourishing the body with food and drink is a basic instinct and human need. Most people have a sense of what is nutritionally healthy or not, although what is eaten varies greatly among peoples and cultures. For example, beef, tofu, rattlesnake, and beetles are each good sources of protein; however, they are not all acceptable in every culture. A healthy diet can vary greatly for different people. Important considerations in choosing a health-promoting diet include eating a predominantly plant-based, vegetarian diet, reducing fat intake, eliminating the intake of refined sugars, reducing exposure to pesticides and herbicides, limiting intake of food additives and coloring agents, addressing food allergies, and determining caloric needs to maintain ideal body weight (Luck, 2000; Murray &

Pizzorno, 1998; Pitchford, 1993). Lynn Keegan's book, *Healing Nutrition* (2002), further describes the benefits of eating healthfully.

REFLECTION 5-5

- What foods do you consider healthy for you? How do you include these in your regular diet? How often and in what ways do you "stray" from eating what is healthy for you?

- How would you alter your dietary patterns to make them more healthy? What is the first step you need to take to do this?

- What is your relationship with the food you eat? What are some of your comfort foods?

- Are there foods in your tradition that are considered sacred? forbidden? healing? Are there foods that must be prepared in a particular way? eaten or avoided at particular times?

The nourishment of food takes into account not only the kind of food eaten, but how it is grown and prepared, and the environment within which it is eaten. Consider the effect on our bodies of chemical fertilizers and toxic pesticides used in growing food we ingest. Within our hectic lifestyles, eating is so often done quickly or on the run, prompting the use of easy-to-fix processed foods with many additives. How often do you prepare and eat your meals with consciousness—bringing the energy of love to your preparation and being aware of your connection with the life forms that are nourishing you? In many households, the art of preparing a meal with loving care seems to be a lost art. Consider the experience of mealtime for you—do you eat alone or with others? Is the environment pleasant or laced with tension? The energetic environment in which we eat affects how our bodies handle the food we take in. Stress affects the digestive system in many ways; for example, increasing acid production and peristalsis, which, in turn, influences the absorption of food. Remember an experience of eating a meal when you were feeling anxious and how you felt physically at that time, and the difference when you are comfortable and at ease when you eat. Eating with awareness is a way of connecting with the body. Consider how often you are really aware of the flavor and texture of what you eat? Because food comes from the earth, coming into relationship with our bodies through food may move us to a different relationship with the earth as well.

SELF-NURTURE: Eating with Consciousness

For the next week, choose one meal each day that you can prepare and eat consciously. As you prepare the food, be conscious of bring loving care to all that you are doing and thank each life form for being willing to give its energy to nourish you. Express your gratitude to the Creator also. When you are eating, do your best to be aware of the flavors and texture of each bite and how they change as you chew and swallow. Be aware of all the parts of your body involved in eating and digesting the food—your lips, teeth, tongue, saliva, jaws, muscles, stomach, intestines, blood, cells—thanking each part of you for its role in nourishing you. Also be aware of your environment and its effect on you as you eat.

Exercise

Our bodies are designed to move—not to be sedentary. Because exercise is vital to our total health and well-being, we nourish ourselves through many types of exercise. We can exercise sitting in a chair, in a pool, at the gym, in our kitchen, lying on the floor, in the park . . . the possibilities are endless! In general, people who participate in regular exercise are happier and have higher self-esteem (Murray & Pizzorno, 1998). Exercise provides a wonderful opportunity for connecting with the physical self, particularly when we engage mindfully in the physical activity. Paying attention to how your body feels during and after exercise is an example of this connection. Listening to your body's cues when you exercise helps you work with your body in ways that promote health and overall well-being.

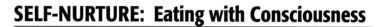

REFLECTION 5-6

- What kind of exercise do you engage in regularly? What motivates you to exercise? What prevents you from doing so?

- How does exercise help you appreciate yourself as a physical being?

- How have you connected with your whole body-mind-spirit self through exercise?

Sleep and Rest/Relaxation

Sleep and rest/relaxation are nourishing and absolutely essential for our body-mind-spirit well-being. We need both the physical rest and the time to dream that sleep provides. Dreams are important for our mental health and are considered significant for spiritual and personal development in many traditions. Giving sleep and relaxation priority time in our lives requires us to attend to our body wisdom—to perhaps view priorities from a different perspective. How often in our busy lives do we pay attention to our physical energy levels and allow ourselves to sleep or take rest breaks when needed? Or do we feel that the many things we must "do" prevent us from giving time for needed rest? Attending to our need for rest helps us respond better to stress and enables our energy and creativity to soar higher. Resting could mean being still, as in napping or meditating, or it might involve activities such as reading, gardening, engaging in a hobby, listening to or playing music, visiting with a friend.

REFLECTION 5-7

- Do you consider sleep a way to nourish yourself, or as something you must do to engage in your busy life, or a mixture of both?

- Do you feel you generally get the sleep you need? If not, how can you take better care of yourself in this regard?

- What helps you to rest or relax? How often have you included this in the past week?

SELF-NURTURE: Permission to Pause

Give yourself permission to take a nap without feeling guilty, and with appreciation for this time of rest and renewal. Sense the recuperative energies and rest that you experience.

Health Challenging Habits

As we reflect on what nourishes us, we do well to consider habits or behaviors that could be harmful to us. We look at these choices, not with judgment, rather with attention to how they contribute to or detract from our sense of incorporating our bodies into our spiritual understanding of ourselves. Habits such as smoking, use of alcohol and other drugs, and over or under eating often muffle our sense of connection with the body. Developing awareness of why we choose to engage in these habits and how they affect us moves us toward more conscious connection with the physical self.

BREATHING

The creation story in Hebrew scriptures tells us that the human that God fashioned out of clay became a living being only after God blew "the breath of life" into the nostrils. Breath, a sign of life, is often associated with spirit. We see this in languages where the words for breath and spirit are the same, for example: Latin, *spiritus;* Greek, *pneuma;* Hebrew, *ruah;* Sanskrit, *prana.* Breath in some traditions is considered the link between our physical body and the world around us, a way of connecting with the universal life energy of the cosmos. Breathing affects our health and well-being. Changes in breathing can increase or reduce sympathetic nervous system activity and trigger either relaxation or fight-or-flight responses. By consciously changing our breathing, we can learn to influence body functions such as blood pressure, heart rate, and digestion. A very simple way of connecting with our physical self is through an appreciation and awareness of our breathing.

REFLECTION 5–8

- How many times have you breathed while reading this?
- What is your breathing like right now?
- When are you most aware of your breathing—when frightened? nervous? congested? rushing? relaxed?
- Do you tend to breathe deeply or shallowly? Are you a chest breather or an abdominal breather?

Our breathing affects our health and our health affects our breathing. The way we breathe gives us information about what is going on in our physical and emotional environments. Tuning into our breathing fosters awareness of what is happening for us in the moment. Choosing to be with our breathing enables us to direct this spirit energy toward health and well-being, to harmonize body, mind, and spirit. Weil (1995) notes that when we understand that breath as the movement of spirit in the body is a mystery connecting us with all creation, we realize working with breath is a form of spiritual practice. Many meditative practices start with attention to breathing. Ancient disciplines such as yoga, t'ai chi and qigong include particular ways of breathing that enhance and direct energy flow for both healing and strength. Attention to breathing is part of many relaxation exercises and stress reduction techniques—often with instructions to merely become aware of our breathing, not trying to change it in any way. Merely paying attention to our breathing is generally followed by our taking slower, deeper breaths.

We can connect to our physical self through attending to our breathing alone or combining breathing with thoughts, vocalizations, or movements. Instructions on the "correct" way to breathe vary in different practices and traditions, and each has merit within its system. The following Self-Nurture offers a few approaches to using breath to bring us into our body.

 # SELF-NURTURE: Connecting with the Body through Breathing

1: Breath Awareness

Do this sitting or lying, with eyes closed or opened and softly focused on nothing in particular. Begin to be aware of you breathing, not trying to change it, just be with how it is in this moment. Pay attention to its rhythm and rate, how deep or shallow, just observing, without judgment. Allow yourself to just be with yourself breathing. After awhile begin to observe the breath as it flows in and out of your nostrils, merely noting what this is like for you. And, after awhile longer, begin to follow the breath from your nostrils to your lungs and back to your nostrils, noting where you feel the breath within you, and the rising and falling of your chest and abdomen as you breathe. Then begin to pay attention to the space between your breaths, allowing the space to be as long or as short as it wishes. Stay with this for a few minutes and return your attention to the breath at your nostrils before returning your awareness to the room.

2: Subtle Breathing Sensations

Begin as in *Breath Awareness*, then move your awareness to the sensation of the air passing in and out of your nostrils. Do not focus on the air as it enters your lungs, but stay focused on the sensation in your nostrils—the touch, where you feel the air when you inhale and exhale, the warmth and coolness of the air when it comes in and goes out. You may be aware that you seem to breathe more air through one nostril than through the other. Be sensitive and alert to the lightest and slightest touch of air on your nostrils as you inhale and exhale. Stay with this for several minutes. (Adapted from de Mello, 1978, p. 23)

3: Breathing Relaxation into Your Body

Begin as in *Breath Awareness* spending a few moments of just being with your breathing. Then move your attention to the top of your head and breath relaxation into the muscles of your scalp. After a few breaths move your attention to your face, breathing relaxation into the muscles of the face, around the eyes, and jaw. After a few breaths, move your attention to the back of the neck and the throat, breathing relaxation into the muscles in these areas. Follow the same pattern, moving your attention slowly to your upper back and chest, down your arms into your hands, to your lower back and abdomen, into the pelvic area, down your legs into your feet. Each time, pause to breathe relaxation into the muscles in that area. Once you have moved through your body breathe a wave of relaxation through your whole body, repeating this wave with 3 to 4 breaths. Then return your attention to the breath at your nostrils and become aware again of the room around you.

4: Letting Yourself be Breathed

With eyes closed and body relaxed, focus attention on your breathing without trying to change it. With each inhalation, imagine that the universe is blowing breath into you, and imagine the universe withdrawing breath with each exhalation. Just allow and receive this process without effort. With each inhalation, let yourself feel the breath of the universe penetrating to every part of your body, even to the cellular level. Experience your connectedness with all creation through this universal life energy. Continue this process for several cycles of inhalation and exhalation. (Adapted from Weil, 1995, p. 205)

MOVEMENT

As long as we are alive, there is movement somewhere in the body. Movement is necessary for general health and well-being. Muscle tone and effective physical functioning require some measure of physical activity. As with breathing, we often move our bodies quite unconsciously. Bringing awareness to our movement is a natural way to connect with the physical self. Conscious movement can take many forms, and can begin as simply as paying attention to what the body feels like and how we move the body when walking. Whether taking a walk for its own sake or walking as part of any activity, listening to the body while we walk brings us into the present moment. Being in the *now* enables us to attend to physical sensations, emotional milieu, and the experiences of all of our senses—feeling the wind and the temperature of the space around us, hearing the sounds and truly seeing our surroundings. Any movement done consciously can help us connect with the physical self and open a door to our deeper self. Take, for example, actions such as lifting a fork from plate to mouth, chewing, swallowing, writing a note, preparing a meal, getting dressed, washing one's face—everyday actions that can help us to become more attuned to the body. Activities such as running, swimming, skiing, bicycling, canoeing, gardening, t'ai chi, yoga, and dancing are all opportunities for connecting with our physical selves through movement as we become aware of the body through which we are engaging in the activity. Such bodily awareness can help us appreciate the wonder of how the physical body works and enable us to more clearly feel where our bodies are not very comfortable with us.

REFLECTION 5–9

- How do you incorporate conscious movement into your life?
- When are you most aware of your body through movement? How can you be more "in your body" as you move through the routines of your day?
- How can you engage in movement that nurtures your body-mind-spirit being?

Many techniques and systems for fine-tuning the body are mental and spiritual disciplines as well. For example, yoga makes use of breath, postures, and gestures to stretch, relax, massage, and open the energies of the body. As a physical exercise alone, yoga has great health benefits. Yoga as a meditative practice enhances the healing potential by opening us to transcendent awareness as well. Forms of moving meditation are practiced in many traditions. The ancient Chinese practice of qigong works with the *Qi (chi)* or vital life energy through breathing, posture, and movement. Developed originally as a Taoist meditative practice, qigong movements and postures connect one with the flow of *Qi* in nature—even the postures derive from movements of animals, trees, and other life forms in nature. qigong's simple, slow movements and breathing open the flow of *Qi* throughout the body, strengthening both the internal organs and muscles. Posture, breathing, and a calm mind are three elements basic to the many styles and techniques of qigong (which includes t'ai chi and other martial arts). In t'ai chi, which is often referred to as meditation in motion, slow movements combined with focused breathing bring one to a centered place, promote relaxation, and enhance the *chi* flow through the body. The breath training is vital to the health benefits of t'ai chi and other martial arts. In fact, one teacher noted that without the breathing, t'ai chi is merely exercise; the breathing makes it t'ai chi. Aikido is another martial art whose practice requires harmonizing with and bringing oneself into accord with the movement of the universe.

 # SELF-NURTURE: Connecting with the Body through Movement

1: Feeling Your Moving

Alone or with others, in a quiet place begin by standing with feet shoulder width apart and slowly shift your weight from one foot to the other, feeling the various muscles in your legs and feet that are involved in this process. After doing this for a few moments begin to walk very, very slowly. With each step, notice each part of the foot—heel, middle, ball—as you slowly take it off the floor and place it down again for the next step. Try to feel each muscle and joint as they move you through the step. Continue walking slowly, feeling the muscles in your legs as you move. What do they feel like? After a few minutes focused on your legs, move to noticing how your hips are involved in your walking. Stay with this for awhile, then return your attention to your feet, and repeat the process, noticing any changes in what you are feeling. Then be aware of as much of your hip-leg-foot as you can with each step. Notice how your breathing is through this process.

2: Body Awareness While Moving

This experience can be incorporated into any physical activity, but is more effective in an activity that does not require much mental attention.

While engaging in activities such as running, walking, swimming, bowling, or working out, be conscious of the muscles and joints you are using for the activity. Just listen to how they are feeling, where they are comfortable or strained, where you feel toned and invigorated, where you feel tired or pain. Be aware of your breathing—is it steady, strained, comfortable? Be aware of your heart—its rate and rhythm. What is your overall feeling during this activity? As you pay attention to your body, what do you notice in your mental and emotional being?

3: Attuning to Senses

This can be incorporated into almost any activity in any location. The goal is to be conscious of what you are experiencing with all your senses—vision, hearing, taste, smell, touch. You can start with any of the senses and attune to each one in turn, or you can choose to focus on only one.

Vision—be aware of what is entering your being through your eyes in as much detail as possible. Note colors, shapes, patterns, textures, light. What feels pleasing or distasteful to you? Where in your body do you feel what you are seeing?

Hearing—listen carefully to the sounds coming into your being, their tone, volume, melody. Are the sounds pleasing or not for you? Which sounds are more prominent or subtle? Are there sounds that seem to be pervasive or intermittent? As you listen, where do you feel the various sounds in your body?

Taste—(this is especially good to do while eating)—start with tasting the air around you, what are you tasting in this moment? While eating, take a small portion of your food, attentive to the texture and various flavors. Does the taste change as you chew and swallow? How do the scents around you affect the taste? Are any particular memories attached to the flavors?

Smell—attend to the scents in your environment, the dominant and the subtle ones. Are they pleasant or not? How do the scents make you feel? Do particular smells elicit memories for you? Where do you experience the scent in your body?

Touch—note the temperature of your surroundings, and its comfort level for you. What does the air feel like on your face or hands? Notice the feel of your clothing against your skin. Notice the feel of the chair touching your back, buttocks, and thighs. How are your feet feeling in your shoes?

4: Prayer or Meditative Walking

When we take a walk for the sake of walking rather than with the goal of getting somewhere, walking can become prayer or meditation. As you walk slowly, focused on being in the body that is walking, become aware of your breathing, and the sights, sounds, textures, and smells of your surroundings. Begin to sense your connection with everything around you and feel the love energy flowing through all of creation. You may feel a sense of joy, awe, wonder, or gratitude. Become aware of the contact between your feet and the earth and walk as if your feet are kissing and bringing peace to the earth (Hanh, 1991). Stay in the present moment, aware that your very walking in openness is prayer.

5: Moving to Music

Play some favorite music and begin to move to the music. Feel the music entering your body and allow the music to move you. Try not to judge or control the movement—let the music express through you. Do this with different types of music, noting how your movements and moods change with the music. How comfortable are you with moving in this way? Does the movement flow freely or does it feel contrived?

Body postures and movements are expressions of our spirit. Think of the dancing or jumping around, waving of hands, and embracing that occur when the favored team has won the game, or the jumping up and applauding in response to a great speech or performance. The experience of joy or elation is a physical, emotional, and spiritual feeling all at once. We pray with the body as well as with the mind and spirit. Our body posture, whether this is standing with hands extended upward, kneeling, bowing, prostrating, or sitting with legs crossed, is part of the prayer. In many traditions, prayer and spiritual ceremony involve dancing, spinning, drumming, or other ritual movement that engages the whole being. Connecting with the physical self enables us to better appreciate how our spiritual essence is expressed and experienced in and through our body. Attuning to the body aids us in discovering and learning to trust our body's wisdom.

REFLECTION 5–10

- How does your moving express who you are—your spirit in various situations?
- How do you express yourself through movement?

WELCOMING OUR SENSUAL SELF

We are sexual beings. Understanding who we are as fully human beings means recognizing our sensual, sexual selves as an integral part of our nature—who we are, our wholeness. We attend to our sexual selves by honoring our sensuality and needs for intimacy. Caroline Myss (1996) notes that each of the seven chakras (major energy centers in our biological system) contains a sacred truth. In the second chakra (the partnership chakra), our sexuality, and our attitudes toward it, are patterned. According to Myss, the creative energy of this chakra is essentially of the earth, the sensation of being physical, giving us our basic survival instincts, intuitions, and desire to create—music, art, life. She describes sexuality as both an avenue of self-expression and as a raw power to form strong bonds and intimate union with another to produce and sustain life. Lesser (1999) speaks of connecting with the sexual self as coming into animal presence. She links the understanding of animal presence with Carl Jung's description of the *Eros* principle that "values the interconnectedness of all life; an ethos that celebrates connection through the pleasure of touch, the sharing of food, the nurturing of relationships, the protection of life" (p.263). The relatedness of the Eros principle is instinctual, personal, and spontaneous. Lesser notes that when the Eros principle is devalued, as it has been in the Western worldview, it grows sleepy and goes underground.

This sleepiness contributes to our lack of connection with our instinctual sense of knowing what is best for our bodies. Myss suggests that the challenge of the second chakra energy is to cherish the sacred unions we form with others while developing and maintaining a healthy, loving relationship with ourselves.

Sexuality is related to our deepest longing for union and communion. Sexual images are used in poems, songs, ritual dance and sacred scriptures to express spiritual ecstasy and the deep inner longing for re-union and communion with God. Rumi, the Sufi poet and mystic, writes, "When soul rises into lips, you feel the kiss you've wanted" (Barks & Green, 1997, p. 52) In the Hebrew scriptures, the *Song of Solomon* begins this way:

> Let him kiss me with the kisses of his mouth. More delightful is your love than wine! Your name spoken is a spreading perfume—that is why the maidens love you. Draw me!—We will follow you eagerly! Bring me, O King, to your chambers. With you we rejoice and exult, we extol your love; it is beyond wine; how rightly you are loved!

Some traditions consider that lovemaking can help to harmonize all realms of the universe when lovers unite with the proper attitude and concentration. The authors of *Chop Wood, Carry Water* note that sex in many ways is identical with the life-force because it "brings us together, serves as an expression of love, creates life, and fulfills our longing for unity and wholeness . . . from the spiritual point of view, we engage in sex not only for physical release, but to merge with the beloved in a state of ecstatic spiritual union" (Fields, Taylor, Weyler, & Ingrasch, 1984, p. 60). When we are connected with our physical selves, sexual expression flows from our deepest, truest selves and reflects our wholeness. However, when we lack a sense of connection with the physical self, sexuality can more easily be viewed as a mere mechanical act, separate from our spiritual self. Societal attitudes that diminish the sacred nature of the physical self and sexual expression make it easier to justify exploitation of the body in many forms, including sexual abuse.

TRUSTING OUR BODY WISDOM

Connecting with the physical self calls us to love the bodies we live in (not those we imagine or wish we had!) There is no condition that I will love my body once I lose ten pounds, after I get in shape, when I overcome my addiction, or if my diabetes goes away. We need to fall in love with our bodies as they are. By embracing and caring for our bodies as they are, we begin to allow room for all parts of us (even the warts) to be included in our life. Often those parts of ourselves that we like the least are most in need of loving attention. Bioscientific medicine has lost sight of the inherent tendency of the body (indeed the whole person) to move toward the balance we call health. Military terminology permeates medical language, treating the body as if it were a war zone where discomfort and dis-ease are enemies. When we have an ache, pain, or illness, our first reaction within the medical model is to eradicate it. A relationship with our physical selves calls us instead to reclaim our bodies as sacred ground, recognizing discomfort and dis-ease as messages that something is out of balance in our body-mind-spirits and needs our attention. When we move our attention to the discomfort or dis-ease and allow ourselves to *feel* what is happening, we gain insight into the imbalance that prompted the discomfort. The first step is to be with what we are experiencing in the moment—a pain, an emotional reaction, stiffness, or other discomfort. We do not have to know why something is happening to give it our attention. Responding to what is happening in a loving way creates a space in which the discomfort is included in our experience, thus opening the opportunity for understanding why it is there. Being present with the whole of who we are, we access the wisdom that the body has to offer, even as we accept what remains mystery.

REFLECTION 5–11

- How do you feel about your body now?
- How do you relate to your body in the face of illness— chronic or acute?
- In what ways do you incorporate attention to your body's wisdom into your self-care?
- Ponder an experience in which you have felt your own body-story—your biography expressed in your biology.
- How can you reclaim your body as sacred ground?

Connecting with and trusting the body may be a particular challenge for someone who has experienced significant physical trauma such as serious injury or sexual abuse. Such trauma often gets pushed into the unconscious and becomes deeply stored in the body, often showing up in feelings and physical responses that might not make sense to us. A personal example is a situation several years ago when I became intensely angry while attending a meeting of a small task force for a project with which I was consulting. My anger was so intense that I felt hot and eventually became feverish. At the start of a massage I had scheduled later that day, the massage therapist even commented on intensity of the heat and energy around me. Although I linked my anger to my reaction to the group leader's attitude and controlling nature, I recognized that the intensity of the physical response I experienced was not warranted by the situation. This prompted me to seek counseling that eventually led to my remembering a childhood trauma that involved being in a situation in which I felt trapped and controlled. Although I did not at first understand what was going on with my physical reaction, attending to my body's messages led to both insight and healing.

The body is so present to what is going on that it organically holds whatever is happening in our experience, both conscious and unconscious, and stores it until we are ready to deal with it. Contemporary scholars and ancient traditions recognize that our bodies tell our history or biography. Our various life experiences, as well as our thoughts about and reactions to these experiences, are carried in our physiology. Thoughts and emotions are energetic forces that travel through our bodies, affecting our biochemistry and resulting in physiological responses that are stored at the cellular level. Graham and colleagues (1998) state that "in restoring wholeness, balance, and harmony within ourselves and in relationship to God, our bodies will communicate to us the imbalance, the disharmony and the brokenness with which we live" (p. 77). As we attune to the body's story we discover parts of ourselves that have been hidden or ignored—secrets held by the body that hold the key to the strength and healing we desire. Lesser (1999) notes that we lose touch with the body when out of fear of illness we doggedly try to prevent or rush to cure it, rather than listening to what the body is telling us it needs. Andrew Weil (1995, 1997) reminds us that healing is a natural power, that the body wants to be healthy and is always trying to restore balance when balance is lost, and that perfect health is not possible. When circumstances of illness, trauma, or injury overwhelm the body's capacity to maintain or restore balance, outside interventions can be helpful and sometimes lifesaving. Weil makes the distinction between treatment (which comes from the outside) and healing (which comes from within), noting that outside treatments support the inner healing process. Connecting with the physical self opens the opportunity for us to heal what we hold in the body through loving release and inclusion in our wholeness.

Our spirits call us to lovingly embracing ourselves as we are, warts, scars, and all. Frank H. Keith beautifully expresses this in a poem, which was distributed at a workshop we attended many years ago. We end this chapter with the thoughts of Keith's poem titled *Imperfect Beauty:*

The rift in the chest of a mountain, the twist in the trunk of a tree,
The water-cut cave in the hollow, the rough, rocky rim of the sea—
Each one has a scar of distortion, yet each has this sermon to sing,
" The presence of what would deface me, has made me a beautiful thing."

REFERENCES

Barks, C., & Green, M. (1997). *The illuminated Rumi*. New York: Broadway Books.

Campbell, P. A. & McMahon, E. M. (1985). *Bio-spirituality: Focusing as a way to grow*. Chicago: Loyola University Press.

Clay, V. S. (1968). The effect of culture on mother-child tactile communication. *Family Coordinator, 37,* 204–210.

de Mello, A. (1978). *Sadhana: A way to God—Christian exercises in Eastern form*. St. Louis: The Institute of Jesuit Sources.

Diekman, G. (1980). The laying on of hands in healing. *Liturgy, 25,* 2–10, 36–38.

Fields, R., Taylor, P., Weyler, R., & Ingrasch, R. (1984). *Chop wood, carry water*. Los Angeles: Jeremy. P. Tarcher.

Gendlin, E. (1982). *Focusing*. Toronto: Bantam Books.

Graham, R., Litt, F. & Irwin, W. (1998). *Healing from the heart: A guide to Christian healing for individuals and groups*. Winfield, BC: Wood Lake Books.

Gwynn, M. B. (2000). *Inner Listening*. Workshop presented at the New River Unitarian-Universalist Fellowship, Beckley, WV, February 5.

Hanh, T. N. (1991). *Peace is every step*. New York: Bantam Books.

Hover-Kramer, D, Mentgen, J., & Scandrett-Hibdon, S. (2002). *Healing touch* (2nd ed.). Albany, NY: Delmar.

Jones, T. (1999). *Awake my soul*. New York: Doubleday.

Keegan, L. (2002) *Healing nutrition* (2nd ed.) Albany, NY: Delmar.

Kollmar, D. (1990). *Coming home to self: Complete self meditation*. [Cassette Recording]. Complete Self Attunement Associates, P.O. Box 1376, New York, NY 10028.

Kollmar, D. (1998). Complete self attunement transformational intensive workshops: Week 1, Boca Raton, FL, January, 1998; Week 2, Beckley, WV, November, 1998.

Krieger, D. (1979). *The therapeutic touch*. Englewood Cliffs, NJ: Prentice-Hall.

Krieger, D. (1993). *Accepting your power to heal*. Santa Fe, NM: Bear.

Krysl, M. (1989). *Midwife and Other Poems on Caring*. New York: National League for Nursing (Pub. # 21–2286).

Lesser, E. (1999). *The new American spirituality*. New York: Random House.

Luck, S. (2000). Nutrition. In B. M. Dossey, L. Keegan, & C. E. Guzzetta, *Holistic nursing: A handbook for practice* (3rd ed., pp. 427–450). Gaithersburg, MD: Aspen.

Mails, T. E. (1988). *Secret Native American pathways: A guide to inner peace*. Tulsa, OK: Council Oak Books.

Mbiti, J. S. (1975). *Introduction to African religion*. New York: Praeger.

Murray, M. & Pizzorno, J. (1998). *Encyclopedia of natural medicine* (2nd ed.). Rocklin, CA: Prima.

Myss, C. (1996). *Anatomy of the spirit*. New York: Harmony Books.

Ostrow, J. (1999). *Ancient ways-modern methods: Accessing inner guidance through cross-cultural healing practices*. Presentation at *Spirituality and Health* Conference, Durham, England, September 29–October 1, 1999.

Pitchford, P. (1993). *Healing with whole foods: Oriental traditions and modern nutrition.* Berkeley, CA: North Atlantic Books.

Seybold, K., & Mueller, U. (1981). *Sickness and healing.* (S. Scott, Trans.). Nashville: Abingdon Press.

Shames, K. H. & Keegan, L. (2000). Touch. In B. M. Dossey, L. Keegan, & C. E. Guzzetta, *Holistic nursing: A handbook for practice* (3rd ed., pp. 613–635) Gaithersburg, MD: Aspen.

Walsch, N.D. (1996). *Conversations with God, Book 1.* New York: G. P. Putnam's Sons.

Walsch, N. D. (1999). *Friendship with God.* New York: G. P. Putnam's Sons.

Weil, A. (1995). *Spontaneous healing.* New York: Alfred A. Knopf.

Weil, A. (1997). *8 weeks to optimum health.* New York: Alfred A. Knopf.

Connecting with Inner Self and Sacred Source

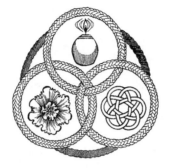

Be still and know that I am God.

Psalm 46

Spirituality flows from the deepest, truest part of who we are. Our spiritual core can become muffled and obscured by constant mental activity, verbal chatter, and a busy lifestyle that allows little time for quiet and inner listening. Connecting with our inner selves requires time and attention to the sacred space within our being. When we turn our attention within, we discover that as we come to know ourselves more fully we also encounter the Divine or Sacred Source within this sacred space. Spiritual teachers remind us that "true wisdom does not come from outside of us, but from within. And it does not come from within simply because we want it. It comes when we live in such a way that invites wisdom . . . through direct experience" (Cooper, 1997, p. 10.) Western societies offer little reward or encouragement for focus on our inner life. In fact, to make time for quiet, centering, and inner listening a priority in our lives is almost counter-cultural! Western societies value and reward our productivity, what we do or can accomplish. There is a sense of busyness that permeates society, where people are always on the go just keeping up with daily activities. When there is space between the activities, it may be viewed as wasted time, and people often search

147

for something else to do. Radios, music from various sources, computers, and televisions provide nearly constant auditory and visual stimulation. Silence is rare. The very thought of sitting quietly for even a few minutes often provokes guilt or discomfort. We long for, yet are afraid of this inner silence that is as vast as the universe (Norris, 1992). Perhaps it is our discomfort with silence that causes us to leave so little room for it. It seems that the place of the soul that is so much the core of who we are, and closer to us than our own breath, is often the hardest place to reach. Yet, when we allow ourselves to experience silence "we remember who we are; creatures of the stars, created from the birth of galaxies, created from the cooling of this planet, created from dust and gas, created from the elements, created from time and space . . . created from silence" (Norris, 1992, p. 9).

FROM DOING TO BEING

Connecting with the inner self calls us to shift from a mode of *doing* to one of *being*. This might seem awkward in societies where there has been so little modeling of, emphasis on, or training in how to *be*. Children are often told to "be still" as a reprimand for bothering adults, rather than being taught how to *be still* as a way to connect with their own spirits—the place of inner knowing and wisdom, the place of encountering self and the Divine or Sacred Source. In some societies, children learn quietness and meditation as a routine part of life. Entering the space of inner quiet is an important consideration in Eastern and many indigenous spiritual traditions. Except for experiences such as monasticism and Quakerism, however, most contemporary Western religious traditions tend to include less emphasis on silence and little instruction on *being still* as a spiritual practice. Kathleen Norris (1992) likens silence to an endangered species, noting that in our culture, experiences of silence are so rare that we must guard and treasure them. Although exploring the seemingly uncharted waters of entering the silence, the inner space of self, is at first disconcerting for many, the process is well worth the risk and effort.

REFLECTION 6–1

- How comfortable are you with stillness, with merely *being* with yourself?

- What have been your experiences of connecting with your inner self? What facilitates this process for you?

- How have you experienced connection with the Sacred Source within your inner being?

Contemporary nursing education gives little attention to self-reflection that leads to deepening connection with the inner self and Sacred Source. Nursing's founder, Florence Nightingale, however, placed great value on this process. Barbara Dossey's (2000) wonderful book on the life of Florence Nightingale illustrates how Nightingale's lifelong quest for understanding the deeper levels of Divine Reality was woven into her work and illuminates her letters of support and encouragement to her nursing students and working nurses. She felt a connection with all things through her deep exploration of experiencing God, and she gained self-knowledge through her intense study of the Bible. Her life provides an example of how important connecting with the inner self and Sacred Source is for the life and development of a healer.

Connecting with the inner self requires that we take the time to be with ourselves in a conscious way. We intentionally choose to be quiet, to be apart, and to pay attention to our souls. We need not seek anything in particular; rather, we attend with our whole being to whatever is in our experience of the moment. Jones (1999) describes such moments as "tiny awakenings . . . almost imperceptible but . . . real," which give him a glimpse of a "deeper spiritual dimension from which something important is trying to make itself known" (p. xiii). Solitude is not essential, but can be helpful. The more familiar we become with our inner self, the more able we are to access this inner space even when with other people and in the midst of activities. As noted in other chapters, there are many paths to the soul. We open to the rich resources of the inner self through intentional practices of mindfulness, awareness, and paying attention. Thus, we nurture what Jones (1999) refers to as "*spiritual* intelligence, a savvy about the issues of life that cannot be measured in gross income or hard disk space" (p. xvi).

SELF-NURTURE: Being with Self

Give yourself time (at least five minutes) each day to merely *be* with yourself, to allow yourself to move gently and effortlessly into your inner stillness. This may be done within the context of prayer or meditation, or may be while you sit quietly with a cup of tea, enjoy a warm bath, or take a leisurely walk. Have no expectations or program other than *being* with yourself *in the moment.*

SACRED SOURCE

Where shall I find God? In myself. That is the true Mystical Doctrine.
But then I myself must be in a state for Him to come and dwell in me.
This is the whole aim of the Mystical Life, and all Mystical Rules

*in all times and countries have been laid down for putting the soul
into such a state. (Florence Nightingale, cited in Dossey, 2000, p. 325)*

Within our own stillness we become aware of our connection with the Sacred Source—the ground of our being through which we know our connectedness with all of life. Quaker Thomas Kelly (1997) describes this experience as "an invasion from beyond, of an Other who in gentle power breaks in upon our littleness and in tender expansiveness makes room for Himself" (p. 25). How we name this Source is influenced by culture, traditions, human needs, and personal experiences. No one name for the Sacred Source captures the view of reality and experience of the Source for all people. Indeed, when we trace the history of any of the world's major religions and spiritual traditions, we see that the Source is called by different names at different times, names that reflect the experience and deep inner values of the society (Armstrong, 1993; Borysenko, 1999; Chopra, 2000; Smith, 1991). Most traditions reflect that the ultimate and essential nature of the Sacred Source is Unity or Oneness. Paradoxically, the Divine Unity contains infinite diversity. All that we see and do not see, experience and do not experience, know and do not know are reflections or manifestations of the Source. The many ways we name and image the Sacred Source are examples of this.

Naming the Sacred Source

Names for the Sacred Source include God, Allah, Brahman, Spirit, Goddess, Sustainer, Most Bountiful One, Tao, Higher Self, Shiva, Lord, Higher Power, Inner Light, Ultimate Reality, the Absolute, The Way, Vishnu, Universal Love, Mystery of Mysteries, Tunkasila, Creator, the One with no name, the life-giving energy, the animating force, the breath of life, and the One before whom all words recoil. For this discussion, we will primarily use the term God or Sacred Source. We must each find and name the Sacred Source in a way that is authentic for us; thus, we encourage you to use whatever term or language best reflects your experience and perspective. An Asian proverb reminds us that it is *better to see the face than to hear the name.* As you read, ponder, and explore, pay attention to what your body, your intuition, and your feelings are saying to you. Attending to your feelings is "your truest guide to the image of God that has the power to draw you into the sweet and mysterious depths of your soul. It is also your guide to healing old images of God that may have hardened your heart" (Borysenko, 1999, p.106).

REFLECTION 6–2

- With what images of the Sacred Source do you feel comfortable? uncomfortable? neutral? angry? empowered? frightened? at home?

(continued)

- Where and how have you learned the names and images by which you know the Sacred Source? Have these names and images changed for you at any times in your life?

- Consider how your images of the Sacred Source reflect and influence your worldview and attitudes about life and life experiences.

Trying to describe both our understanding of God and our experience of connection with God has been a challenge for people through the ages—both sages and common folk alike. In attempting to describe God, great spiritual teachers of many traditions ultimately echo the ancient saying that those who know do not speak, and those who speak do not know. We borrow from the wisdom of great spiritual teachers and mystics in acknowledging that whatever we say here about the Sacred Source reflects our limitations and understanding. The story is told that, when the well-known Christian theologian, Thomas Aquinas, finished his massive theological work *Summa Theologica,* he sadly said that all he had written was as straw compared to what he had seen. Ultimately, what is essential for the spiritual journey is how we know and experience the Sacred Source with our hearts and souls rather than how much we think we understand about this Source.

We cannot *think* God. Our rational minds cannot conceive or grasp God, and any words or descriptions we use are sorely lacking. Aquinas reflected that what we can know of God is to recognize that we cannot know God. None of our images of God are big enough to contain all that God is and is not. Huston Smith (1991) reminds us that the human rational mind has evolved to survive in the natural world, to deal with finite things, not the infinite. He notes that we cannot avoid the use of words and concepts because they are the only equipment our minds have to move us toward God, and we need a name or description on which to hang our thoughts. Although words and descriptions point us in the direction of God, God is far more than anything we can conceptualize. Because God cannot be contained within our words or concepts, it is wise to avoid mistaking the pointer (the name or image for God) for that to which it leads. It is like the student who asks the master to show him the moon. The master points with her finger to a round yellow object in the night sky saying that is the moon. The student then becomes really excited and goes to tell his friends that he has seen the moon. When they ask him to describe the moon, he says it is about three inches long and round like a small tree branch. The master, overhearing this, tells the student he has missed the point, and what he is describing is only her finger, which was pointing to the moon, not the moon itself. Smith (1991) notes that both Hinduism and the writings of many Western mystics suggest that the most accurate way of describing God is to recognize that God is far beyond even our greatest and grandest descriptions. Ultimately, our souls yearn not for words and descriptions, but for relationship.

The ideas and concepts or icons of God that our rational minds develop may be personal or shared within a group. Every image of God tells us something about the truth of ourselves. Joan Borysenko (1999) suggests that our icons for God arise in the left brain while the right brain creates the stories that give the icons life and provide the context for giving meaning to life. In seeking to understand the mysteries of the universe and the rhythms of life, people throughout the earth have created ideas of God, which vary in different times and places. God has many faces. Different religions and spiritual traditions create their own icons of God, as do individuals within these traditions. Some people relate to a personal God, whereas others feel God is impersonal. God may be viewed with human traits, or as a Presence or Energy that is far beyond and void of human likeness. God may be experienced as transcendent or far away, or immanent, closer than one's own heartbeat. Borysenko notes that people with similar religious backgrounds can develop idiosyncratic ideas of God related to their own life experiences. For example, people with higher self-esteem and more positive life experiences tend to believe in a more merciful God, whereas those with more negative experiences often imagine God as punitive.

In his book *How to Know God,* Depak Chopra (2000) reminds us that the God of any religion or tradition is but a fragment of God, yet so complete that it creates a complete world. He suggests that there are seven versions or stages of God, which relate to activities of the brain and biological response and are associated with organized faith. Each of these stages meets a particular human need and implies a different relationship with God; however, no stage is absolute in its claim to truth. The conceptions of and characteristics attributed to God in each of these stages influence our perceptions of who we are, our life challenges and gifts, how we fit in, what the world is like, how we find God, and the nature of good and evil. Chopra proposes that

- God the *Protector,* who may be vengeful, jealous, judgmental, and sometimes merciful, is found through the *fight-or-flight response* of fear and loving devotion.

- God the *Almighty,* who may be sovereign, omnipotent, rule giver, and answerer of prayers, is found through the *reactive response* of awe and obedience.

- God of *Peace,* who may be detached, calm, conciliatory, and meditative, is found through the *restful awareness response* of meditation and silent contemplation.

- God the *Redeemer,* who may be understanding, tolerant, forgiving, and accepting, is found through the *intuitive response* of self-acceptance.

- God the *Creator,* who may be open, generous, abundant, and willing to be known, is found through the *creative response* of inspiration.

- God of *Miracles,* who may be transformative, mystical, healing, and magical, is found through the *visionary response* of grace.
- God of *Pure Being,* who may be unborn, undying, intangible, unchanging, and infinite, is found through the *sacred response* by transcending.

SELF-NURTURE: Personal Connection with Sacred Source

Consider your relationship with, and the place in your life of, the Sacred Source. Spend some time each day in communion or conscious connection with the Sacred Source, as you know and call this Source. Explore how this connection affects your awareness of who you are.

God and Gender

Although our images of God reflect our experience of both masculine and feminine traits, God is beyond gender, being neither male nor female, yet paradoxically containing both. The mystics teach us that the mystery of God contains all of life—light and darkness, beauty and ugliness, cruelty and compassion, *yin* and *yang.* Referring to the Sacred Source as He or She is a human convention that has historically been associated with power and the value placed on the role and gifts of each gender. Assigning God a gender is not only limiting, but potentiates an imbalance in society where those of the gender not like God are devalued. In a patriarchal system, it might be hard to remember that God has feminine qualities. History shows us that, in contrast to the more subservient place of women in societies with a patriarchal God, in cultures and societies in which God is viewed as a woman or androgynous, women are more respected and valued (Achterberg, 1990). Achterberg particularly notes the impact of the societal image of God's gender on the value placed on the healing activities of women, and on the treatment of women healers. This inequity also occurs when our icon of God reflects human traits that are limited to a specific race or culture.

REFLECTION 6–3

Consider how images of God influence relationships with ourselves, others, and the earth when

- God is experienced as loving contrasted with a God that is judgmental

(continued)

- God is seen in all life contrasted with being distant and not involved
- God is viewed with human traits contrasted with God as mystery
- God is a personal companion contrasted with God as a majestic mover

INFLUENCES OF BELIEFS AND EXPERIENCES ON THE SPIRITUAL JOURNEY

Spiritual teachers and scholars remind us that our conception of the nature of God is critical to our spiritual life, and the kind of God in which we believe makes all the difference in how we relate to others, ourselves, and the world. Scriptures and sacred teaching from different traditions reflect various facets of the same Unity and different experiences of the Sacred Source. These are guides for the spiritual journey that speak to different hearts, different peoples, at different times. Florence Nightingale appreciated that, to know God, we must learn about religious traditions other than our own (Dossey, 2000). Borysenko (1999) echoes this sentiment as she remind us that, while finding and following our own way to God, we need to know and appreciate the paths of others, and recognize that God's household has room for all to live and grow. We can appreciate the wisdom that is associated with the various expressions of God and better understand how our own concept of God unfolds as we make more space within ourselves for that which we can experience yet never understand.

The experience of interior silence of "resting in God" is beyond thinking, images, and emotions. This awareness tells you that the core of your being is eternal and indestructible, and that you as a person are loved by God and share his divine life. (Keating, 1995, p. 114)

As we mentioned previously, there is a difference between *beliefs about* and *experiences of* God or Sacred Source. How we *experience* God or Sacred Source is ultimately more important for the spiritual journey than our intellectual understanding or *belief about* God. Because we cannot "think" God does not make God unreal. It only means we must use more than the rational mind. We must do more than *think about* God if we are to truly *know* God. Rabbi David Cooper (1997) reflects that as we explore the spiritual path we often learn a great deal of information without integrating it into our daily experience. He notes that wisdom teachings about God or any aspect of spirituality remain abstract if we remain content to learn about the experiences of others rather than bring meaningful practice and experience into our own lives.

We experience our connectedness with God within our inner being. Our inability to adequately express the experience does not negate or limit our ability to experience connectedness with God. Spiritual teachings from many traditions help us to transcend the knowledge of the rational mind and access the "deep yet dazzling darkness of the mystical consciousness" (Smith, 1991, p. 60). The Sacred Source may be experienced as a person, a presence, as mystery, or that which is beyond words. The Sacred Source is often experienced as a power greater than the self, yet wholly the self, both within and beyond the self. Teachings of different religious and spiritual traditions offer their own perspectives of, and guidance for how to be in relationship with the Sacred Source. Connecting with God leads us to connection with the inner self. As we come to know more fully who we are, we discover more of the Sacred Source within our being. Encountering the God of our inner hearts enables us to better understand the meaning and reality of our own lives. The processes that foster these connections are as varied as people, might or might not be part of religious and spiritual traditions, and lead along many paths. Our encounters with God, which open us to the fullness of who we are, can come in surprising ways and in unexpected places, as Tammy's journey illustrates.

 ## Journey Away from and Back to God: Tammy's Story

My life thus far can best be described as a journey away from and back to God. The journey back began in February 1990. Lying in bed in a treatment center, I was thinking about what might happen to me. No, better yet, what actually did happen to me?

I went to church on a regular basis throughout my younger years. I tried to differentiate between what was imposed on me and what I thought my own relationship with God should be. As my teenage years approached, there was a restlessness that settled within me. There was something not quite right. I felt different, maybe because there were no other kids from my neighborhood in my grade at school, my brothers were much older than me, my parents seemed older than most parents, and I thought my parents were much more strict than most parents. I resented having to go to church and not be able to stay home to watch Wizard of Oz at 7:00 P.M. on Sunday.

I remembered thinking for a long time that all I wanted out of life was to be happily married with a loving husband and to have children. As the years passed, along came a college degree in nursing, a good job, a new car, and a long-term relationship that resulted in marriage. There was also the use of alcohol and drugs that was becoming more than social recreation. Church and God eventually faded into the background. I believed I was self-sufficient and didn't need anyone in the world, except my mother. I thought I was getting what I wanted out of life. Why then, did I feel like I was dying inside? My outlook on life was very bleak; I viewed everything in shades of gray. The act of living day by day became a chore. I didn't recognize it at the time, but I was slipping into a deep depression. Isolation and withdrawal became very comforting. I would wake up in the morning and couldn't wait for it to be night. At night, I would lie awake and think about all the sins I was committing. I would vow to change my actions the next day, but sadly enough, the next day never came. Alcohol and drugs became my number one attraction. I would not do anything at all without considering how it would affect my ability to use, conceal my use, or hide my stash. I knew I was heading for a downward crash, but I could not do anything to stop it.

After the crash and two weeks in the treatment center, I was still minimizing. I didn't want people to think badly of me. The blame was on everything and everyone else. I couldn't be such a bad person. It just wasn't my fault. Lying in bed, dozing on and off, I awakened with a start. The realization jolted me forcefully. The question in my mind was "What is going to happen to you? You're nothing but a liar, a thief, a drug addict, and an alcoholic. You have been so suave through the years, always managing to slide right out of any sticky situation or avoid any trouble." But, it was very clear to me that I had been backed right into a corner with no possible way to escape—checkmate. Something had finally got the best of me. I was no longer self-sufficient. My wings were broken.

Slowly, a revelation happened before my very eyes. I saw an image of a huge white banner floating across the room. On it read "The truth will set you free!" The next two weeks were incredible. My eyes were opened. The blinders were gone. Like a butterfly breaking free of a cocoon, a baby bird breaking out of its shell. The shades of gray were gone. I started to see the most gorgeous colors—the green trees, blue skies, red cheeks of a small child. All of a sudden I knew what spirituality and God was all about. It was so simple to understand. The years of struggling with religion and my salvation were over. God, creative being, universal power, spirit of nature. My journey back to God had begun. I did not experience an outward reformation but an inward transformation. My life is full of gratitude and appreciation for God, nature, and His goodness. I marvel at the creation of each human being, an animal, the growth of a tree, the seasons, etc.

Today, daily, ongoing prayer and meditation is a priority. A prayerful life is a powerful life. My faith has intensified. I can go to any church I want and worship anywhere with anyone. Religions are irrelevant to my ability to be spiritual. My load is light; my heart wants to sing. The healing has been so very enriching. I try not to sweat the small stuff. I look at the Big Picture and ask what really matters? What is most important here? I know that my worst day today is in no way as bad as my best day when I was bound to the chains of addiction. And I have to work on my spiritual condition on a daily basis. If I am not moving forward, then I am moving backwards. I feel an enormous sense of gratitude for recovery and the program of Alcoholics Anonymous.

The Serenity prayer has been a wonderful guide for living my life each day. It makes so much sense. I have also learned that I have to give away what I have in order to keep it. My favorite thought and saying is "I shall travel through this life but once. If there is any good I can do, let me do it now. For I shall not pass this way again."

AWAKE AND AWARE

In her book, *Awareness in Healing*, Lynn Rew (1996) notes that in common usage, awareness generally means to be cognizant and informed about a subject or event. She points out, however, that *cognitive* awareness, though very important, is only the most concrete of three dimensions of awareness in human experience. *Intuitive* awareness moves beyond the logical and rational focus of cognitive awareness and includes other ways of knowing. Intuitive awareness is a direct knowing experienced by a person that might be difficult to explain or validate to another. *Transcendent* awareness is the most abstract of the three dimensions. It is direct, and often sudden, knowing that is not bound by time or matter, an exchange of energy occurring without rational thought or analysis. Transcendent awareness encompasses our spiritual sphere and our relationship to the universe as a whole, permitting the closest and most intimate communication among beings. Although each of these dimensions plays a role in the spiritual journey, transcendent awareness reflects the deepest and most intimate connection with the inner self and Sacred Source.

REFLECTION 6–4

- Be aware in this moment not only of *what* you are reading, but *that* you are reading.
- Be aware of *who* is reading in this moment.
- As you are reading, what is your awareness of your body, your feelings, the environment around you?
- How aware are you in this moment of what is going on in your inner self?

Sometimes, noticing the moment, I simply remember God. The remembrance does not take me out of the moment, because God is in the moment. It is what Brother Lawrence called the little interior glance, just a simple recognition of divine presence whenever immediate awareness happens. (May, 1991, p. 71)

When people questioned what manner of person the Buddha was, he would tell them "I am awake." Spiritual literature and teachings across traditions reflect that "waking up," "seeing clearly," "developing awareness" are at the core of the spiritual journey. Our spirits call us to awaken and to be aware, to remember that in essence we *are* awareness. Awareness opens us to the space of our innermost being where we know ourselves as whole and connected to everything else. Awareness is *being*—totally present in each moment to whatever is going on within and around us. Being in the present might seem difficult because we live so much in our minds, which tend to focus on the past or future and are seldom in the present moment. Another barrier to awareness is the belief that the key to our inner fulfillment lies outside of us—in material possessions, outer achievements, and what we do and accomplish in life (Russell, 1992). This belief is part of the illusion that we are separate and incomplete and must have something outside of us to make us whole. It is as if we are in a trance or seeing through cloudy glasses. Spirit calls us to awaken from the trance, and reconnect with our wholeness and remember that the source of our deepest fulfillment is within.

Living in awareness is possible for everyone, although waking up is not always easy! As with so many experiences of life, learning to live in awareness requires commitment and patience. Anthony de Mello (1982) illustrates this with the story of a Zen student, Tenno, who became a teacher after completing the requisite ten years apprenticeship with the Master. One rainy day Tenno went to visit the Master, leaving his clogs and umbrella on the porch of the house. When Tenno entered the house, the Master asked whether he left the umbrella on the right side or left side of the clogs. With this question Tenno became confused and had no reply. Realizing he had not been able to practice constant awareness, he became the Master's student for another ten years! This story reflects that learning to live in awareness is a life journey, not necessarily a fast and easy process. This can be a challenge, particularly in fast paced Western society that is so focused on the quick fix and instant gratification. You might have heard the joke about a person trying to get to a symphony concert in New York who asked a man passing by "How do I get to Carnegie Hall?" The man responded "Practice, practice, practice!" The same directives are true for being awake and aware! However, this is not, as Jones (1999) reflects "a massive self-improvement project." Rather than our usual mode of striving to accomplish something, we are asked to be open to receive the grace that is offered.

Lest you feel discouraged, or wonder if you really have the energy and time needed for waking up, remember that this is what the spiritual journey, indeed the life journey, is truly about—re-awakening and living in awareness. Although we need to be serious in our commitment to the process, and the path can be rocky at times, we are wise to approach the journey with compassion and light-heartedness. There is no failure! You are likely to already be practicing mindfulness at some level in your life. Every event and experience of our lives is an opportunity for opening more to awareness. Even when we recognize that we have not been living in the present, this realization is itself awareness that calls us to the now. Engaging in mindfulness helps us become more conscious in all aspects of our lives.

Mindfulness

It is important to realize that the place to which we are going is one in which the knower, the knowing, and that which is known are all one. Awareness alone remains. (Keating, 1995, p. 74)

Concepts of awareness and mindfulness are the basis for many spiritual disciplines or practices that call us to pause in the midst of our activities and busyness to attend to matters of spirit or soul. The practice of spiritual disciplines requires both intention and attention. Intention implies that we are acting consciously rather than unconsciously. We nurture the ability to be centered and aware by making the intentional decision to pause and be mindful of the present moment and all that it holds. Taking the time to observe what is going on within ourselves, without judgment or elaboration, noting thoughts, feelings, physical sensations, and distractions, provides valuable experiences in the practice of awareness. Observing what is going on in the environment, attending to all of our senses and experiencing our sensations, enhances our full presence in the moment.

Mindfulness is a process through which we reach within ourselves to find and acknowledge our own specialness. Practicing mindfulness has many faces and forms. Many traditions emphasize the importance of mindfulness as a way of life. Among traditional indigenous people, mindfulness is evident in the consciousness with which they live in relationship with all of life. Prayer, ceremony and ritual punctuate daily cycles and the cycles of life—acknowledging the presence of Creator in life's gifts and events, honoring the earth for her nurturing, and honoring plants and animals who give their lives for our well-being. People who are aware of their relationship with the earth are often very conscious of subtle shifts in the wind, taste of the air, sounds or activities of birds and wild life, energies of plants, patterns of the clouds—all of which reflect being awake to the world around them. Practices such as qigong, yoga, t'ai chi, and aikido develop consciousness of breathing and movement. The mindfulness that is basic to the practice of these disciplines affects one's life as a whole. The process of attending to the body sense discussed in Chapter 5 is a practice of mindfulness, as is the centering that is integral to Therapeutic Touch (Krieger, 1979; 1993), Healing Touch (Hover-Kramer, Mentgen, & Scandrett-Hibdon, 2002), and other healing modalities.

For him [the old Indian] to sit upon the ground is to be able to think more deeply and to feel more keenly; he can see more clearly into the mysteries of life. Standing Bear, Lakota. (Hifler, 1996, p. 257)

The term "*mind*fulness" refers to more than a cognitive process or thought. Mindfulness brings the attention of our whole physical-mental-emotional-spiritual being to the present moment in a way that focuses yet expands our awareness. Our minds can actually be a stumbling block to focusing in the present because of the incessant mental chatter regarding the many concerns of our lives. Mindfulness enables us "to transcend the junk pile of information and our emotional overlay through focused concentration. To dwell in the immediate now, without consideration of anything outside of being mindful . . ." (Umlauf, 1997, p. 27). As we develop mindfulness we learn to allow stimulations such as thoughts, emotions, noise, light to pass through our awareness without needing to analyze, name, interpret, or in any way give them meaning. Mindfulness is the way we look and see, listen and hear, touch and feel, open our senses and presence to every moment. Jean Pierre de Caussade refers to the "sacrament of the present moment" which is the divine potential in each instant (Jones, 1999, p. 59).

In moving us to a deeper place of awareness mindfulness includes, yet goes beyond, our intellectual and emotional experience. Rabbi Cooper (1997) likens this to the different ways we might experience a garden. He writes,

Most of us experience deep pleasure when in a garden. We encounter sensory delights: colors, shapes, and odors. Intellectually we may appreciate the process of preparing the land, planting the seed, caring for the sprouts, fertilizing, watering, and all of the work that a well-tended garden requires. Emotionally we may be touched by the vibration of the blossoming life, the tenderness of fragile plants, the calmness and serenity of the garden during some moments, and the busyness and vitality during others.

A mystic [one who is mindful] in the garden experiences all this, but is drawn to other contemplations as well. He or she attempts to connect with the soul of each plant, the other beings that live in this garden, the angels that hover everywhere, and the interactions of plants with one another. A mystic contemplates the sparks of holiness that reside within every plant and insect, knowing that these sparks are raised to new levels of consciousness when the fruits or vegetables are ingested by beings with higher consciousness. In the mystic's holistic view, every garden—every aspect of creation, for that matter—is a microcosm of the Garden of Eden and a reflection of everything happening in the cosmos (p. 10).

Thich Nhat Hanh (1991) writes that the way we practice mindfulness is to be in touch with life, looking deeply as we engage in everyday activities such as walking, doing dishes, driving, observing a flower. The secret, Hanh says, is to be really ourselves, because only then can we encounter life in the present moment. As we connect with our inner selves, we can be who we are, as we are. Many paths and processes can assist us in re-awakening to ourselves, and different ones might resonate in us at various points on our journeys. We need to recognize and honor our own paths and honor those of others as well.

SELF-NURTURE: Practicing Mindfulness

Approach each of these self-nurture suggestions with a sense of playfulness. There is no need to get anywhere in particular. The goal is to *be* where you are! Whatever you find yourself feeling, just acknowledge the feeling and embrace with loving compassion the part of you that is feeling that way. Journey well. There is no pass or fail—the journey is what is important.

- Choose a "mindless" activity of your daily life such as dressing, folding laundry, doing dishes, or bathing and begin to bring more mindfulness to the activity. Be aware of how you move, what you are thinking, how you are feeling while doing the activity. Each time your thoughts move away from focusing on your involvement in the activity in this moment, gently acknowledge the part of you that became distracted and return your focus to the activity. Do this as often as you are aware that you are not in the present moment, merely acknowledging, without judgment. At first you may find that you are calling yourself back to focus every few seconds or minutes, but as you continue the practice the time in awareness may increase. Commit to this activity for three days, then three days more, and three days more . . .

- Choose a sound in your environment. It can be a clock ticking, the traffic moving by, a bird singing, or music playing. Focus your attention on this sound without needing to describe or analyze it, merely listen and hear the sound. Do this for five minutes. When you find your mind wanders to something note your awareness of this shift and gently bring your awareness back to the sound, without judgment. As you become more conscious with your listening for five minutes, you might want to gradually increase the time to 10 or 15 minutes.

- Select an aspect of your work to which you can bring mindfulness each day. You might bring your attention to your posture as you work, or spend five minutes in which you really look at and listen to a co-worker, or be conscious when you eat your lunch, or be aware of your emotional reactions to situations, without needing to analyze or judge them. You might just pause for a moment in the midst of your work to take a breath and bring your full attention to being in your body, aware of being in the present moment.

- Take a moment to gaze at the sky, a flower, a plant, a picture on the wall, and allow yourself to really see that to which your gaze is directed. No need to describe or label, merely look with consciousness of what you are seeing in the moment. As your mind wanders, return it to the object in your vision, being aware that you are looking at the object.

- As you walk or sit outside feel the breeze or warmth of the sun on your skin. Focus your attention on your feeling, without analysis or judgment. Stay with your awareness of feeling the breeze or sun's warmth for several minutes, then begin to be aware of who is feeling these sensations and be with you who is feeling the touch of the breeze or warmth of the sun.

PATHS TO CONNECTING WITH INNER SELF AND SACRED SOURCE

You can change and save the world by changing yourself. And that begins with waking up to the power of life in the present, and finding there the presence of your Creator and all creation. (Hartman, 1998, p. 220)

Many different paths help us access and connect with inner self and Sacred Source. We might find that certain paths call to us, open to us, or even descend upon us, at various phases of our journey. Waking up to the power of Life in the present can come through our regular spiritual practices of prayer, meditation, and participation in religious worship or spiritual ceremony. Serving people in need, working for social justice, or being involved in environmental issues can lead us to deeper connection with our inner self and Sacred Source. Illness or any crisis can be a powerful way of waking us to ourselves and the Sacred. As Ram Dass (2000, p. 113), who lives with limitations resulting from a stroke, writes "illness (and aging in general) contains the seeds of great opportunity in terms of spiritual growth. By making stillness *necessary*, it slows us down to here-and-now." However, we might not initially appreciate illness as a spiritual path. Our initial reaction often is that we are not ready for or desirous of this slowing down. Esber Tweel (2000) reflects this in saying "when illness comes, you are consumed by the moment; but it is not where you want to be. You want to either take your time machine to the past or fly to the future. Our brain scurries to the past and to the future because if we were in the moment, we feel as if we would like to climb the highest hill and scream with every breathe of life within our lungs, or cry, or yell 'Out, out, damn spot.'" He notes that his illness continues to teach him how important it is to learn to be present to the moment "having eyes to see and ears to hear, which are opened to the beauty and healing of the moment . . . experiencing the reaction to the internal and external surroundings within and around us. If we miss this, we may miss the hopeful signs even in the state of hell. We may miss the acknowledgment of someone standing beside us, walking with us in the present. Not trying to lead us anywhere, but being there. We may miss the patch of blue sky or butterflies wings. We are always so quickly wanting to jump into tomorrow without knowing today. To have hope, we've got to find it in the present, and be aware of it tomorrow, after we are aware of where we are today."

A common thread found in various paths to inner self and Sacred Source is the process of paying attention and being focused in the present moment, listening more carefully to the experience of our inner space. These paths help us to "begin to enter the present moment and break the time-binding traps we've set for ourselves," freeing ourselves from "worrying about the past and from anxiety about what's to come in the future by fully entering the present moment" (Dass, 2000, p. 113). These processes help us to recognize our interconnectedness, and that "all these things in a moment can become mystical doorways for the Soul" (Dass, p. 113). Consider what approaches have been part of your experience over time, whether or not by conscious choice. How have experiences of illness or crisis opened you more to your spirit and connection with God or the Sacred? What processes have felt congruent with your worldview and personal style? How might you be called to explore a different path at this time?

Prayer and meditation often come to mind first when we think of spiritual practices through which we connect with our inner self and Sacred Source, and certainly they are some of the primary paths to this connection. Approaches to prayer and meditation vary within and among different traditions, and the distinctions among them sometimes blur. Other practices that can assist us in this journey include relaxation processes, guided imagery, working with dreams, walking the labyrinth, writing and journaling, artistic expression, counseling of various types, religious services, and spiritual rituals and ceremony.

Prayer

I have told you that prayer is a virtuous act. However, the soul and spirit of prayer are more virtuous than the form. Through them we arrive at Union with God, in a way that only God knows. (Rumi, in Harvey, 1999, p.50)

Prayer is an expression of spirit that is a fundamental way of connecting with our inner self and Sacred Source. It is a deep human instinct that flows from the innermost part of who we are, reflecting our awareness that life is a sacred journey. Prayer is a place of both longing for and awareness that we are already connected with the Sacred Source. A reminder of our nonlocal, unbounded nature, prayer is infinite in space and time. It is Divine, the universe's affirmation that we are not alone (Dossey, 1993; 1996). Prayer invites us to live in the *now*, at least for a few moments. As Nouwen (1997, pp. 20–21) writes

> To live in the present, we must believe deeply that what is most important is the here and the now. We are constantly distracted by things that have happened in the past or that might happen in the future. It is not easy to remain focused on the present . . . Prayer is the discipline of the moment. When we pray we enter into the presence of God whose name is God-with-us. To pray is to listen attentively to the One who addresses us here and now. To pray is to listen to the voice of love . . . if we could just be, for a few minutes each day, fully where we are, we would indeed discover that we are not alone and that the One who is with us wants only one thing: to give us love.

Prayer represents our deep desire for communication and communion with God or the Sacred Source. It is one of the ways we seek insight into universal questions related to where we came from, where we are going, and why we are here. Prayer is mystery and a journey through which we come to know more of who we are and with whom we journey. The path for this journey is created by walking it (Farrell, 1972). In essence, prayer is the most fundamental, primordial, and important language that we humans have. Prayer begins and ends without words, flowing from yearnings of the soul that arise in a place too deep for words and move to a space beyond words.

We do not know what we ought to pray for, but the Spirit . . . intercedes
for us with groans that words cannot express. (Romans 8:26)

Prayer is intrinsic to religious and spiritual traditions and rituals worldwide. In ancient times and in many non-Western societies today, there is no division between secular and sacred. In these traditions, prayer is a continual experience, inseparable from the daily awareness of the Divine Presence in all aspects of life (Ameling, 2000). Prayer flows through all of life, associated with common daily acts such as dressing, gathering and preparing food, eating, planting, encounters with others, doing chores, and bathing, as well as being intrinsic to spiritual ceremony or religious services, and special occasions. Prayer, in this perspective, is a way of being, of approaching life with awareness, trust, and gratitude.

Forms and expressions of prayer are as varied as the people who pray and can be public or private, individual or communal, engaged in consciously or with limited awareness. We pray in stillness and through activity. Prayer includes praise and adoration, petition, intercession, confession, lamentation, invocation, thanksgiving, being, and showing care and concern for others. Speaking (aloud or silently), singing, chanting, moaning, listening, waiting, being with what is going on in the present moment, and silence can all be elements of prayer.

Processes and techniques such as relaxation, quieting, breath awareness, attention training, focusing, imagery, and visualization can be incorporated into prayer. Prayer is also expressed through postures and movement such as walking, dancing, swaying, or drumming (Burkhardt & Nagai-Jacobson, 2000). Whatever form our prayer takes, Dolan (1991) encourages us to be who we are, allowing the openness, spontaneity, and trusting of the child within us to have full expression.

REFLECTION 6–5

- What are your earliest memories of prayer?
- What is prayer for you? How do you pray?
- How has your understanding and experience of prayer changed throughout your life?
- With what form(s) of prayer do you feel most at home?
- How do you create space in your life for prayer?

PRAYER AND HEALING

Across time and cultures, prayer and healing have been integrally linked. Although people in general do not need research to affirm the efficacy of prayer in healing, many in the scientific community require verification to accept the truth that people have known for ages: Prayer does affect healing. Larry Dossey (1993, 1996) discusses studies conducted on prayer, documenting that both directed and nondirected methods can affect healing and other outcomes. His extensive review of research on prayer suggests that nondirected prayer that focuses on the greatest good of the organism might be more effective than directed prayer that focuses on a specific outcome. The research also documents that prayer at a distance alters processes in a variety of organisms, including plants and people, and that observed effects of prayer do not depend on understandings or beliefs about prayer held by the one prayed for.

What we believe about prayer and the meaning that prayer has in our lives influence how, when, and even whether we pray in a conscious way. Although prayer is a basic way of connecting with the inner self and Sacred Source for many or even most people, some people object to any considerations of prayer. For example, persons who are atheists or agnostics might not consider prayer a viable path to the inner self. Dossey (1997) notes that along with evidence of the positive aspects of prayer, there is evidence of prayer's potential to harm, terrify, and offend. He discusses the power of negative belief to influence our health and well-being, whether such thoughts are directed toward ourselves or others. Citing research on the powers of consciousness and distant intentionality, he notes that if a person can influence the physiology of another through prayer or focused intention, such influence can be harmful as well as healing. Negative prayer includes hexing, cursing, conveying harm through the *evil eye,* and any prayer or ritual that wishes harm to another. Dossey suggests that prayer can also be negative when we direct our prayer toward what we feel is "best" for another without knowing or honoring that person's wishes, use prayer to manipulate or control someone, or pray for someone who does not want it. Noting that negative intentions, though common, are often unconscious, Dossey suggests that we can protect ourselves from the harmful intentions of others through personal prayer, protective images, aromas, and love.

SELF-NURTURE: Ways of Praying

Although prayer often arises spontaneously in response to needs, incorporating prayer consciously into our lives requires commitment and discipline. For this, we need to schedule prayer into our lives just as we do for other activities that we consider important (like eating, bathing, or watching our favorite TV show!) The following are a few examples of ways of praying. Consider what immediately feels most comfortable for you. Consider experimenting with approaches that are less familiar. Incorporate into your life a way of praying that nurtures you.

- Read a passage of your sacred scripture or another inspirational reading. Just sit with and ponder the passage, allowing yourself to think about and feel its meaning or message within your whole being.

- Take a prayer walk. As you walk outside, be aware of the thoughts and emotions that arise within you in response to what you observe around you. Perhaps you feel joy in the singing of birds, gratitude for a coat that is keeping you warm, concern as you pass a neighbor's house where you know there is strife, wonder at the beauty of the setting sun, pain regarding the mistreatment of the earth. Listen to these feelings with your heart and reflect on what your heart is calling forth from you. You may also just use this walking time to converse with your God, sharing the joys and frustrations, blessings and concerns, and questions and wonderings of your life.

- Practice the presence of God. Be conscious of inviting God into your life, and being in God's presence, recognizing how God is present in every moment of your day.

- Pray with your body. Use your body to express the prayer of your heart through dance, spontaneous or ritual movement, or posture.

- Listen to the still, small voice within you. Just be in the quiet with your Soul, with your God. Silence makes room for God.

- Write your own psalm, prayer, hymn, or chant. Create a sacred image or mandala.

Meditation

> *The true power of meditation—and the true reason for meditating—*
> *is to become awake in this very moment. And from that place—*
> *that here-and-now touching the power of life—we can find the*
> *ability to transform ourselves and others in ways which can and will*
> *transform the world (Hartman, 1998, p. 221).*

Meditation, which can also be a form of prayer, is a practice of mindfulness that flows from and leads to connection with our inner self and Sacred Source. Dolan (2000) reminds us that meditation is both a practice that we engage in consciously and something that happens organically when we are in a place of awareness. Meditation has many forms rooted in both spiritual traditions and secular practice. Meditation can be done while being physically still or when active. Some approaches to meditation give directives about how to sit and breathe, whether to have eyes open or closed, whether to focus on a word or object or let thoughts flow freely through our awareness. Whatever the directives of a particular approach to meditation, the goal is to bring awareness to the present moment through focused concentration, facilitating body-mind-spirit balance and connection with the Sacred within us. Relaxation is a beneficial response to meditation. Even when meditation involves physical movement, an inner stillness promotes relaxation. In our fast-paced world, where we are valued for what we do and accomplish, where we often feel the stress of being always in a hurry, of having too much to do with too little time, the importance, for our health and well-being, of connecting with our inner stillness cannot be over emphasized!

Meditation, an ancient process through which we can experience expansion of consciousness and deep connection with the Sacred, has positive physiological effects and overall health benefits. Research documents that meditation leads to a deep state of relaxation in which there is a slowing of both breathing and heart rate and an overall decrease in metabolic rate similar to that of the sleep state, but the meditator is neither sleeping nor in a trance (Chopra, 1990). The beneficial effects of meditation include decreasing hypertension, chronic pain, anxiety, and blood glucose levels, improving cardiac outcomes and reversing heart disease, and reducing stress (Benson, 1984; 1997; Kabat-Zinn, 1994; Ornish, 1990). The deep relaxation gained through meditation affects the physical body in numerous ways. Relaxation increases peripheral blood flow, electrical resistance of the skin, and production of slow *alpha* waves and enhances overall immune system function. Relaxation decreases oxygen consumption, carbon dioxide elimination, blood lactate levels, respiratory rate and volume, heart rate, blood pressure, skeletal muscle tension, epinephrine levels, gastric motility and acidity, and sweat gland activity (Anselmo & Kolkmeier, 2000). Overall stress reduction is another significant benefit of meditation that promotes general well-being, facilitates rest and sleep, and enhances mental alertness and creativity. Research suggests that long-term meditation might retard the physiological aging process (Chopra, 1990).

CONSIDERATIONS REGARDING MEDITATION

Meditation must be done on a regular basis to realize the long-term benefits and move to deeper and more expanded levels of consciousness. Connecting with our inner self and Sacred Source through meditation requires commitment and practice. In the same way that we would plan times for physical exercise in our lives, scheduling a time and place for meditation helps to encourage us in the practice. Because meditation takes concentration, choosing a space that is relatively free of distraction helps. Using the same place for meditation, even if it is merely the chair in the corner of the room, marks that as *sacred space.* Over time, our body and our person become conditioned, so that merely going to this place begins the process of entering into meditation. In addition, we become familiar with the routine sounds of that space, making it easier not to be distracted by them. The environment for meditation should be comfortable for you; thus, you might consider the lightening, temperature, furnishings, presence of plants, and the like. Incorporating sounds such as music, chant, chimes, drums, flowing water, or scents such as flowers or incense might enhance meditation for some but be a distraction for others. Establishing a regular time for meditation sends the message to ourselves and others that it is a valuable part of our lives. Consider the time of day that will be most conducive for you. Among the many excellent books and resources available regarding meditative practices of various traditions are *Healing Meditation* (Umlauf, 1997) and *The Nurse's Meditative Journal* (Kahn, 1996). These authors discuss basic considerations for meditation practice of many forms and provide guides for developing personal meditative practice and for incorporating meditation as a healing intervention in clinical settings.

The goal of meditation is to experience more fully who we are in this moment in relationship with the Sacred Source and with all of creation. In considering whether meditation is supporting us along our spiritual paths, Kahn (1996, p. 8) suggests that we consider, not whether we are enlightened but, rather, whether through meditation "Am I more compassionate and loving? Am I less judgmental? Do I feel more unified with everything and everyone around me? Am I more forgiving? Am I more flexible? Is my happiness less affected by external events?" (p. 8).

Prayer and Meditation

Because practices of prayer and meditation have many similarities, we discuss types or approaches to these practices together, recognizing also that there is overlap even within these approaches. Recalling that there are as many ways to pray and meditate as there are people, of prime importance is to use the approach that suits you best. Prayer and meditation practice includes devotion, visualization or imagination, concentration, contemplation, conversation, awareness of presence, movement. One of the goals of all these practices is to move us from the head to the heart. In talking about getting out of the head de Mello writes,

> The head is not a very good place for prayer. It is not a bad place for **starting** your prayer. But if your prayer stays there too long and doesn't move into your heart it will gradually dry up and prove tiresome and frustrating. You must learn to move out of the area of thinking and talking and move into the area of feeling, sensing, loving, intuiting. That is the area where contemplation is born and prayer becomes a transforming power and a source of never-ending delight and peace. (1978, p. 13)

Devotion, found in all traditions, can be practiced in different ways. Through focusing on a word or passage from a spiritual source, on images of divine or sacred figures, or on a spiritual teacher or guide such as a guru or saint, devotion opens the heart to a feeling of love, joy, or gratitude toward God or another who represents divine qualities. Devotion is a path of the heart, not of the mind. We allow the object of focus to sink into the heart and mind until it becomes part of us. Devotion can be silent or include vocalized prayers or chants. An example of devotion is the ceaseless repetition of God's name with one's heart and soul such as the Jesus Prayer in Christianity and the Hindu practice of the Remembrance of the Name.

Visualization or *Imagination* involves an interior process of focusing the mind. One way of quieting the mind is to imagine one particular object in the mind's eye. The object should be something easy to connect with, may have spiritual connotation, yet be without strong emotional charge such as a word, a symbol, a number, a tree, a rock, or a chair. With eyes closed, this object becomes the focus of one's inner attention. Whenever the mind drifts to other thoughts or images, attention is brought back to the image of the chosen object. Another approach is to use the imagination to recapture a scene of a favorite place or to fantasize a place where we feel love, peace, and connection with self and Sacred Source. With this process, we use all our senses to experience the sights, sounds, scents, and feelings of the imagined place. Through imagination we can create and discover our inner sacred space. We can use imagination to revisit places where we have experienced or encountered God, other spiritual figures or guides, or in some way connected with our spiritual self. With our imagination we can enter into the events of stories from sacred texts or other sources that serve as guides along our paths, interacting with and sharing the experiences of those in the stories. Imagery is a powerful way of connecting with our inner guidance and the Divine Source within.

Concentration, which is basic to meditative practice, refers to the ability to focus our attention on a particular task or process. Within meditation, concentration fosters relaxation of the body while keeping the mind focused, yet relaxed (Kahn, 1996; Kaplan, 1986). Several practices or techniques are helpful in nurturing and developing concentration. One practice is to hold an object softly in your vision, such as a mandala, a candle flame, or a flower. There is no need to describe or analyze the object, merely maintain the focus. Whenever thoughts or sensations enter as distractions, gently return your focus to the object. In a similar way, paying attention to your breathing, or to the feel of the air on your skin, or to a particular sound in your environment foster concentration. Repeating a word or phrase over and over (often called a *mantra*) is another approach to focusing attention. Through repetition, our consciousness merges with the content or intent of the word or phrase. Although the Sanskrit word *mantra* comes from Eastern traditions, the practice of repeated vocalization of a word or saying is common to many spiritual traditions. Examples in Christianity include the Jesus Prayer, the rosary, repeating a line from scripture or a short prayer such as "the Lord is my Shepherd." In Judaism this practice is seen in repeating the *Sh'ma* "Hear, O Israel: the Eternal One is our God, the Eternal One alone." The central prayer of Islam *Insha'allah* "There is no God but God" is yet another example. A well-known Eastern mantra is the Sanskrit word *aum* or "om," meaning one. Either a spiritually significant or secular word can be used as a mantra. As Kahn (1996) points out, however, ancient spiritual traditions use spiritual words as mantras for both their meaning and vibrational tones, suggesting that mantra meditation can contribute to attuning the whole being while quieting the mind. Ancient Sanskrit and Hebrew are two such sacred languages in which the tone or sound of words used in prayer facilitates spiritual deepening even when we do not understand the meaning of the words.

Contemplation is another process for quieting the mind and opening the heart that uses few or no words. Contemplation is a way of being with an image or inspirational passage that opens us to the life beyond the form or the words. There is no need to describe or analyze; rather, we allow the image or passage to speak to the deeper place of knowing within us. Being present with and experiencing the energies of nature where we observe without comment or thought, is a form of contemplation. Sitting in a church or temple gazing on a sacred symbol or stained glass window can be contemplation. The Zen Buddhists use a seemingly nonsensical word riddle called a *koan* as a focus of contemplation. These riddles have no answer, for example, "what was your face like before you were born?" Gazing at a sunrise, a starlit sky, or one's sleeping child may be moments of contemplation.

The practice of *Presence* is a form of contemplation—just being in the presence of God, the Holy One, Universal Love, without thoughts or words. Practicing presence is a way of communing or communicating with God, the Divine, or Sacred Source using few words, concepts, or images. The mystics tell us that experiencing the presence of God takes us to a place that is beyond words. Presence within the stillness of our own hearts or inner space draws us into the deeper places of our own knowing and is a doorway to connecting with our Sacred Source.

Conversation can be considered more prayer than meditation, but it can flow from the centered place of meditation. In conversational prayer, we speak with God directly as we would talk with anyone and listen for the response within our hearts. Attending to our inner sense or gut sense is one way of listening to the "still, small voice" of the Sacred within.

Movement can be a form of prayer and meditation. Practices such as yoga, t'ai chi, aikido, and qigong incorporate focused breathing with movement. Mindfully doing these practices or repetitive exercise such as jogging, walking, and swimming makes them meditation in motion. The body can also be used to express prayer in many ways by bringing focused concentration to the movement and allowing the body to express that which flows from the heart. Ceremonial and sacred dance and postures are but a few examples. Connecting with our inner self through movement is discussed further in Chapter 5.

Ritual and *liturgical prayer or meditation* are often shared and have particular meaning within the traditions of a community. These prayers may be recited, chanted, sung, or expressed through movement. The prayer of religious services and spiritual ceremony and ritual (both silent and vocalized) are examples of this form of prayer. People might include recitation of these more formal prayers as part of their regular spiritual practice.

Relaxation Response

Meditation and certain types of prayer elicit what Benson (1997) calls the relaxation response. A significant decrease in the body's oxygen consumption is a prime characteristic of this response, leading to slowing of the metabolism and reducing the internal wear and tear on the body that is brought on by stress. The relaxation response can also be evoked through processes such as progressive muscle relaxation, jogging, yoga, t'ai chi, walking, and certain types of breathing exercises.

Eliciting the relaxation response requires no particular religious or spiritual focus but can include individual spiritual context. The two basic steps for eliciting the relaxation response are to repeat a word, sound, prayer, phrase, or muscular activity and to passively disregard everyday thoughts that come to mind, returning to the repetition (Benson, 1997). The word(s) chosen can have either a secular or religious focus depending on personal preference and meaning. Benson generally suggests doing this process sitting in a quiet relaxed place with eyes closed but notes that we can do it with eyes open, while standing, kneeling, or being in other postures. When done while exercising, the focus becomes the repetitive movement such as paying attention to the right, left cadence of the feet when walking.

Using Imagery

> *Imagination is the source of everything we have done or achieved*
> *as a species; every idea we have ever brought into expression . . .*
> *was first born as an imagining and was only brought forth*
> *into reality "after the fact" (Taylor, 1982, p. 17).*

Processes of creative visualization and guided imagery are particular approaches to connecting with the inner self. These processes use the power of our minds and imagination for body-mind-spirit healing (Shames, 1996). Through exploring our inner world, imagery helps us to provide a safe space for being with emotions, thought forms, and past hurts that can seem to be barriers to moving along our spiritual path. Imagery also enables us to connect with the inner guidance that helps us to heal the hurts and gives us a sense of direction for our journey. Through song, chant, ritual, and story, imagery is used in many cultures as a way of connecting with the spirit world. An example is a Navajo *Sing,* which is a complex spiritual and healing ceremony of several days duration incorporating ritual, sand paintings, herbs, chants, and family and community presence. The chant recounts the story of a spirit being whose experience relates to the person's problem, describing the spirit being's journey to healing. This provides sick persons with an image for their own healing process as well as the healing powers derived through connection with the spirit being. The images and energy of the sand painting are integral to the healing.

Dream Work

Ancient cultures knew, and modern science affirms, that, whether or not dreams are remembered, dreaming is a universal human experience. Many cultures and spiritual traditions consider dreams an important resource for inner knowing and for receiving messages and guidance from the Divine and the spirit world. Some cultures believe that dreams are the experiences of the soul as it journeys from the body at night to seek wisdom in the spirit world. Indeed, ancient Egyptian, Babylonian, Greek, and Roman cultures all placed great value on dreams as a vehicle for receiving knowledge from the spiritual world. Indigenous peoples today continue to honor the importance of dreams as a source of wisdom from a place beyond ourselves and for their insight into the truth about our own life and soul's path. For Australian Aboriginal people, the dreamtime represents the place of their deepest connection with their origin, from which they know who they are and their place in the world. Among Native American traditions is a strong belief that wisdom comes through dreams, giving direction for the individual dreamer and for the community as a whole. Sun Bear (1994) suggests that one thing that contributes to the imbalance on earth today is that people cannot remember and work with the material that comes to them in their dreams. Accounts of dreams or similar experiences are found throughout the Hebrew-Christian scriptures, documenting how God or God's messengers visited people in their dreams. In the West, attending to dreams is given emphasis within some psychotherapeutic approaches and in some spiritual traditions. Paying attention to the symbolic language of our dreams enables us to access creative ideas, important insights, and conscious understandings related to our life experiences, purpose, and direction.

Creativity and Art as Windows to the Soul

> *Art is not something that stands in opposition to science; it is a part of science. Indeed, it is a part of all human experience. Art expresses what words usually fail to express. Art brings wholeness to human consciousness (Chinn, 1994, p. 20).*

The creative impulse is an expression of the divine within each of us, both doorway to and reflection of the soul. Art in its myriad forms helps us connect with the place of Soul or Spirit. Creative expression is a path that may lead us to God, and may reflect our experience of the Sacred. In her book *Walking on Water: Reflections on Faith and Art,* Madeleine L'Engle (1980) shares her hard won understandings and recurring wonderings about faith and art in her own life. She reflects that her personhood embraces various forms of expression—Christian, daughter, wife, mother, grandmother, artist, writer. In her understanding, creativity is a way of living, not dependent on one's vocation or way of earning a living. In her words "creativity is a holy act because it opens us up to God's creativity in our lives. Using our creativity reminds us that there is something about us that not only mirrors God, but also incarnates God's spirit . . . It is that God-shaped place inside of us that is the authentic shape of our human soul" (p. 13–14).

Creative expression often takes us beyond words, connecting us with universal truths and experiences, and enabling us to express the agony, the ecstasy, and the ordinary of what is going on in our inner and outer lives. We infuse spiritual energy into what we create. In the broad sense, anyone who creates is an artist—the dad who decorates cookies, the weaver at her loom, the painter, the photographer, the gardener, the carpenter, and the chef—the list is endless. Whether creating a work of art or experiencing and appreciating the work and talents of another, we find our souls engaged and enlivened by creative expression. Such expression gives voice to the soul when words fail.

Art has an energy that speaks to various levels of our being. When standing before a painting, lost in its colors, textures, and images, we may feel our eyes fill with tears or our hearts sing. We heard a jazz pianist recall that when he first heard jazz it was like hearing and feeling the wonder of all creation, and he wanted to learn to play jazz to participate in it. For a jazz musician to "swing," he explained, was to be in touch with a deep truth and rhythm, a creative source of life experienced in music. Artists often reflect that they see themselves as channels, receiving their creative expression from places deep within and beyond themselves (Cameron & Bryan, 1992).

The creative arts experienced via our senses and moving through our whole being bring us in touch with the spiritual. An artist's whole being is involved in the creative process. In learning the art of calligraphy, the artist soon realizes that although the hand moves the brush across the paper, the whole body is attuned to and involved in the creation of the strokes on the page. We dance with more than our feet and sing with more than our voices. The whole being is engaged in the magic of creation. Like a ritual, a work of art provides an experience of our inner being both in its creation and in its completion.

SELF-NURTURE: The Arts in My Life

Spend time with art in a form that is meaningful to you. You may want to read a single poem, visit a museum, admire a single work of art, spend time with a special object of art in your own home, read a favorite story (how about a childhood favorite), listen to music, or visit a studio. Be fully present with the art and receive what it brings to you.

WRITING AND JOURNALING

> We write to taste life in the moment and in retrospect . . . We write
> to be able to transcend our life, to reach beyond it. We write
> to teach ourselves, to speak with others, to record the journey
> into the labyrinth. (Anaïs Nin, quoted by Albert, 1996, p. 14)

As one form of creative expression, writing can afford an opportunity for connecting with ourselves and the Sacred Source. Keeping a journal, writing prose or poetry, or recording our thoughts, feelings, and experiences make us more aware of our inner world and the flow of our lives over time. Norris (1998) writes, "poetry, like prayer, tends to be a dialogue with the holy" (p. 379). At times the process of writing becomes meditation. Deep prayer and meditation may prompt us to record and reflect on the images, insights, and the knowing that come from the intuitive right brain. Learning to write freely, allowing ourselves to be honest and spontaneous without censoring, we gain deeper insight into our soul's knowing. As Baldwin (1977) aptly states, "the journal is a way of connecting. The journal is a connection of the self with the self . . . The journal is a river . . . is a mirror . . . is an anchor . . . is myself . . . The journal is a process of survival" (p. xiv–xvi).

In her book, *Amazing Grace—A Vocabulary of Faith,* Norris (1998) writes about the process by which she moved from feeling "bombarded by the vocabulary of the Christian church," which she experienced as a tremendous weight of baggage from both her family history and childhood, to a living faith in which the words "had become real to me, in an existential sense" (p. 2–3). Her book affords readers the opportunity to accompany her on the spiritual journey of exploration and discovery with all its questions, wonderings, and observations, reminding us of our own continuing journey filled with wonderings and questions, new understandings and explorations.

> *Though writing may be painful, there is a joy and power in writing,*
> *even though you're dealing with something that is hard to live through*
> *day by day. You're trying to understand what you're living through*
> *by using the tools of words and images and the beautiful inner structure*
> *of language (McPherson, cited in Moyers, 1995, p. 288)*

Writing affords the opportunity to re-live or re-visit experiences, to think about their meanings for us at the time of their happening, and in retrospect. Journaling may take as many forms as there are writers to conceive them. We can reflect on something we have read, events, persons, objects, passions, struggles, questions, or feelings. Writing is one way we listen to our lives, whether it be writing in a journal, letters to friends, or the creation of a poem or story. Albert (1997) reminds us that "in writing, we become more reflective, more deeply aware of the meanings that were obscured by the chaos and excitement of the lived experience" (p. 1).

Cameron and Bryan (1992) offer two tools for reawakening creativity that they call *morning pages,* which they liken to prayer, and *the artist's date,* which they consider a time of release and creativity. Morning pages are "three pages of longhand writing, strictly stream-of-consciousness . . . not meant to be art or even writing . . . pages are meant to be, simply, the act of moving the hand across the page and writing down whatever comes to mind . . . just write three pages . . . and three more the next day" (p. 10). Persons who have written morning pages find surprising experiences from the practice. The artist's date is just that, a period of time (two hours a week is suggested) when you and "your inner artist, a. k. a. your creative child" spend time together, uninterrupted by anyone else. Their book offers a full and readable discussion of both of these practices that help us to "fund the creative reserves we will draw on in fulfilling our artistry" (p. 20).

Our list of references contains some of our favorites from the variety of books available on the subject of writing. You will discover others to suit your own particular needs and style as you explore writing as part of your journey.

REFLECTION 6–6

- What is the place of the arts in your life and how can you honor this place?
- What is the gift of arts to your life?
- How do you connect with your inner self and Sacred Source through creative expression?
- Consider how certain music can enliven you and uplift your spirits.
- Consider how books, poems, or plays that you have written or read have drawn you to deeper awareness of who you are.
- Consider a time when you have received insight from or have become "lost" in a painting or photograph that speaks to a your inner being.
- Consider the experience of sharing your creative expression with someone you love.

SHARING THE JOURNEY WITH OTHERS

Although connecting with the inner self and Sacred Source is something that we each do ourselves, our nature is to seek support, encouragement, and companionship for the journey. As embodied souls, we experience God as we journey within our inner space and as we share our outward journey with others. Norris (1992) reminds us of the importance of sharing silence as well as activities with our companions, noting that sharing silence with another creates a bond that cannot be compared to ordinary exchanges. It helps us know that each of us is essentially, a vibrating essence. When we sit quietly together we sense that vibration. We can feel it singing in our cells . . . when we support the silence in one another, we discover what we each have been given to be. The silence in each of us is the medium through which the words we are may be spoken, clearly and purely. In silence we are revealed. (p. 24–25)

Across time, cultures, and traditions, people have found a door to the inner self and Sacred Source through religious and spiritual teachings, tradition, ritual, and ceremony. Religious services and sacred ceremony bring people together as community. Noting that individuality and community are inexorably linked, Hawkins (1987) writes that approaching God requires that we also approach our very human brothers and sisters. We must include not only our carefully selected close spiritual friends, but also the mixed multitude of friends, strangers, and acquaintances that we encounter in various experiences of our lives.

As we engage with others in prayer, meditation, study of sacred texts, ritual, or ceremony, we often receive insight and support for our own journeys. Rituals help us to order and find meaning in our life experiences as we express shared beliefs, understandings, and values related to the spiritual path. Within the religious and spiritual community we can access the wisdom and guidance of spiritual leaders and guides, those who we consider to have knowledge and experience of the spiritual path—the shamans, priests, priestesses, rabbis, imams, gurus, ministers, monks, nuns, medicine people. Our connection with others and with our spiritual tradition informs and illuminates our path toward deepening connection with inner self and Sacred Source.

Counseling

Counseling, a particular way of sharing our spiritual journey with another, is a path to the inner self and Sacred Source. Whether meeting with a licensed therapist, or discussing concerns with a trusted friend, we can gain deep personal insight through the counseling process. This process can help us to reconnect with parts of ourselves that have been hidden away for any number of reasons and provides an opportunity for healing at many levels of our being. Although some approaches to counseling more readily include acknowledgment of the spiritual than do others, all can bring us to a deeper appreciation of who we are in our innermost beings.

REFERENCES

Achterberg, J. (1990). *Woman as healer.* Boston, MA: Shambhala Press.
Albert, S. W. (1996). *Writing from life: Tell your soul's story.* New York: Tarcher/Putnam.

Albert, S. W. (1997). Opening our stories, sharing our lives. *Story Circle Journal, 1*(1), 1, 3.

Ameling, A. (2000). Prayer: An ancient healing practice becomes new again. *Holistic Nursing Practice, 1*(3), 40–48.

Anselmo, J., & Kolkmeier, L. G. (2000). Relaxation: The first step to restore, renew, and self-heal. In B. M. Dossey, L. Keegan, & C. E. Guzzetta, *Holistic nursing: A handbook for practice,* (3rd ed., pp. 497–535). Gaithersburg, MD: Aspen.

Armstrong, K. (1993). *A history of God.* New York: Ballantine Books.

Baldwin, C. (1977). *One to one: Self-understanding through journal writing.* New York: M. Evans.

Benson, H. (1984). *Beyond the relaxation response.* New York: Berkley Books.

Benson, H. (1997). *Timeless healing: the power and biology of belief.* New York: Simon & Schuster.

Borysenko, J. (1999). *A woman's journey to God: Finding the feminine path.* New York: Riverhead Books.

Burkhardt, M. A., & Nagai-Jacobson, M. G. (2000). Spirituality and health. In B. M. Dossey, L. Keegan, & C. E. Guzzetta, *Holistic nursing: A handbook for practice,* (3rd ed., pp. 91–121). Gaithersburg, MD: Aspen.

Cameron, J. & Bryan, M. (1992). *The artist's way: A spiritual path to higher creativity.* New York: G. P. Putnam's Sons.

Chinn, P. L. (1994). Developing a method for aesthetic knowing in nursing. In P. L. Chinn & J. Watson (Eds.), *Art & Aesthetics in Nursing.* New York: NLN Press (pp. 19–40).

Chopra, D. (1990). *Quantum Healing.* New York: Bantam.

Chopra, D. (2000). *How to know God: The soul's journey into the mystery of mysteries.* New York: Harmony Books.

Cooper, D. A. (1997). *God is a verb: Kabbalah and the practice of mystical judaism.* New York: Riverhead Books.

Dass, R. (2000). *Still here: Embracing aging, changing, and dying.* New York: Riverhead Books.

de Mello, A. (1978). *Sadhana: A way to God—Christian exercises in Eastern form.* St. Louis, MO: Institute of Jesuit Sources.

de Mello, A. (1982). *The song of the bird.* Anand, India: Gujarat Sahitya Prakash.

Dolan, J. R. (1991). *Meditations for life* (2nd ed.). Syracuse, New York: Scotsman Press.

Dolan, J. R. (2000). *Communion meditations.* Anand, Gujarat, India: Gujarat Sahitya Prakash.

Dossey, B. M. (2000). *Florence Nightingale: Mystic, visionary, healer.* Springhouse, PA: Springhouse Corporation.

Dossey, L. (1993). *Healing words.* New York: Harper Collins.

Dossey, L. (1996). *Prayer is good medicine.* San Francisco: Harper San Francisco.

Dossey, L. (1997). *Be careful what you pray for.* San Francisco: Harper-Collins.

Farrell, E. (1972). *Prayer is a hunger.* Denville, NJ: Dimension Books.

Hanh, T. N. (1991). *Peace is every step.* New York: Bantam Books.

Hartman, T. (1998). *The last hours of ancient sunlight: Waking up to personal and global transformation.* Northfield, VT: Mythical Books.

Harvey, A. (1999). *Teachings of Rumi.* Boston: Shambhala.

Hawkins, T. R. (1987). *Sharing the search: A theology of Christian hospitality.* Nashville, TN: Upper Room.

Hifler J. S. (1996). *A Cherokee Feast of Days,* volume II. Tulsa, OK: Council Oak Books.

Hover-Kramer, D., Mentgen, J., & Scandrett-Hibdon, S. (2002). *Healing touch.* (2nd ed.). Albany, New York: Delmar.

Jones, T. (1999). *Awake my soul.* New York: Doubleday.

Kabat-Zinn, J. (1994). *Wherever you go, there you are: Mindfulness meditation in everyday life.* New York: Hyperion.

Kahn, S. (1996). *The nurse's meditative journal.* Albany, New York: Delmar.

Kaplan, A. (1985). *Jewish meditation: A practical guide.* New York: Schocken Books.

Keating, T. (1995). *Open mind, open heart: The contemplative dimension of the gospel.* New York: Continuum.

Kelly, T. (1997). *The sanctuary of the soul.* Nashville, TN: Upper Room.

Krieger, D. (1979). *The therapeutic touch.* Englewood Cliffs, NJ: Prentice-Hall.

Krieger, D. (1993). *Accepting your power to heal.* Santa Fe, NM: Bear.

L'Engle, M. (1980). *Walking on Water: Reflections on faith and art.* Wheaton, IL: Harold Shaw Publishers.

May, G. (1991). *The awakened heart.* San Francisco: Harper San Francisco.

Moyers, B. (1995). *The language of life: A festival of poets.* New York: Bantam Doubleday Bell.

Norris, G. (1992). *Sharing silence: Meditation practice and mindful living.* New York: Random House.

Norris, K. (1998). *Amazing grace: A vocabulary of faith.* New York: Riverhead Books.

Ornish, D. (1990). *Dr. Dean Ornish's program for reversing heart disease.* New York: Ivy Books.

Nouwen, H. (1997). *Here and now.* New York: Crossroad Press.

Rew, L. (1996). *Awareness in healing.* Albany, New York: Delmar.

Russell, P. (1992). *Waking up in time: Finding inner peace in times of accelerating change.* Novato, CA: Origin Press.

Shames, K. H. (1996). *Creative imagery in nursing.* Albany, New York: Delmar.

Smith, H. (1991). *The world's religions.* New York: HarperCollins.

Sun Bear, Wabun Wind, & Shawnodese (1994). *Dreaming with the wheel.* New York: Fireside Book.

Taylor, J. (1982). *Nurturing the creative impulse.* San Raphael, CA: Dream Tree Press.

Tweel, E. N. (2000). *Unpublished personal journal of illness experience,* Charleston, WV.

Umlauf, M. G. (1997). *Healing meditation.* Albany, New York: Delmar.

READING–JOURNALING

Adams, K. (1990). *Journal to the self.* New York: Warner Books.

Broyles, A. (1988). *Journaling: A spirit journey.* Nashville, TN: Upper Room.

DeSalvo, L. (1999). *Writing as a way of healing.* San Francisco: Harper.

Goldberg, B. (1996). *Room to write: Daily invitations to a writer's life.* New York: Tarcher/Putnam.

Goldberg, N. (1990). *Wild mind: Living the writer's life.* New York: Bantam Books.

Heart, R. D., & Strickland, A. (1999). *Harvesting your journals: Writing tools to enhance your growth and creativity.* San Cristobal, NM: Heartlink.

Killen, P. O., & DeBeer, J. (1995). *The art of theological reflection.* New York: Crossroads.

LeGuin, U. K. (1998). *Steering the craft: Exercises and discussions on story writing for the lone navigator or the mutinous crew.* Eight Mountain Press.

Jean Watson's Story

Dr. Jean Watson shares with us part of her personal journey. Her story eloquently reflects the many phases, moods, and paradoxes of the spiritual journey, a journey that includes suffering and joy, darkness and light, mystery and meaning. She speaks of presence and caring, about connecting with inner self, with Sacred Source, with others, about taking time out, about daily rituals, about ways of expressing pain and joy. Her story is, as she reflects, the story of us all, a journey of the soul, the spirit. (Story, poem, and psalm copyright 1998, Dr. Jean Watson, reprinted with permission of the author.)

———

I begin with a personal paradox, my own being and my own becoming. I live in pain, Yet I dwell in a semblance of peace. I know fear, yet dwell in love. I know terror and life's horror's, yet I glimpse joy. I live in darkness; yet I experience light. I know despair, yet I live in hope. I know doubt, I reside in faith.

I live with and witness gut wrenching suffering for myself, my two daughters, my grandchildren, family, friends, and loved ones.

I learn about deep self-caring and healing. I am asked to learn how to bear the unbearable.

I live with a broken heart which may never mend. Yet the blood of life still flows through my veins and my life, reminding me of the sacred flow.

I am blind in one eye. Yet I see. I move at the speed of sound. Yet I am still. I weep, yet I rejoice still.

I am alone and lonely. Yet I am never alone.

I am sad; yet I laugh and cry. I lose my eye. Yet I am sighted

I lose my husband. Yet I am wedded.

I lose my home. Yet I am housed.

I lose my balance. Yet I still dance.

I lose my identity. Yet I am finding myself.

I lose my life as I had known it for almost 37 years with my husband, who is now gone, leaving me full of tears. Yet I now seek and glimpse another, deeper, inner life.

I lose my "I" as I have lived it for 57 years. I find a greater "I"—the divine I AM.

I am fragile, vulnerable, and labile. Yet I am softened and purified, opened, strengthened by my wounds and my wonder at life and death.

I will never be cured. I may be healed. I am being changed. I AM.

I can never reveal or explain my story through logic or modern science. Through my journey I find words I never thought to speak. I offer my story as a mantra and a meditation, as another way to find our presence. I do so after my own time out, and time in, and my own journey into these uncharted territories and unknown domains . . . I am present from another time and place . . . from my own inner journey of healing in search of holy communion, blessings and lessons in the midst of personal pain, loss, and suffering. Here is part of my personal story, which may serve as a microcosm for others.

My experiences fall into two or three areas: lessons for being present, evoking the sacred, and learning to bow down, to surrender, to be still, to wait, to listen, to see anew, to be open, and to be becoming. I begin with a journal entry, late June, 1997: "Every day seems like Sunday." This I wrote as I was learning how to "be" still, to be present, to be held in my so-called cradle of suffering and healing during the long hot summer and fall, and approaching winter of 1997. In a freak accident where I was hit by a golf club in my eye—an unbelievable accident, when my adorable nine-year-old grandson swung before I knew he was going to, and I stepped right into his line of fire. My life changed irrevocably in one flashing mini-second. In that instant, I suffered a traumatic eye injury, so severe that the surgeon said it was parallel only to some of the injuries of the Vietnam era.

After emergency surgery and hospitalization, and more surgery and hospitalization, I was required to lie, face down, 24 hours a day, on a massage table, with my head in the cradle. It became my sacred cradle, hanging upside down like the ancient story of Odin, who hung upside down, and later discovered the ancient wisdom of the Runes. Except, my eye could not be saved—and I still seek ancient Runic truth . . . which is part of my search for the present.

There is not only this story. It continues, as does all of life's mystery. You see, my husband, who lovingly cared for me during my recovery, and during which we experienced the pinnacle of our love—through creation of sacred space, meditation, giving me daily massages, reading poetry and love stories, serving all my meals, bathing me—found my experience somehow unbearable. After my eye could not be saved, he, a peaceful, loving romantic, did the unimaginable, the unthinkable. He committed suicide. So I shudder and reel with the losses and the pain that I have, and am, learning to endure . . . learning to bear the unbearable, to seek meaning in the mystery, to dwell in the unknowable, the mysterious, the impossible. Yet, I have to honor this too, enter the dark and the void—and we all do—and acknowledge this, too, as part of my learning and healing.

One of the privileges during this time was that I got to experience my own theory, because he took care of me. So I have all this theory out here, but I've never had the experience. And another thing about entering into the void or mysterious, there are some levels of this that we can never understand. I was talking to a Native American elder, and he said to me that we all come from the Spirit world, and we come with a soul's purpose. And when that purpose is fulfilled, we return to the Spirit world. And I said to him "What about somebody going home prematurely?" He said, "What do you mean 'prematurely'? That's your terminology." And, I said, "Well, take somebody committing suicide." He said, "Well, we're all committing suicide in our own way. When we are spiritually satisfied, and our soul's work is done, we return home." And that has probably been the most helpful thing for me to grasp in terms of making sense out of something that's ineffable. There's no way to make sense of it.

But, the other thing I want to share is that from the mystery of this, and from that broader spiritual perspective, my husband said something to me during the time he was taking care of me, and he put it like this, "I feel like I've been preparing all of my life just for this." What a gift! And when that was finished, his work was done, I guess. So it's been quite a journey here. So, as a result of this so-called tragedy or gift, depending on how you view it, I now have many stories of caring and healing to tell, and many experiences to share from the inside out, and the upside down, from my early work . . .

One of the other more recent experiences I had . . . because I went into retreat for a couple of months back in the winter, I returned home and was sitting at the airport, and a bus with a huge billboard came by. The sign on the bus said "*Up Close and Personal*," and it was advertising Loveland ski area. And, for some reason, that hit me directly. That is exactly what we have to do to get to Love-land, to get into this space, this kind of territory. Because we are the instruments of healing, we must be up front, and personal. We can use theory and be informed by theory, but we cannot hide behind the mask of the professional that we have had. It is through our personal story, our personal being, our personal presence, that we become the tool for healing.

I also want to say that my accident taught me, and continues to teach me, about learning to be still, to stop and to surrender to the flow of pain and sweet joys of each moment, each day, one merging into the other in a seamless line of Sundays. Second, in having always to hold my head down, I was at first embarrassed, because, as a part of the healing process, even as I was able to be up, I still had to hold my head down. And as we would go for walks in the neighborhood, I felt embarrassed and ashamed. As I continued to walk, I learned that when you look down, you look inward with reverence, more of a contemplative place, an inwardness. It became a walking meditation. I experienced a sense of bowing down with gratitude and inner stillness, humility, and praise for all that life continued to offer me in the midst of this.

So being stopped in my tracks, as I was, left me stopped on the spot, with no agenda but to be still, feel the pain, and surrender to what followed. But during the first instance of my experience of my eye injury, even in the deepest unbearable pain that cannot be described, I felt an indescribable outrush of love and peace. It felt as if my soul was given space to catch up with me, and teach me at some deeper level still about caring, and healing, and soul care, from the inside out and upside down, that removed me from external theories and writings. I also discovered that what I was experiencing was not just my pain. I learned that going into the dark, along with being in the light, was shared by hundreds, if not thousands of others. I received an outpouring of love and prayers and healing energy, and cards and letters, and gifts and blessings from around the world. So all the love and care became a significant part of my healing. I don't think I could have gotten through this had I not felt that.

And so, one of my lessons has been learning to receive and be connected with others, even though I was alone in my personal pain. So all of this had allowed me to understand that my personal experience was mirroring others. At some deep level my experience mirrored the pity, terror, and oneness of the human condition that Shakespeare talks about. And, during this time of learning to be present, I also had what I would call some mystical experiences where I began having Biblical dreams. They were dreams, for example, about being in the Holy Land, being led by someone in a long robe who was taking me to the cradle of Christ's birth, and I said, "But, I didn't think people were allowed to go there." He said, "Well, they aren't ordinarily, but I've been instructed to take you there." I have an accumulation of dreams from this time. In one dream I am on a sacred journey and climbing mountains in Tibet, going with a group into a holy space, making it sacred space. As I reach the space, I say, "I've made it, but it wasn't as hard as I thought it was going to be." In another dream I am in a monastery with a group of people, leading them to lunch. I go to the back door of the dining room, which looked like it had been hermetically sealed for a long time, and when I barely touch the door, it opens. There is a large, Christ-like figure (in this case Matthew) and there is a beautiful banquet in this very heavenly dream. I don't understand these dreams, but they were quite amazing, and very Biblical.

One morning I heard a voice, just as I was waking. The voice said, "Who wrote the Psalms?" I answered to myself, "I don't know." Then I leaned over to my husband and said, "Doug, who wrote the psalms?" My husband, with his quick wit, said, "The psalmists." I persisted, "Well, who were the psalmists?" "They're everyday citizens . . . common people who bowed down with praise and thanksgiving, and gave expression to all the suffering and pain, along with the joy and song for the holiness of all of life's experiences." Thereafter, I began to write psalms to give voice to all the holy and horrific that I was experiencing, because along with the outrush of love and peace, I also had this other part that was unbearable that I'm dealing with. The psalms gave me an outlet, which I didn't ordinarily have, to express this. Now I have a collection of almost one hundred psalms. The dark shadow side of my pain, as well as the light needed to be expressed with reverence, being present to both the holy and the horrific of all life's experiences. I share one of my psalms here:

Blind, maimed, wretched with pain. I come before Thee.
My heart of darkness, fill with light of day.
Come before me with Thy Comfort.
Deliver me from Sorrow and suffering.
Hold me in the bosom of Abraham, Ruth, the communion of Saints.
Surround, enfold, and cradle me with Thy loving Mercy.
Thy grace sustain me.
Matthew speak to me of Christ's healings.
Saul blinded for a reason.
Give me hope for the other side of mine affliction.
Fill my heart with Thanksgiving, my head with Praise.
Thine alone knows of my grief, my silent inner torture.
I seek Thy grace and relief.
AMEN

And, like the Buddhist practice of Tonglen, where one meditates and breathes in a way that is opposite common sense or natural tendency (wherein we seek pleasure and avoid pain), I would breathe in pain (not only mine, but of all the world), and breathe out compassion, caring, peace, and relief. The practice of Tonglen is a way of awakening the compassion and caring that is inherent in all of us.

In my cradle, I felt like it was a crucible where my impurities were being burned off. That is what has to happen as part of transformation. The path is one of being truly present to the holy in the midst of the profane and horrific. It is a path of heart, dwelling in harmony with nature. If we are truly in the present, we are in sacred space, a place of healing and caring. From my journey I offer you some tentative words of guidance: Listen to the call, what it is you *must* do; listen to the heart beat; listen to the sound between the beats; connect with the in-betweens, the silence between the breaths, the rising up and falling away of each moment; be aware of mind and heart, and when mind and heart are shutting down; learn to walk through fire; follow your inner light; develop a practice of introspection; work to awaken; become conscious of what you believe and why; keep an open mind and heart and *become*; receive guidance through dreams, wisdom, insight; release thoughts of self-pity, anger, blame of self and others for any reason; practice mindful presence and detachment from specific outcomes; take time to slow down and pause; bow down; consider the ground beneath your feet; let go of how you thought life should be; rest in the present; ponder hopes and dreams. As we let our own lights shine, we give others the right to let their own light shine.

CHAPTER 7

Connecting through Cycles of Rest and Re-Creation

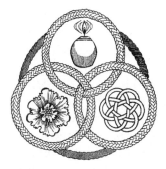

Cultivating a peaceful, compassionate heart,

making time to relax and tend to our well-being,

is a gift we give to ourselves

and impacts everything we do, every life we touch

Our Spiritual path calls for nothing less.

DOSSEY, KEEGAN & GUZZETTA, 2000, P. 495

The pace of life in our world today continues to speed up. People, at least in industrialized societies, have many labor saving devices that are supposed to make life easier and give us more free time. Yet, we often complain about having too much to do and being too busy. How often have you heard people say they wish they had more time—to read, to cook, to spend with family or friends, to do so many things they would like to do. How often have you said this yourself? When we do have free time, however, we often "fill" the time by finding something to do. The work ethic, still prevalent in society and many religious traditions, suggests that hard work brings success and that "idle hands are the devil's workshop." This ethic suggests that we should fill each moment doing something productive, and sitting idle is looked on as laziness. Our down or nonwork time is often filled with other activities, and even our "leisure" or play happens according to a schedule. Although *doing* and *activity* are necessary parts of life that have their place, *rest* and *re-creating* times are also essential for our health, well-being, and general survival.

Nature provides a prototype for the cycles and rhythm of rest and activity. We see this in the solstice and equinox cycles and in the gifts of the seasons. The letting go of autumn and the dormancy of winter are necessary for the new growth of spring and the full life of summer. The "simple" act of breathing includes a pause between inhalation and exhalation. Our physical bodies need the recuperating time of sleep to function and remain active. Physical fatigue affects our emotional, mental, and spiritual beings as well. We think less clearly when we are tired, our emotions become more labile, and it is more difficult to connect with our inner self.

Society's emphasis on work and productivity contributes to emotional and mental stress in many areas of life. Many people work in jobs that provide little personal satisfaction, in which they feel constant pressure to produce more and more with less, in which they feel manipulated by forces outside their control, and in which they feel treated as objects rather than persons. The expectation of long hours of work, imposed either by self or others, limits time with family and important companions, causing strain in relationships. Emotional and mental fatigue affect us physically, give rise to mental and spiritual distress, and contribute to use of numbing agents such as drugs and alcohol.

OUR NEED FOR AUTHENTIC LEISURE

In today's world, we need more than ever to reconnect with our creative and re-creative self, the self that can rest and be still, and experience the joy and beauty of life. Acknowledging that stress is a significant factor in the major diseases of industrialized societies, we also recognize that lack of authentic leisure contributes to stress. Work is not the villain; our inability to balance work with leisure is what throws us out of wack! Leisure and rest are a necessary part of our wholeness, our holiness. We must become sensitive to our own cycles and seasons—our time to work and our time to rest. Moving deeply into the present moment, we attune to the cycles of our own lives and bring ourselves into harmony with the rhythms of these cycles. We need to be aware, not only of when we are stressed or when we are fatigued, but of the rhythm of leisure that we need to promote and maintain balance in body-mind-spirit. Leisure is more than taking time off from work, or going on a vacation. Vacations, in fact, often offer little rest or true leisure. Vacation time is often filled with work on projects, participating in other activities, traveling and being constantly on the go—affording little or no time to just sit and be present in the experience. In describing the consequences of not attending to the necessary rhythm of rest in our lives, Wayne Muller (1999) notes that when we do not rest, we miss the pointers that show us where to go with our life, and thus, lose our way. We also miss that which would nourish us, the quiet that gives us wisdom, and "the joy and love born of effortless delight" (p. 1). We cannot sustain ourselves if all we do is "do." Without a place of being as well as of doing, we will destroy ourselves. Esber Tweel illuminates this in sharing his own struggle between pushing on with his usual "doing" and making time for the rest needed for his healing:

> In George Lucas' new *Star Wars,* drones act out what they are programmed to do, without question. Many times we, as humans, become like drones due to the "shoulds" and "should nots" in our lives. The purpose of our lives starts to fade away, like a morning mist, and our identity begins to take on a new form by being molded by another hand and not by our own. Even when illness inflicts our mind and body, we erect walls like those around a castle to protect our "shoulds" and "should nots," and this creates a stone monstrosity as if we are being shackled with a ball and chain . . . The enemy is ourself who is not willing to give permission for our well-being to evolve . . . On my release from the hospital things were very bad, and I needed to be away from everything for at least two months. The dear people of this parish graciously wanted me to take a leave of absence, and I was so, so sick. But, the voices inside me would not allow it. It was a battle between strength and weakness. The voices within the caverns of my mind would not give me permission to let go. The price of not doing this was costly, both physically and emotionally. When we don't give ourselves permission for the development of our wellness, we become smothered by the heaviness of the expectations which mold us in the likeness of the voices we hear. (Tweel, 2000)

Authentic leisure nurtures not only the body-mind, but our deeper self, our soul as well. Indeed, rest and leisure are essential elements of spiritual care. Leisure is an attitude of the heart, a way of being, that opens us to reflect on and re-vision our life of doing, indeed our whole way of living. Connecting with our inner self and Sacred Source requires that we be still, become quiet. The word *quiet* derives from the Latin *quietis,* meaning rest. The rest and quiet of leisure is a space in which we encounter Sacred Source, God, the Holy, and through which we can remain open to each new experience of God in our lives. Doohan (1990) reflects that lack of leisure leads to loss of a sense of mystery, of wonder and appreciation of something beyond ourselves, of seeing the value in simply "being with" God. In the Psalms, we read "be still, and know that I am God." Leisure provides the space and time for connecting with this stillness, the place of receptivity where we open to our own gifts and capacities, allow our inner selves to expand, and become more aware of the fullness of who we are.

Leisure is an attitude toward life that is not so much related to the amount of free time we have as to the way we approach our doing and being in every moment. Muller (1999) speaks of Sabbath time, the time of rest as "whatever preserves a visceral experience of life-giving nourishment and rest," whether this be an afternoon, an hour, or a walk (p. 6). Having a leisured approach to living is an important element of the spiritual journey. Only when we allow ourselves to pause, can we experience wonder, beauty, joy, and God and feel how these nourish our spirits. Doohan (1990) believes that leisure is essential for spiritual development. He suggests that time for reflection is necessary for our image and sense of God to develop beyond our childhood concepts. To *know* God, we must spend time with God, experiencing who God is in our lives and in all creation now, in this moment. Processes that enable us to connect with our inner selves and Sacred Source, such as prayer, meditation, centering, mindfulness, all require that we step aside from our busyness and give ourselves leisure time.

Authentic leisure means relaxing into another level of being that leads to personal enrichment and deepening self-awareness, not merely recuperating from our frenetic activity. Entering into authentic leisure can include giving ourselves time to rejuvenate at various levels of our being. I have experienced this when I have taken several days away for retreat. The first day or two I often sleep and nap a lot—perhaps time for letting my soul catch up with my body! Only by allowing this can I then relax into deeper levels of being. Leisure does not necessarily mean doing nothing. Activity can be part of leisure, but the focus is on *us,* not the activity, choosing to *do* that which renews and refreshes us.

Rest and leisure have no particular formula or shape and will look different for different people. What is leisure for us is influenced by personal values as they interface with those of family, society, and culture. How we understand leisure, Doohan reminds us, relates to our understanding of the human person and how our worldview looks at the relationship between work and play or rest. He notes that leisure is more than the rest needed to maintain intense work and cautions us against confusing the true pleasures of leisure with focusing our time and energy on leisure goods and activities that ultimately turn leisure into work. Doohan comments that leisure includes rest, creative self-development, and personal discovery of what renews and re-energizes the inner self intellectually, psychologically, emotionally, and spiritually. He also believes that genuine leisure culminates in religious or spiritual expression because it "enables an individual to focus on the truly human, religious dimensions of his or her personal integrity and wholeness" (p. 32). He goes on to say,

> We claim to believe that God is near to us, in us, in others, in the wonders of the world. Only in leisure do we act on this belief by giving time to developing attitudes necessary to meet God . . . it is not by work that we earn salvation, but in leisure we appreciate it as gift. Leisure is the corrective that puts work in perspective and expresses faith. (p. 33)

Authentic leisure, then, is an expression of our spirit that nourishes our wholeness and helps us deepen our connections with God or Sacred Source and those around us.

SABBATH

Sabbath is a way of being in time where we remember who we are, remember what we know, and taste the gifts of spirit and eternity. (Muller, 1999, p. 6)

Most religious and spiritual traditions include Sabbath time—time set apart from the routines of life for sacred rest that includes personal reflection and community celebration. In the Judeo-Christian tradition, the Ten Commandments include only one ritual observance: to remember the Shabbat (Sabbath) and keep it holy (Wieder, 2000). Within the spiritual precept of Sabbath is the wisdom that rest is essential for our health, our holiness, our wholeness. Muller (1999) reflects that the admonition to "remember the Sabbath" essentially is a reminder to appreciate that all is gift and is a blessing, to delight in our lives and what we do and accomplish, to celebrate the beauty and sacredness of life, and to pause to express our joy and gratitude for the wonder of it all. This joy and gratitude are natural states of the heart.

Within the Hebrew tradition, Sabbath is a time to take delight in God—a joyful time to pause from work and celebrate God's redemption and covenant. From the prophet Isaiah (58:13–14) we hear that

If you call the Sabbath a delight, and the Lord's holy day honorable, If you honor it by not following your own ways, seeking your own interests, speaking with malice—Then you shall delight in the Lord, and I will make you ride on the heights of the earth.

The Judeo-Christian creation story tells us that the six days of creation ended with God resting on the seventh day, providing the basis for Sabbath as the climax of creation. Wieder (2000) notes that the Hebrew meaning of rest in this account reflects that God *ensouled* the seventh day. The completion of the creative process is the place of *being*, that is, the creative process is not finished until we receive what we create. Sabbath, then, is about how we receive the creative process (Wieder, 2000). We follow God's example by giving a day of the week for rest, refreshment, and re-creation of soul, mind, and body. The writers of Deuteronomy reflect that the call to rest and observe the Sabbath is also a celebration of God's covenant and redemption.

For remember that you too were once slaves in Egypt, and that the Lord, your God, brought you from there with his strong hand and outstretched arm. That is why the Lord, your God, has commanded you to observe the Sabbath day (Deuteronomy 5: 15).

Sabbath is not so much a day of the week as a state of consciousness, a place of stillness, like the space between our breaths. Sabbath, a place of receptivity, of beingness, is the feminine aspect of God (Wieder, 2000). The practice of Sabbath provides a sanctuary or refuge from the busyness of our lives in which we can be "available to the insights and blessings of deep mindfulness that arise only in still-ness and time" (Muller, 1999, p. 7). Sabbath creates sacred time and sacred space wherever and whenever it is observed, whether in a church, temple, mosque, home, office, or somewhere in nature. Within this space and time we are able to be attentive to what is most true, nourishing, beautiful, sustaining, and graced in our own lives. As we surrender to the space of our inner God-nature, we align with our innate nature of love, of wholeness. Muller notes that for Buddhists this means taking refuge in the Buddha nature, which includes the wisdom of the Buddha and the family of the Buddha. From this space, we are more able to expe-rience our natural perfection and to cultivate right action, right effort, and right understanding. Christians find refuge in the person of Jesus who taught that the kingdom of God is within each of us, inviting us to "Make your home in me, as I make mine in you," and inviting those who labor and are burdened to find rest in him. Jesus' own life reflects the rhythm of rest and activity that grounds Sabbath living. He relaxed with and shared meals and conversation with friends, saw and delighted in the beauty and wonder of creation and saw the hand of God in all of this, recognized his need for time apart and retreated to the seashore or the hill-sides, and invited people to share in joy and gratitude for all the gifts of life and creation. The Judeo-Christian traditions teach that Sabbath is a gift from God, that we are not made for the Sabbath, but the Sabbath is made for us. Indeed, throughout the Hebrew scriptures, references to Sabbath, including the story of creation, suggest that rest is a divine way of living.

Sabbath living calls us to pause, to reflect, to joyfully celebrate life with all its light and shadows, to remember and deepen our connections with self, others, God, and nature. Sabbath rest is a re-creating time that brings necessary rejuvena-tion for body, mind, and spirit. In turn this rest enlivens our relationships and pro-vides a grounding for living in a healing way, a holy way in all of our life. The nourishment and refreshment of our Sabbath time helps to bring more balance, not only into our lives, but into our world as well. We are more able to be with the suffering and joy of others and ourselves, and to be with wonder, awe, and mystery.

REFLECTION 7-1

- How do you include rest and leisure in your life?
- What is your experience of the relationship between rest and work?
- What is rest or leisure for you?
- How do you rest or relax?

(continued)

- How would you describe a real vacation?
- If you had 30 minutes in the cycle of your day for rest or leisure, what would be included in this time?

Our times of leisure or Sabbath provide an opportunity for developing attitudes that enable us to bring leisure more consciously into our daily life. These attitudes include

- *rest:* allow yourself to just sit, put your feet up, or lie down and rest
- *read:* something you enjoy, that nourishes your mind and spirit
- *relax:* be attentive to the stresses in your being and make sure you are truly relaxed
- *recreate:* engage in recreation that is pleasant, enjoyable, and re-energizing for you
- *re-think and refocus:* reflect on personal values and approach to life; reevaluate what is truly important to you and define your priorities
- *rejoice:* in who you are as person, as member of family or community, in your challenges and opportunities, in your blessings
- *renewal and rejuvenation:* focus on what you need to be re-energized in various areas of your life, nurture your playful self (Doohan, 1990, pp. 88–90)

CONNECTING WITH THE CREATIVE, PLAYFUL SELF

Rest and leisure is a way of making space for ourselves, space to be with the fullness of who we are. When we make space for ourselves, we honor and open ourselves more to the gift that we are, a reflection and manifestation of the Sacred Source. In letting go of our need to be doing and allowing ourselves to *be* in the moment, we provide the space for our creative and playful selves to emerge. Play both flows from and enhances our creativity. In true play, we step outside constrictive ways of thinking and being and allow our imaginations to put a different spin on reality. Play expands our limits. Play fully engages us in the present moment. Plato reminds us that we can discover more about a person in an hour of play than in a year of conversation. Children show us that a stick can become a horse, a baton, or a broom. A hat creates a queen; a cape creates a super hero. In play, what we consider reality can become absurd and distorted, opening us to humor and laughter. Play, as much an attitude as something we do, brings our focus to the present moment. Wooten (2000) describes play as "a spontaneous or recreational activity that is performed for sheer enjoyment rather than to reach a goal or produce a product. Playfulness is a mood or attitude that infuses the individual with a sense of joy and positive emotions" (p. 471). True play enlivens and energizes us in body, mind, and spirit. Even though some forms of play result in some physical fatigue, this is a fatigue of satisfaction rather than of exhaustion. Play requires leisure; we need to give ourselves time and space for play. We may engage in play alone or with others. Quilting, cooking, woodworking, pottery, walking, fishing, singing, dancing, playing an instrument, story telling, spending time with children, visiting with a good friend, reading, perusing a photo album, weeding the garden, engaging in a team sport—all can be play. The way we approach the activity determines whether or not it is play. A playful spirit connects us with others and with all creation.

Our spirit is nourished and enlivened by play. This is the imaginative, creative, spontaneous self, where we experience joy, wonder, delight, and beauty. Children help us to remember how to connect with our creative and playful self. They take delight in the wonders of the world around them, are able to laugh without being self-conscious, and generally know when they need rest. Children (who have not had to grow up too quickly) so readily connect with the playful self. They delight in watching, touching, and experiencing the world around them. Their laughter is spontaneous and not strained; their tears also are spontaneous. Simple things bring them joy and pleasure—a cardboard box, kitchen utensils, crinkly paper, a song. Perhaps this is why Jesus invited the children to come to him, and is part of what he meant when he said "the reign of God belongs to such as these . . . whoever does not accept the kingdom of God as a child will not enter it" (Luke 18:16–17). Our playful selves open us to the life of God within us—the imagination, creativity, and spontaneity of our own being, the joy, and the wonder that flow from the infinite love from which we come.

REFLECTION 7–2

- How do you connect with your playful self?
- Describe a recent experience of play. Relive the feelings!
- When have you experienced joy, wonder, awe in your life? What brings joy to your life? Where do you find beauty? What causes you to wonder? When have you experienced awe?
- In what ways do you experience and express your creativity?
- Where do you allow your imagination to carry you?

There is no one way to connect with the playful self. What is restful, brings joy, gives pleasure, brings insight, and calls forth the imagination might be different for each of us. Leisure for some means not having to think or put forth much mental effort; for others, the greatest joy of Sabbath time is the opportunity to ponder or explore an area of interest. The same activity can be restful for one but work for another, and what is leisure at one point in our lives might not be so at another time. Although Jocelyn once took great delight in tending to her gardens, gardening has become more like work and a burden to her because of physical limitations. For Joe, a busy physician, gardening, though physically demanding, is restful and a way of expressing his creativity, a change from his usual mental intensity. Cooking for Wilheim is a work of art in which he takes great pleasure. Preparing tasty meals is relaxation for him. Seraya, on the other hand finds cooking one of those unfortunate necessities of life, and preparing meals for her family is by no means a way to rest. Doing building and remodeling around the house is recreation for Marge and for Ray. Leisure time for Ruben and for Juana is sitting by the river fishing. We each need to listen to what our bodies, our minds, and our souls need for rest and play.

REFLECTION 7–3

- What nourishes your creativity?
- What activities are restful, relaxing, re-creating for you? Have these changed at different times in your life?
- Where do you find joy, laughter, and humor in your life?

HUMOR AND LAUGHTER

A joyful heart is the health of the body, but a depressed spirit dries up the bones.
(Proverbs 17:22)

We have heard the saying "laughter is the best medicine," and hear more and more about the healing power of humor. When the medical system offered Norman Cousins only a very grim prognosis concerning his diagnosis of the progressively degenerating disease of ankylosing spondylitis, he chose to pursue activities that would encourage and support positive emotions. In his now-classic book,

Anatomy of an Illness, Norman Cousins (1979) described how laughter and humor helped him to heal. He watched comic films, played practical jokes, had people read humorous books to him, and told jokes. Although sages have told us that a joyful heart is healthy for the body, science is helping us to understand how this happens. Research in the field of psychoneuroimmunology (Pert, 1996) demonstrates patterns of connection and communication that link our immune, nervous, and endocrine systems. This research suggests that our emotions are stored in the body as chemical messengers, particularly neuropeptides, which have a strong influence on our health. In response to our emotions, neuropeptides are released from the brain and travel through the blood stream to plug into receptors of immune cells, altering the metabolic activity of the immune cell in either a healthy or not so healthy way. Because viruses use these same receptors, having more of the natural peptides for the receptor around will make it harder for the virus to get into the cell.

Laughter causes physiological responses that interact with the cellular elements of emotions. Laughter is a full body experience that is often preceded by emotional, physical, or cognitive tension (Wooten, 2000). Recall a time when you had a really hearty laugh, how it began with the muscles of your face around your lips and eyes, your eyes twinkling and your breathing changing, your throat and vocal cords becoming involved as noises of snickering, giggling, and hooting come forth. The muscles of your chest and stomach became involved as the noises got louder and deeper, and your breathing might have become almost gasping as the laughter got deeper. You might have started crying or felt like other body functions might be hard to control. After hard laughing for a while, you may have felt like you had a real workout and needed to just sit and rest. While this was going on you were probably not as aware of all that was occurring at the cellular level. In summarizing findings from research on laughter, Wooten (2000) notes that mirthful laughter modulates particular immune system components, increasing the number and activity of cells that attack virus-infected and some cancer cells, increasing antibodies that help ward off upper respiratory infections, increasing biochemicals that activate the immune system, and decreasing levels of stress hormones. So as laughter lifts our spirits, it is also contributing to healing vibrations throughout our whole being.

Have you noticed how effective speakers and teachers often interject humor into their presentations? Humor can facilitate the process of connecting with others. Humor gains our attention, helps to dissolve tension, is an acceptable way of expressing emotionally charged or uncomfortable feelings, and helps people to begin to feel comfortable with each other. James (1995) reflects that, through holding absurdities of life and the human condition up in jest, humor can rescue the human spirit from a sense of despair. She notes that some of the spiritual benefits of humor include helping us accept reality with its inherent contradictions, helping us maintain a sense of proportion about ourselves and our importance in relation to life and a higher order of being, and increasing our sense of connectedness to others and life as a whole.

As with play, humor also brings us into the present moment. This is evident in a story we heard about a person who was invited to participate in a Native American ceremony. When gathering with the others before the ceremony he was surprised by all the joking and laughing that was going on and tried to stay focused to prepare for the sacredness of the experience. With one joke he could not help but laugh, and shortly thereafter the ceremony began. Later his host reflected to him how important it is that people who are engaging in their ceremonies be in the present moment, and that humor and laughter bring one into the present moment. The ceremony could not begin until he too was in the present moment, signified by his laughter. Humor is a common element across cultures; however, how humor is expressed varies among different cultures. Cultural context determines what is considered humorous, situations and relationships that call for humor, when humor is appropriate, and the overall intent of humor.

Wooten (2000) considers humor as "a flowing energy, involving and connecting the body, mind, and spirit" (p. 473). She describes three types of therapeutic humor:

- *Hoping humor:* provides courage to face challenges, provides laughs despite overwhelming circumstances, sustains the spirit during shock and natural disaster, and reflects accepting life with its contradictions, incongruity, mystery.

- *Coping humor:* enables release of tension and supports the ability to change perspective and regain control in a situation, expresses frustration and anxiety related to feeling out of control, and can be used to deal with embarrassing or uncomfortable experiences or to express hostility in a socially acceptable way.

- *Gallows humor:* provides release in the midst of intense situations of dealing with suffering, death, and horrific situations, and provides a way of distancing and protecting self from the suffering and pain.

A patient who kept leaning to one side because of paralysis following a severe stroke provided us with an example of coping humor when she shared this joke: An elderly woman who was wheelchair bound was visited by her son after she had been in a nursing home a few days. The son asked how she was adjusting and liking the place. She told him that she liked the food, the other residents were friendly, and the staff members were generally nice. She just had one complaint. Any time she would start to lean to one side in the chair, a nurse would come and prop her back up with a pillow. When she would start to lean the other way the same thing would happen. Thinking that this showed that the staff was quite attentive, her son asked her what was the problem with that. She replied, "How is a person supposed to pass gas in this place!"

Esber provides an example of how he used humor to deal with some of the dynamics of his illness:

Medication might save your life, but it kills you at the same time. Some days you feel like the mule you rode in on decided to collapse while you are in the Mojave Desert, and you are surrounded by 1500 archers who decided to use your body for target practice as you huddle behind this fallen jackass. Looking at this predicament, you might figure you are having a bad day, and something has definitely broken the flow. You think to yourself, "It can't get any worse than this." But sure enough, it does!

Prednisone, Prednisone, flowing through my veins.

Prednisone, Prednisone, causes my nose to drain (like the bloody Nile).

Prednisone, Prednisone, causes my eyes to react, and later forms a cataract.

Prednisone, Prednisone, causes you to tremble and quake, and later causes your bones to break.

Prednisone, Prednisone, you are making my kidneys and liver to go haywire, without even having a drink to numb the fire.

Prednisone, Prednisone, you are putting a hole in my gut, like a burning fire you erupt.

Prednisone, Prednisone, you make my nervous system flip and flop, and my heart pounds like a jackhammer on top.

Prednisone, Prednisone, make this polymyositis to heal, and get me back on even keel.

There is another big drug that dances in your vein,
That keeps your body from chewing you up and spitting you out the drain.
God help you if you catch a cold, as cyclosporine won't let you defend it and keep it under reign.

. . . Now back to that old fallen mule. The best thing to do at a time like this is to lie back on this fallen beast, and put aloe lotion and cocoa butter all over your body. Make sure you use a hypoallergenic sun block all over your skin. Open that umbrella, put your favorite tunes in your Walkman, and order a piña colada with a lean corn beef sandwich, and visualize the images that you see in the clouds overhead. (Tweel, 2000)

Although all humor can uplift and support the spirit, not everyone responds to humor in the same way. When, either consciously or unconsciously, humor is used inappropriately, it can be hurtful and dis-spiriting. Regarding appropriate use of humor, James (1995) offers three criteria: timing, receptiveness, and content. She cautions that sexist, ethnic, or ridiculing humor should be avoided and that humor in general is more therapeutic when used in a warm, caring, and trusting environment. We can explore whether humor might be appropriate for a patient through questions such as—Do you like to laugh? What things make you laugh? Do humor and laughter make you feel better? Can you recall a painful past experience where humor may have soothed you? Has humor ever made you feel hurt or embarrassed? (James, 1995, p. 244). Observing a person's responses to humor provides another insight into the person as a whole being.

INCORPORATING SABBATH TIME AND LEISURE TIME INTO LIFE

Leisure time does not just happen, we must plan for it. We need to listen to our bodies' and souls' rhythms and need for rest and provide space for including this in our lives. Many religious and spiritual traditions call us to observe Sabbath one day each week—a day for resting from our usual work and focusing on our connection with our inner self and Sacred Source. The religious observance of this time generally includes prayer, ritual, and communal celebration. There is much to Sabbath rest that can take place beyond religious observance. In our research on spirituality, some people commented that they are not religious, but do believe in God or a Higher Power. Their Sabbath time might be spent observing the birds, or walking among the trees, or sitting in a quiet spot listening to the yearnings of their heart, or gathering wild flowers to fill the house, or visiting a special friend. Teresa gets up about an hour before the rest of the family so she has quiet, undisturbed time for reflection and inspirational reading. A morning walk with her dog provides Sabbath moments for Michelena. Scott sits in meditation twice daily. Johanna schedules periodic days for reflection and retreat with spiritual companions. John plans special time with each of his children each week. Every couple of months Liz and Rob go away for the weekend to have focused time together.

 ## SELF-NURTURE: Creating Space for Sabbath and Leisure

Leisure means more than taking a vacation and Sabbath refers to more than religious observance. Consider what is a true holiday, holy day, for you. What renews, rejuvenates, refreshes, re-creates you? Make space in you life in the next week for the leisure your body, mind, soul needs by scheduling an appointment with yourself on your calendar. This may be for an hour, an afternoon, or a day. Commit yourself to keeping this appointment and planning something that nurtures your playful self, remembering that doing nothing is perfectly acceptable!

Consider whether you need time alone or to be with others to refuel and renew your spirit. You might need a combination of both, or your needs might change in different circumstances. Are you able to make your needs known and make the necessary arrangements to meet your needs? Connecting with the re-creating self draws us into deeper awareness of and calls us to honor our own rhythms and cycles. This might mean saying no to another's request for support to attend to where we are feeling depleted. We might need to take time away and be unavailable to others to reconnect with our own inner core. Continuing to give without replenishing our own inner stores leads to having nothing more to give. Such depletion is a major factor contributing to emotional and spiritual distress and burnout among nurses and other health care providers.

REFLECTION 7–4

- How and when does time alone support your renewal, rejuvenation, re-creation?
- How and when does time with others support these processes for you?
- What is dis-spiriting or causing a depletion of energy in your life right now? How can rest, Sabbath time, connecting with your re-creating self help you regain balance in this area?
- Some people help us to relax . . . who does that for you? How often do you connect with those who help you relax?
- What helps you to relax?
- What gets in the way of your relaxing? What blocks your joy and playfulness?
- Within the past week when and how have you experienced authentic leisure? How do or can you make this part of your regular pattern of living?

SELF-NURTURE: Stop and Rest

In his book *Sabbath*, Wayne Muller (1999) offers many examples of ways we can include Sabbath more consciously into our lives. He suggests some simple ways to stop to rest and connect with the creative and playful self:

Choose one pleasurable activity that is easily done and takes little time. Leaf through a magazine and tear out a picture that you find appealing; put it somewhere you will see it, and notice how you respond to it throughout the day. Write a short poem about nothing of any importance. Put a new flower in a cup by your bed. Take a walk around the block, sing a song you know from beginning to end. Do something simple and playful like this everyday. Take a crayon and make a simple drawing of your bedroom. Let the power of a simple act of creativity stop you, slow your pace, interrupt your speed. Notice how willing you are to be stopped. Notice how it feels when you are. (1999, pp. 145–146)

Our creative and playful self needs leisure—the time for being present to the moment—time focused on care and nurture of self. Our relationships need this same time and presence. Relationships with our children require time and the ability to be playful, imaginative, and creative and to connect with the deep places within us. Relationships with lovers are nourished with play and leisure. Playfulness and leisure help us to connect with the holiness, wholeness of our sensual self. This includes our sexual selves, but also means what we experience with all our senses. The truest and deepest expressions of sexuality flow from the playful self—grounded in love and wonder, joy, and appreciation for who we are as individuals and together. Our sexuality and sensuality are sacred gifts, to be enjoyed, honored, and delighted in. How hurtful and dis-spiriting when experiences of our sensuality bring pain instead of delight or are demeaning rather than nourishing for our being. Consider how infants and young children explore the world of touch, texture, taste, sound, scent, and vision with curiosity and wonder. They want to smell the flowers, feel as well as taste their food, roll in the sand and splash in the water, and use their voices to make all kinds of wonderful sounds. And they find delight in these experiences. When was the last time you felt the grass or the sand with bare feet? Have you felt the freedom and joy of having your body caressed by the water during a leisurely bath or while skinny dipping in a warm lake? Consider the anticipated enjoyment that accompanies the aromas of your favorite foods, the wonder and gratitude you feel when viewing a beautiful sunset, the way certain music seems to energize you, or the way your whole being responds to caring touches and caresses from someone you love.

REFLECTION 7–5

- **How does your sensuality help you connect with your playful self?**

(continued)

- Through what experiences of your senses do you find joy, delight, rejuvenation, a deepening sense of who you are?
- Has your sensual self been a source of joy, delight, wonder, gratitude, or of pain, shame, fear, confusion?
- How do you nurture your sensual self?
- How do you experience play in relation to sexual intimacy?

SELF-NURTURE: Bringing Play into Your Life

Although play means different things to different people, it includes common characteristics of focus on enjoyment for its own sake, positive emotions, joy, spontaneity, and being present in the moment. Consider how you bring play into your life.

- Listen to your favorite music. Sing along if it has words. Express yourself through moving spontaneously as the music draws you. You might consider accompanying the music with some drumming. Write a few lines to express your feelings as you listen to the music.

- Make time to be with a friend with whom you can be and express yourself. You might just sit and visit, take a walk, go fishing, have coffee or tea, share a meal, shoot some hoops, whatever allows you to share the joy of being together.

- Do something that is low technology fun with your family—children, spouse or partner, siblings, parents. Plan something interactive such as a board game, playing hide-and-seek or Frisbee, singing or telling stories, bicycling, going to a park, or sharing a sunset.

RELAXATION AND LEISURE

All Life requires a rhythm of rest. (Muller, 1999, p. 1)

As we reflect on how rest and leisure are, or are not, part of our lives, we bring these aspects of life into more conscious awareness. Such awareness makes these areas available for intentional evaluation, and, if desired, change. We can explore this aspect of spirituality by asking ourselves (or our patients) questions such as "What is a real vacation like for me (you)?" "What time of the day (year, season, week) is most restful or peaceful for me (you)?" When you cannot seem to rest, consider when you have been able to rest, what has helped you at those times, and how you can make these a part of your life now. Perhaps you find reading restful. Perhaps doing something physical like walking, exercising, yoga, or t'ai chi helps you to unwind. Meditation, centering or relaxation exercises, or guided imagery could provide the focus you need for moving to a more restful place. Relaxation may be prompted by doing something repetitive that requires minimal concentration, such as folding laundry, weeding the garden, dusting a bookshelf, or chopping wood. We are more likely to provide for the important element of leisure in our lives when we plan a specific time for rest and quiet and commit to incorporating these experiences into our daily lives.

The intensity and constant change in life and professional responsibilities makes it especially important for us to attend to our need for relaxation, leisure, and play. Anselmo and Kolkmeier (2000) remind us that regular practice of deep relaxation of the body-mind-spirit offers a refuge, a self-awareness foundation for deepening our spiritual journey. Regularly incorporating leisure and relaxation into our lives helps us to more easily and consciously bring this presence into our care with others, making everything sacred because we come from this place in ourselves. We are also better able to appreciate how lack of leisure relates to health concerns of our patients and how challenging it can be to make lifestyle changes that provide space for connecting with our playful selves.

 # SELF-NURTURE: Daily Relaxation or Centering

Choose a deep relaxation practice that you can incorporate daily into your life. You might use an audio tape of a guided imagery meditation, progressive muscle relaxation, or breath awareness meditation. You might follow a practice from the many books that offer processes of centering, relaxation exercises, and meditation. Your spiritual tradition may include practices of contemplative prayer or meditation. Yoga, t'ai chi, or qigong can become meditative practices. The mindfulness, meditation, centering, and prayer processes included in this book can be used to foster relaxation and deepening into the self. The following practices can also be used.

Progressive Muscle Relaxation

You can do this sitting or lying down. Adjust yourself and your environment so you are as comfortable as possible—consider how your body is positioned, the temperature of the room, the light and noise in the environment, and the like.

Listen to your body throughout this process and do not go beyond your personal limits in any area. Begin by lifting your right leg slightly and tightening all the muscles of that leg and foot. Flex your right foot and feel the muscles become even tighter—only on the right leg, let the rest of your body stay relaxed. Maintain that position for another few seconds, tightening even more—then gently release and relax your right leg, letting it melt into the surface that is supporting it. Now begin the same process on the left by lifting your left leg slightly and tightening all the muscles of that leg and foot. Flex your left foot and feel the muscles become even tighter—only on the left leg, let the rest of your body stay relaxed. Maintain that position for another few seconds, tightening even more—then gently release and relax your left leg, letting it melt into the surface that is supporting it. Now begin to tighten the muscles of your buttocks, your pelvic muscles, the muscles in your abdomen and lower back. Push the small of your back toward the surface that is supporting you. Keep breathing and relaxed in the rest of your body as you tighten these muscles even more, tighter, and still tighter, holding for a few more seconds. Then release and feel the tension in this area melt into the surface that is supporting you. Take a breath and feel the letting go of tension from the lower part of your body. Move now to your upper back and shoulders. Bring your shoulder blades back as if you are trying to touch them together. Feel the muscles in your chest also contracting and stretching. Continue to breathe consciously while tightening these muscles even more, and a little more. Then take a deep breath and release, feeling your upper back and chest letting go of the tension. Now lift your right arm and hand, making a fist, and tightening all the muscles in the arm and hand. Continue tightening all the muscles even more, and a little more (only in the right arm and hand), and even more. Hold this a few more seconds, then release, and feel all the muscles let go. Turn your attention to your left arm and hand, lift it slightly and make a fist, tighten all the muscles in the arm and hand. Continue tightening all the muscles even more, and a little more (only in the left arm and hand), and even more. Hold this a few more seconds, then release, and feel all the muscles let go of the tension. Note how much more relaxed your upper body now feels. Finally, bring your focus to your head and neck. Bring your chin toward your chest, tightening your neck as much as you can, also squeeze your eyes and mouth tightly shut and crinkle up your face as tightly as you can, hold this a moment more, then gently and carefully release back to your neutral position. Now open your eyes and mouth as wide as you can, and stick out your tongue as far as you can. Hold this a moment or two, then relax into a comfortable expression for you. Take a few deep breaths and feel how relaxed your body is feeling. Be aware of any areas that may be somewhat uncomfortable and adjust yourself to allow any remaining tension to flow into the surface that is supporting you. Send love and gratitude to every part of your body, letting it know that you intend to be more aware of when it is feeling tense, tired, or needs attention. Honor and thank yourself for giving yourself the time and space to relax.

Guided Imagery Relaxation

Get into a comfortable position, either sitting or lying down. Begin by paying attention to your breathing, not trying to change it—just become aware of yourself breathing. Stay with your breath and allow yourself to tune into its rhythm. Observe how you are feeling as you breathe. Are there any areas in your body that are uncomfortable? Adjust your position to be as comfortable as possible. Return your focus to your breathing and begin to follow it. Let it lead you to yet a deeper place within you, a place where you feel safe, where you feel loved, supported, at peace. Just be there and allow yourself to deepen even more into this space. This is a sacred place where you connect with your inner wisdom. With your inner eye, look around this place. What do you "see" there? What is the place like? This may be a place where you have been before, or it may be a new place. Observe any colors, textures, and sensations you are experiencing. Perhaps you hear sounds. Perhaps you are aware of certain scents. Just be in this space and let the love and peacefulness enfold you. After a while you become aware of another presence there, the presence of a very wise being. Invite this being to sit with you for awhile. You may just want to be in the presence of this wise being, or you may wish to talk to this wise one about concerns or questions you have. Listen within your heart to what messages this wise one has for you. Spend as much time as you would like in this space. When you are ready, thank the wise being in any way that seems appropriate. Acknowledge all that makes this space sacred for you, the sights, sounds, scents, sensations, and tastes. Take your leave, knowing it is a place you can return to any time you wish. Return your awareness to your breathing, begin to gently stretch your body, open your eyes, and return your awareness to the room you are in, feeling refreshed and grounded in your own inner wisdom.

Quieting Response Exercise

Anselmo and Kolkmeier (2000, p. 513) offer this brief quieting response exercise as a way of becoming aware of external stressors. Because it takes only a few seconds, it can be done in various circumstances periodically through the day.

Check your breathing. Notice what is bothering you at this moment. Smile at yourself and say to yourself, "What a silly thing to do to my body!" Take a slow, deep breath to a count of 1–2–3–4, and breathe out slowly to a count of 1–2–3–4. Again, slowly breathe in. As you breathe out, let your body, particularly your lips and jaw, go as limp as possible. Imagine warmth and heaviness flowing down your body to your toes. Allow your eyes to dance and inwardly smile. Go on with your activities, alert and relaxed.

REFERENCES

Anselmo, J., & Kolkmeier, L. G. (2000). Relaxation: The first step to restore, renew, and self-heal. In B. M. Dossey, L. Keegan, & C. E. Guzzetta, *Holistic nursing: A handbook for practice* (3rd ed., pp. 497–535). Gaithersburg, MD: Aspen.

Cousins, N. (1979), *Anatomy of an illness.* New York: W. W. Norton.

Doohan, L. (1990). *Leisure: A spiritual need.* Notre Dame, IN: Ave Maria Press.

Dossey, B. M., Keegan, L., & Guzzetta, C. E. (2000). *Holistic nursing: A handbook for practice* (3rd ed.). Gaithersburg, MD: Aspen.

James, D. H. (1995). Humor: A holistic nursing intervention. *Journal of Holistic Nursing, 13*(3), 239–247.

Muller, W. (1999). *Sabbath: Restoring the sacred rhythm of rest.* New York: Bantam Books.

Pert, C. (1996). *Emotions: The mind/body connection.* Paper presented at the First Annual Alternative Therapies Symposium: Creating Integrated Healthcare, San Diego, CA, January 20, 1996.

Tweel, E. N. (2000). Unpublished personal journal of illness experience, Charleston, WV.

Wieder, K. (2000). *Meditation and Teshuvah: Exploring the Jewish contemplative tradition.* Centers of Contemplative Living, Gassaway, WV, September 8–10.

Wooten, P. (2000). Humor, laughter, and play: Maintaining balance in a serious world. In B. M. Dossey, L. Keegan, & C. E. Guzzetta, *Holistic nursing: A handbook for practice* (3rd ed., pp. 471–493). Gaithersburg, MD: Aspen

CHAPTER
8

Connecting with Nature

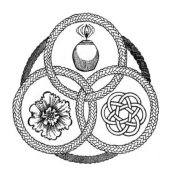

Such nearness to nature as I have described

keeps the spirit sensitive to impressions not commonly felt,

and in touch with unseen powers.

<small>OHIYESA, SANTEE DAKOTA, 1852—QUOTED BY HIFLER, 1996, P. 71</small>

People from various traditions worldwide express and experience spirituality through a sense of connectedness with nature, the earth, the cosmos, the environment, and the universe. Awareness of the life forms of the earth and the celestial bodies of the heavens, and their place within the natural order, often fosters appreciation of and connection with our spiritual selves. Relationships with animals, plants, water life, and rocks and merely being in and experiencing nature can be a source of strength, inspiration, and comfort, all of which are attributes of spirituality. Sensing awe at the wonder of life and feeling in relationship with all things, with or without a belief in a Divine being, is an experience of spirituality. For some, connection with nature flows from the experience of finding God or Creator in all things. For others the earth reflects the handiwork of God. Relationship with the earth for others can also be experienced as an energetic connection. Throughout this chapter, we use the term *nature* in the broad sense, referring to the universe and all its phenomena. Within the context of particular traditions or writers, nature can also be described as the natural world, the environment, earth, universe, cosmos.

Ancient wisdom and indigenous spiritual traditions teach that we are part of the earth and the earth is part of us. People who live close to the earth recognize that all life is sacred and that our lives are intimately connected with all the life forms in nature. Indigenous people see the world as a seamless garment in which there is no separation between sacred and secular, humans and nature. We are part of the same story. What we do to the earth, we do to ourselves. Connecting with the earth, with nature, then is a way of connecting with ourselves and with the Source of life—God, Creator, Tunkasila, Life Force, Great Spirit. As we become more conscious of our interconnectedness with the earth, we also recognize the interconnectedness of our health with the health of the earth and the environment.

REFLECTION 8-1

- How is awareness of the natural world a part of your every day living?
- When you think about nature, what meanings, thoughts, images, and experiences arise?
- Recall your childhood experiences of nature and the feelings associated with those memories.

ALL IS SACRED

In symbolic terms, the earth is not just our home, to be kept clean and properly managed, but is indeed, as every ancient civilization recognized, our "Mother," a living planet, a sacred place. (Porritt, 1991, p. 185)

Nature is always around us. For many people, living in relationship with nature is a way of life. Some people periodically experience their connection with nature in a conscious way, whereas others have little awareness of this connection with nature. Our sense of relationship to our environment derives from our worldview. The Western scientific perspective is grounded in a worldview in which there is a radical distinction between humans as subject and world as object. The more primal or indigenous worldview, which is echoed by mystics in many traditions, understands that the soul is embedded in a universe permeated by spirit or soul (Fox, 1991; Schuster & Keegan, 2000). "Before the Age of Reason and the advent of modern science, our ancestors invariably ascribed a special spiritual significance to their rivers and lakes, the oceans and seas. It was a sacrilege to defile a pure spring or beautiful river, not only as a source of aesthetic satisfaction, but as a source of natural, God-given wealth on which their lives depended" (Porritt, 1991, p. 144). Indigenous peoples do not separate spirituality from life. They recognize all things as sacred, and, hence, that life and well-being of individuals and the community are inevitably bound to living in right relationship with the earth and universe.

REFLECTION 8–2

- Describe your relationship to the earth, to nature?

- How do you like to be in nature? Observe nature? Interact with nature?

- Consider the ways in which you feel comfortable with nature. In what ways are you uncomfortable with nature? Recall a time when you felt appreciative of nature.

- How have you learned to relate to nature as you do?

A speech given by Chief Seattle of the Duwamish and Suquamish people in 1854, when the United States government wanted to negotiate the purchase of his people's land, reflects the relationship with, and love and respect for the earth that is common to many indigenous or native cultures (Jeffers, 1991; Seattle, 1992). Even the concept of someone wishing to "buy" the land was incredulous in his understanding because the land was so much a part of who they were. He asked how one could sell the air or the warmth of the earth because we do not own these. The earth does not belong to us; rather, we belong to the earth. The air is precious because it breathes its spirit into the life it supports. All parts of the earth are sacred—the pine needles, the insects, the woods, the clearings, the rivers, the shores, the rocks. The plants and animals are viewed as sisters and brothers, each with their own gifts and purpose in being. The sap in the trees, the waters, the rocks all hold the memory of the people. We do not weave the web of life. We are each but a strand in this web that connects us all; thus, what we do to the web, we do to ourselves. Contemporary authors echo this understanding, writing about the intercommunion of the universe (Berry, 1998; Fox, 1991; Schuster & Brown, 1994; Swimme, 1998), and noting renewed awareness of the interconnectedness and interdependence of all of life (Ornish, 1998). Ancient wisdom and contemporary scholars call our attention to the need for living in balance with and healing the earth, reminding us that human health depends on the health of the earth.

Sacred Circle—Web of Life

The sun is my father; the earth is my mother; on her bosom I will repose
(Tecumseh, Shawnee—quoted by Hifler, 1996, p. 9).

Indigenous cultures teach us that the earth is our mother—that we belong to the earth, to the universe. Their teachings recognize the implicit balance of nature and call us to live in harmony with all beings. For the Navajo people in the United States, this is living the *Beauty Way*—walking in balance or harmony with all creation. Traditional Navajos understand that disease and illness occur when we have somehow become out of harmony with nature (which includes many levels of our relationships) and that healing requires reestablishing this balance. Implicit in this understanding of interconnectedness is the awareness that we must take care of the earth, and she will take care of us. The Lakota Sioux of North America express this concept as *Mitakuye Oyasin*—meaning, we are all related. Lakota tradition teaches that the great Circle of Life (of all Earth Creation), the Sacred Hoop, is the Spirit way of life that sustains and binds all things (Neihardt, 1972). The center of the Circle of Life is *Tunkasila*—Grandfather (God). The seventh direction, which is in every one of us, is in the center of the circle (God). However, because people stopped listening to Spirit, and nations pulled away from the center of the circle, this hoop has been broken, and Mother Earth is no longer honored, resulting in the torture and pollution of the Earth and the suffering of her people (Two Elk, 1998).

Eastern philosophy basic to oriental medicine teaches that all life occurs within the circle of nature in which all things are connected and mutually interdependent (Beinfield & Korngold, 1991). Because all things are connected within this circle, to nourish a part nourishes the whole and, conversely, to harm a part harms the whole. The way we treat nature is ultimately the way we treat ourselves. Within the indivisible unity of nature, the Tao, are complementary and polar aspects of *yin* and *yang*. Congruent with the Native American worldview, the oriental system holds that life is harmonic and flourishes when the elements of nature are in balance, and disease and disaster occur when the balance of nature is upset. The Eastern worldview holds that the human being is a microcosm of nature. "Human beings represent the juncture between Heaven and Earth, the offspring of their union, a fusion of cosmic and terrestrial forces . . . Sustained by the power of Earth and transformed by the power of Heaven, humanity cannot be separated from Nature—we *are* Nature, manifest as people" (Beinfield & Korngold, 1991, p. 29). Other traditions, such as the Lakota Sioux, hold that God is nature and nature is God. Buddhism teaches that the natural world and humankind are intimately connected, and Hinduism emphasizes that the world of nature is grounded in God (Smith, 1991).

The creative Life Force, or vital energy that animates all of life is known as *Qi* (pronounced *chee*) in the oriental tradition. Beinfield and Korngold (1991) note that the invisible substance and immaterial force of Qi has palpable and observable manifestations. In essence, "matter is *Qi* taking shape. Mountains forming, forests growing, rivers streaming, and creatures proliferating are all manifestations of *Qi*. In the human being, all functions of the body and mind are manifestations of *Qi* . . . It is fundamental mystery and miracle" (p. 30). Our health and well-being at all levels depends on our being in beneficial relationship to Qi both within our bodies and in our external environment.

SELF-NURTURE: Sitting with Nature

Sit with a plant, a tree, flowers, a special stone, a pet, or any object or element of nature. Begin by being in your own inner stillness in the presence of the natural element. As you are in that space of inner quiet, begin to be aware of the presence of the object and the experience of looking at the object, without thinking about or analyzing it. Merely be with how you are experiencing being with the object or element. You may sense the object as something separate from you, or you may begin to feel a subtle sense of connection with the object. Just stay with the experience without having to name what is going on.

LIVING IN BALANCE—BELONGING TO THE WHOLE

Taoism, Native American, and other ancient traditions teach that observing and following the ways of nature enables us to remain in sacred balance. In the Judeo-Christian story of creation, God formed humans from the clay of the earth and gave them life by breathing God's spirit into their nostrils. The Genesis story tells us that humans began earthly existence in a garden where they experienced connectedness with nature, living in harmony or balance with all plants and animals. Alberto Villoldo (1999) notes that in many respects, only in Western spiritual traditions have humans been thrown out of the Garden. The spiritual traditions of indigenous peoples are still grounded in awareness of our basic interconnectedness with nature. Fields and colleagues (1984) suggest that rather than humans being sent out of the Garden by God, perhaps it was God who was kicked out of the Garden by human society's attitude that reason and ingenuity were sufficient for it to prosper and survive. These authors quote Wendell Berry in saying, "If God was not in the world, then obviously the world was a thing of inferior importance, or of no importance at all. Those who were disposed to exploit it were thus free to do so. And this split in public attitudes was inevitably mirrored in the lives of individuals: a man could aspire to Heaven with his mind and his heart while destroying the earth and his fellow men, with his hands . . ." (p. 222). Industrialism, urban living, and large-scale agriculture remove people from immediate connection with the natural world, thus continuing to foster the myth of separation between humans and the earth and things of nature. This sense of separation perpetuates viewing the natural world as "Other," as Habito (1993, p. 9) notes "to be tamed and controlled and brought into submission for our human purposes." He reflects that our way of seeing the natural in opposition to us, rather than as the very source of our being and nature that it truly is, "has resulted in our destructive attitudes toward it." When we destroy that which sustains us, our health suffers. Our healing, then, "depends on our coming to a *right view* of the way things are" (Habito, p. 2).

REFLECTION 8–3

Think about the relationship you have with nature—as you
- notice what the weather is doing
- decide whether to wear a coat or take an umbrella
- decide to take a walk to relax and think
- plan a picnic or a day's outing
- plan to travel for work or pleasure
- orient yourself to the direction you are facing or traveling

Contemporary scholars (Fox, 1991; Habito, 1993; Webb, 1998) echo what indigenous elders and holy people have been teaching—that we in industrialized societies need to reconnect with a cosmology that understands we belong to a whole universe, not just to a city, culture, or nation. In their book *The Natural Step for Business,* Nattrass and Altomare (1999) discuss the link between healthy business and ecological sustainability and the need for cyclical industrial processes of business to mimic and integrate with natural cycles. They remind us that even our economy depends on the natural world—that all our basic life needs of breathing, eating, and drinking depend entirely on the natural world to provide us with clean air and water and uncontaminated food.

We must learn anew a sense of "being at home in the world, in the earth household, in the God household" (Steindl-Rast, 1998, p. 104). Although science provides many benefits, particularly in the area of health, the cosmology of science teaches that we are separate from nature—nature is an object "out there" to be studied and manipulated. Berry (1998) notes that, in contrast to the cosmology of science, natural phenomena have meaning for indigenous peoples the world over. For those who live in awareness of and relationship with nature, "the dawn and the sunset are mystical moments. You know where you are in the context of north, south, east, west, and in relationship to the sky above and the earth below. You have to know where you are. You have to read the natural phenomena. Because if you don't interact creatively with natural phenomena, you are dead." (Berry, 1998, p. 39). The collective wisdom of ancient and indigenous peoples reflect a clear sense of living in and belonging to a sacred universe, and of recognizing that "everything is hitched to everything else" (Swimme, 1998, p. 139).

Because nature is a source of sustenance and nurture for our whole body-mind-spirit being, connectedness with nature is integral to our total health. Several years ago singer and songwriter John Denver noted that, in nature, he felt *listened to* as no where else—a listening that occurs at a level that is deeper than words. Our understanding of and relationship to the world around us flows from our deepest essence of spirit as well as from our cognitive knowing (Burkhardt, 1994a, 1994b, 1998; Burkhardt & Nagai-Jacobson, 1994, 2000). When we allow ourselves to become quiet and enter our space of inner stillness, we begin to experience that which our spirits know—that all things are connected. Nature offers a space for our being that requires only that we show up and be there. When we give ourselves time and opportunity to be with nature we can experience healing at many levels—physically, mentally, emotionally, and spiritually (Burkhardt, 2000).

SPIRITUALITY AND NATURE

REFLECTION 8-4

- How does relationship with nature fit into your life and spirituality?
- What would you like to do to live in more conscious relationship with nature?
- How have you experienced nature's nurturing of your spirit?

As with any relationship, intent, commitment, and time are essential for deepening our connection with nature. Quietly and carefully observing the natural world around us helps us reconnect with the spiritual in nature. We have an example in great spiritual teachers such as Jesus, Buddha, Moses, and Patanjali who found inspiration for their instructions from and in nature—sitting under a Bodhi tree, on a mountain, near the sea (Fields, Taylor, Weyler, & Ingrasci, 1984). Connecting with nature does not mean we need to move to the country and work on a farm (although that would be a wonderful way to reconnect with the earth!) We are always in relationship with nature, although we might be less than conscious of this interaction.

We can observe the natural world from wherever we are—an urban high-rise, a neighborhood flat, a suburban house, or a country cabin. Simple things such as watching the sunrise or cloud patterns in the sky, the birds in the park or in the tree next door, the flowers in our garden or the neighbor's window are all ways to open us to greater awareness of nature. Another approach is to choose to love one thing well. This may be a river that flows through town, an animal friend, a tiny tree, a nearby mountain, a rock along your walking path, or special plant.

REFLECTION 8–5

- What in the natural world do you love?
- Consider what it means and requires for you to love one thing well.

Relatedness or connection with nature or the environment has emerged as a common theme in our research on spirituality (Burkhardt, 1993, 1994a, 1994b; Burkhardt & Nagai-Jacobson, 1995, 2000). In describing personal understandings of spirituality, study participants indicate that being close to the earth and in nature often brings them more in touch with their spirituality. Participants describe finding peace of mind when walking in the woods or being at the ocean, and often experiencing God there. One woman noted, "the times I feel most spiritual are when I am alone and when I'm outside and walking or sitting . . . it happens outside usually in connection to the earth or sun." One of the men commented, "It is really important for me to spend time out of doors. I just walk, I observe, I look at things, I try to be aware of things. I like to be around running water. I notice all forms of life, animal life, insect life, just the wind blowing on me. Watching the lightening, taking time to smell things, to listen, just being quiet. Being with nature gives me a sense of awe and a sense of order." Other study participants described their spirituality as feeling connected to and grateful for everything in the universe and having a sense of purpose here; feeling that something makes this world go round that relates to the universe—that some call God, Higher Power, or Life Force, and that ultimately we are all one substance and more like all other creatures than we are different from them.

SELF-NURTURE: Consciousness of Nature

Consider how nature is always in your life and make time each day to be with nature in a more conscious way. For instance, you might

- Listen to the sounds around you when you walk outside, or bring the sounds of nature into your environment via audiotape, or open window.
- Observe cloud patterns, the rustling of leaves, the feeling of the air on your skin, or the activity of birds, insects, or other wildlife.
- Work in the garden, sit in the park, or feel the texture of a rock.

Because we are part of the natural world, we are continually interacting with nature at one level or another. The air we breathe, the food we eat, the clothes we wear, the places we live and work all involve participation with nature. (Even things that are synthetic or human-made derive from molecules that are basic to "natural" life forms.) Connecting with nature in a way that reflects and nurtures our spirituality requires that we be more conscious of our relationship. We can consciously interact with nature in a multitude of ways: Gardening, bird watching, fishing, hunting, identifying wild flowers, sitting in the park, hiking in the forest, walking in the desert, camping in the mountains, nurturing pets and house plants, cleaning up the local river, or spending time at the ocean are but a few. Whenever we are conscious with any part of nature, we have an opportunity for deepening our relationships. Taking in a beautiful sunset, listening to the sound of the wind, marveling at the power of a lightening storm, feeling the warm or cool air on our faces—all draw us to be aware of the life and energy of our environment and can call us to that still point deep within us.

EXPERIENCING GOD OR LIFE FORCE IN AND THROUGH NATURE

Many people, regardless of their religious backgrounds, discover and experience closeness with their God or their sense of the Life Force through the wonder and beauty of nature (Burkhardt & Nagai-Jacobson, 2000). Gazing at a starlit sky or feeling the energy of an old-growth forest can open us to consider our places in the cosmos and sense a deeper connection with creation and Creator. Seeing the handiwork of God in creation calls forth awe and praise from the psalmist:

Bless the Lord, O my soul! O Lord, my God, your are great indeed! You are clothed with majesty and glory, robed in light as with a cloak. You have spread out the heavens like a tent-cloth; you have constructed your palace upon the waters. You make the clouds your chariot; you travel on the wings of the wind. You make the winds your messengers, and flaming fire your ministers! You fixed the earth upon its foundation, not to be moved forever . . . How manifold are your works, O Lord! In wisdom you have wrought them all—the earth is full of your creatures (Psalm 104, vs 1–5, 24).

Throughout the ages and across traditions, people recognize the Source of Life, the Creator, in the natural worlds of earth and heaven. People express an awareness that creation itself praises the Creator. From the mystic, Hildegard of Bingen we hear:

Glance at the sun. See the moon and the stars. Gaze at the beauty of earth's greenings. Now, think. What delight God gives to humankind with all these things. Who gives all these shining, wonderful gifts, if not God? . . . The blowing wind, the mild, moist air, the exquisite greening of trees and grasses—In their beginning, in their ending, they give God their praise. (Uhlein, 1983, pp. 45, 47)

Connecting with God or the Absolute through nature calls forth gratitude for the gifts of all living things that nourish and sustain us in many ways. As we become more deeply aware of our connectedness with nature, we appreciate even more that honoring and caring for nature, the earth, is a way of connecting intimately with our God. As the artist writes:

> Earth is God's handiwork, "a work in progress." To know and love Earth is a way to know and love God. To collaborate in Earth's self-creativity, self-healing process . . . is to participate in the very life of God, the work of God, the Great Work, (Southard, 2000)

Connecting with God through Nature: Beth's Story

My connection with God that is mystical, beyond words, and beyond doubt, rose out of my experience with the trees in the woods behind the house we moved to when I was five. At first, I'm sure I just explored the woods out of natural curiosity—we had come from the city. When I found it could be a refuge, I fled to it to escape what was happening in my house. Very soon, I went just to "be" with the Presence there, though at that age, I know I had no name for it. The Presence had different aspects or flavors—individual trees, the wind, various mossy nooks and crannies, the stream, the open fields—all expressed this Presence, as a felt sense, but with various nuances. The underlying sense was the same, however—alive, flowing, healing, nurturing, sacred and "full."

The most active nurturing and healing came from individual trees in the woods. It was blissful to allow myself to become "attuned" to each one, to experience myself as part of this flow of Spirit through Nature. But even more, I knew at age six that these trees were helping to keep me whole, psychically whole, in the midst of the violence in my house. Through connecting with the trees, I experienced unconditional love, safety, and the "more" to life than was apparent on the surface. Connecting with that "more" within myself through the trees kept me whole. Later, at age seven and eight, I found I could let myself connect with more than just the Nature in the woods behind the house. If I could find the interior privacy and space, I could join with the ocean, the mountains and storms.

Our family were practicing Roman Catholics, and my sister and I attended Catholic grade and high schools. Like many children abused by a father, I had a hard time knowing what to do with God the Father, and the male person of Jesus was tricky too. Not only did I not have a relationship with them, I didn't really want one either. But I never for a moment doubted the existence of God, as the Spirit, the Living Presence, that flows through all things. I had direct experience of this God; it wasn't a matter of belief. In trying to find a way to fit this into

Catholic grade school theology, I decided this Living Presence must be the Holy Spirit. All through grade school my connection with God was through Nature. Church and religious school were just part of what I did in the rest of my life.

I faced a crisis at age 12 as I was desperately struggling to "hold it together" on the outside, to look normal, in spite of the abnormal circumstances of our family life. Communing with trees was not going to "further" my blending in with the rest of my classmates, so I made the choice to give up my connections with the trees and entered adolescence with grim resignation. I remember the day I made that decision. Though a terrible loss, for me it was matter of survival.

Two decades, graduate schools, a job overseas, an early failed marriage, then one that "took," and the birth of our first child passed. I never doubted the existence of God through all of this, but no longer experienced the immediacy of the Presence. In spite of this, my childhood experiences in the woods remained the most "real" experiences of my life. Knowing I needed emotional healing, I sought and found a psychotherapist. One criteria for selection was that the therapist had to be willing to allow for the possibility of the reality of my childhood experiences with Nature, rather than to dismiss it out of hand as magical thinking. In my thirties, I faced another spiritual crisis. With no little trepidation, I decided to begin the spiritual training as a Complete Self Attunement © facilitator. During the first week-long training intensive, we received instruction in opening to the experience of "Life behind the form" of Nature. We opened to the consciousness of trees, and other aspects of Nature, and participated in that consciousness at deeper and deeper levels. This was the beginning of my return Home, to Wholeness.

Speaking of the wonder, beauty, awe, and mystery of nature, or finding a sense of peace, meaning, and support in nature reflect our spiritual selves. However, this spiritual connection need not include religious language or belief in God or Higher Power. An example is the scientist who claims no belief in God, yet speaks with awe and wonder regarding the evolution of the universe and all that has led to her being alive at this particular time, giving her a feeling of belonging in the universe (Burkhardt & Nagai-Jacobson, 2000). The sense of awe, wonder, and feeling at home in the universe reflects our spiritual connection.

REVERENCE FOR CREATION

Prayers and sacred rituals of many traditions express awareness that God's presence is disclosed in the beauty, variety, splendor, and wonder of the natural world—the mountains, sea, flowers, sky, animals, birds, insects, colors, changing seasons. When we take time to carefully observe the world around us, we discover that the earth is a sacred scripture, continually revealing the simplicity and complexity, gentleness and power, majesty and wonder, healing, care, and balance that reflect God's presence and show us how to live our earthly existence. In the Christian Scriptures, Jesus often used experiences in nature to illustrate his teachings: you can tell a tree by its fruit, the sound tree bears good fruit; have faith as a grain of mustard seed; behold the lilies of the field that neither toil or reap, yet are cared for by God. Fields and colleagues (1984) quote Chief Fools Crow of the Oglala Lakota saying, "the Creator gave to us all the living things so that we would know how to act. The natural world is our Bible; by watching the chipmunk and the meadowlark and even the tiniest flower we learn the lessons that the Creator has put before us. Everything is sacred. This very land is our church" (p. 224). Without reverence for the earth and all creation, our spirits and our spiritual quest are incomplete. Recognizing the Divine in all creation calls us to a different relationship with the world around us. We are drawn to honor, respect, and care for the gifts of the Creator, with a greater awareness of our interdependence with all of creation. Chief Jake Swamp's (1995) book, *Giving Thanks: A Native American Good Morning Message,* beautifully expresses an ancient message of peace and appreciation for Mother Earth and all her inhabitants from the *Haudenosaunee* or Iroquois Nation. He tells us it is an honor to be human and to offer thanksgiving for all the gifts of life. This prayer thanks Mother Earth for giving us everything we need—the deep blue waters, the green grasses, good foods, fruits and berries, good medicine herbs, all the animals, birds and trees in the world, the gentle Four Winds, Grandfather Thunder Beings, Elder Brother Sun, Grandmother Moon, twinkling stars, Spirit protectors of our past and present. And most of all, thanks is given to Great Spirit, for continually giving all these wonderful gifts for our happiness and health.

 ## SELF-NURTURE: Expressing Appreciation for the Gifts of Nature

- Consider the gifts and wonder of nature, or focus on one particular gift of nature, and write your own psalm, prayer, song, or love note to the earth expressing your feelings and appreciation.
- Listen to your body and attend to its needs.
- Taste the life energy and love in your food.

NATURE AND SPIRITUAL EXPRESSION

We include nature in our expression of spirituality in many ways. Consider how we use flowers and plants to decorate places of worship. In some traditions, incense is used in spiritual ritual for purification, honoring the deity, and as part of prayer. The Judeo-Christian scriptures tell us to let our prayers rise like incense. Smudging with plants such as sage and cedar for cleansing and balancing is part of many Native American spiritual ceremonies. Use of tobacco, corn meal, various herbs, and other plants, special stones and crystals, and feathers are integral to spiritual ceremony and prayer in many indigenous traditions. Fruits of the earth, bread and wine (or grape juice), are blessed and shared in Judeo-Christian religious services, and foods of various kinds are included as part of sacred ritual in other traditions. Various spiritual purification rituals require wood, water, and herbs. Water is a basic element of Christian baptism and purification rituals in other traditions. Candles and other sources of fire used in many spiritual ceremonies are yet another gift of nature.

The cycles, seasons, and rhythms of nature are evident in spiritual ceremony in many traditions. Judeo-Christian liturgical calendars relate to the cycles of the moon. Acknowledging the spirits and energies of the directions (north, south, east, west, heaven above, and earth below) is integral to rituals and ceremonies of many indigenous people, as is facing the rising or setting sun to greet or end the day with prayer. The direction one faces when praying is important in some traditions. Elements of earth, air, fire, and water are often important components of spiritual ceremony. The ancient Chinese art of *Feng Shui* is rooted in the Chinese worldview in which all things are categorized into five basic elements of fire, metal, earth, wood, and water and take on implications of positive or negative (*yin* or *yang*) energy (Too, 1999). "Literally translated, Feng Shui means wind and water and refers to the earth, its mountains, valleys, and waterways, whose shape and size, directions and levels are created by the interaction of these powerful forces" (Too, p. 8). Drawing on the directions, the energy and natural flow of nature, and other elements, *Feng Shui* helps create homes and work places of beauty, of life, of harmony—sacred places that inspirit us.

REFLECTION 8-7

- Many traditions recognize that certain herbs and elements of nature are gifts of the creator that enhance prayer and spiritual practice. They consciously acknowledge the energy of the life form as part of the ceremony or ritual. Consider how nature enters into your expression of spirituality. How consciously do you include the gifts of nature into your spiritual practice with awareness of their energy and purpose? How might you develop a more conscious relationship when including nature in your spiritual expression?

- What rhythms or cycles are you aware of in your own life and spiritual expression?

(continued)

> • What lessons, insights, wisdom do the seasons bring to your life?

ECOLOGY AND SPIRITUALITY

Relationship with nature is a two-way process—a partnership in which nature shares many gifts and in which we offer care and nurture. Caring for nature involves personal, community, and global awareness and action. In our contemporary world, we speak of care of the earth as ecology; ancient traditions understand this care as our responsibility. Spirituality and ecology share the same basic understanding that all things are related. David Steindl-Rast (1998) suggests that ecology and religion interface in our sense of belonging to the whole universe and being at home in the world—which he refers to as the earth household and God household. The universe story and our place within this story has been told by religions and spiritual traditions through the centuries. The story that is told gives us a cosmology within which we develop ethical and spiritual values that inform how we think about and relate to nature. When our cosmology views God or Creator as distant from the world, we are more likely to see ourselves as separate from the rest of creation. We feel less responsibility toward and value of that from which we feel alienated or separate, allowing us to more easily treat the other (the earth) as object and inflict harm. When we see the Divine as the deeper center of the world, however, we come to realize that we find God through our relationship with all life and recognize our responsibility to respect and care for this community of life as a whole (Rockefeller, 1998). Ultimately, we recognize the intrinsic wholeness, integrity, and value of all phenomena in the universe.

SELF-NURTURE: Creativity with Nature

Be creative with the gifts of nature: gather flowers, work with clay, dig in the garden, attend to houseplants, make something with wood, sand, shells, or seeds.

Oral teachings and sacred scriptures in various traditions help us understand our role as earth keepers. An example is the second account of Genesis in the Hebrew Scriptures in which Adam is expected to till and keep the Garden. (In

Hebrew, *Adam* is also the name for the whole human race, and *Adaama* is the word for earth.)

> So we have the whole human race, which is of the earth, being told to till and keep the Garden. But when you look at the word "till," it's the Hebrew word *'abad,* which means "to serve." So the human race is asked to serve the Garden, God's Earth. The idea here is that since the Earth serves us with oxygen, food, etc., we need to serve the Garden by taking care of it and protecting it. This calls for reciprocal service, con-service, conservancy, conservation—a service that runs in both directions. Then we come to the next critical word in this request and expectation of Adam. We come to the word "keep." the human race is asked to serve God's Earth and keep it. The word "keep" is transliterated from the Hebrew word *shamr,* means "to preserve." (DeWitt, 1998)

We are called to remember that the earth is our home, our dwelling place, the place of our sustenance and nurture. Being at home in the world calls us to respect and care for our surroundings as we do our homes. Our personal choices reflect our relationships with nature. What we do to the earth, we do to ourselves and our children. Traditions of many Native peoples caution us to consider the effects of our decisions on our children for seven generations to come.

Choosing to recycle, to avoid littering, or to help clean up a local stream express our care for nature. "Good science and informed spirituality lead to the same conclusion: that the destiny of humankind is inextricably linked with the well-being of the rest of life on earth" (Porritt, 1991, p. 185).

REFLECTION 8–8

- Consider how the packaging of products we buy or the choices we make regarding transportation affect the environment, and reflect our relationship with nature.

- Think about what actually happens to all the packaging once it leaves your house.

- How do decisions and actions at the community or corporate level affect the purity of air, water, and other essential resources?

- How does your sense of service to the Earth Garden call you to respond to these decisions so as to foster a healthy environment now and for seven generations to come?

- What are some of the decisions you make to be a good steward of the earth?

Health care workers are faced with a particular dilemma regarding concern for the environment because of toxic waste and use of so many disposable items prompted by the need for disease prevention, cost reduction, and efficiency (Schuster & Keegan, 2000). Shaner (1994) notes that even in medical institutions, solid waste can be source-separated and much can be recycled and that hazardous waste can be minimized and disposed of properly. Health care practitioners must be actively involved in this process, however, if it is to work.

SELF-NURTURE: Caring for Earth

Recognizing our interconnectedness with all life calls us to appreciate that whatever we do to care for and heal the earth is also caring for and healing ourselves. The following are a few ways you can nurture yourself through your caring for the earth:

- Make every effort to recycle all that you can and support community recycling.
- Take a bag with you wherever you walk to collect litter along the way.
- Compost.
- Work on developing a community garden.
- Use energy efficient light bulbs.
- Decrease your overall water use and consumption.
- Consider the environmental impact of products you buy and support companies that work toward corporate responsibility and sustainability.

NATURE AND HEALING

Creation is to serve humankind in its bodily needs, and to be for the health of the soul as well . . . the earth should not be injured, the earth should not be destroyed. (Hildegard of Bingen, quoted in Uhlein, 1983, pp. 68, 78)

Because we breathe, eat, drink, wash, and have to move from one place to another, we are constantly interacting with nature within the environment of our daily lives. We know that the environment affects our health in many ways. Basic things like the quality of air, water, and food available to us influence our overall body-mind-spirit well-being. Florence Nightingale recognized the essential role of the environment in healing. Some of the first instructions given in her *Notes on*

Nursing (1859) relate to ensuring that sick persons have pure air and water, light, clean rooms, and no unnecessary noise. Although these instructions refer to the particular environment of home or hospital, it is implied that the necessary natural elements such as clean air and water exist within the global environment. In our contemporary world, however, pollution of air and water, and thus of our food sources, has become dangerously prevalent. Industrialized societies have lost a sense of spiritual connection with the earth and awareness of the earth as a living organism. Porritt reflects on the legacy of this disconnection:

> For much of the history of humankind, in all its different cultural manifestations, Mother Earth was held to be a living planet. But the Protestant Reformation and the intellectual revolution set in motion by 17th-century philosophers like Descartes and Bacon progressively turned nature into something inert, more like a machine than a living organism, stripped of its sacred values. (1991, p. 184).

We need to remember the primacy of our environmental connection, appreciating that it is basic to our life on earth. Porritt again reminds us that

> the healing of the Earth and the healing of the human spirit have become one and the same. As we struggle with the implications of pollution control, environmentally friendly technologies, green consumerism, or "sustainable development," it is that overwhelmingly powerful convergence between our human needs and the needs of the rest of life on Earth that now begin to offer real hope for the future. (1991, pp. 183–184)

REFLECTION 8–9

- How can you align with nature to create more healing environments in which to live, work, play, and worship?

- How healthy is the air, water, and food that you take into your being?

- How do you see your destiny linked with the rest of life on earth?

- How does your own spiritual, religious, or philosophical perspective call you to relate to the earth, to nature. How does this draw you to more of a sense of your own wholeness?

- What can you do to more consciously integrate your relationship with nature into your spirituality?

Conscious relationship with nature can make our environment more healing in many ways. Florence Nightingale's directives concerning pure air and water, light, cleanliness, and noise are a basic starting point. Bringing elements of nature such as plants, pets, fresh flowers, decorative rocks, or small water fountains into the environment help to create a healing atmosphere. Pictures of nature scenes enable people to visually connect with natural settings. Attention to color, temperature, light, and overall atmosphere helps to create a nature-sensitive environment. Incorporating therapies provided by nature into personal care or care with patients in various settings is a way of bringing a more conscious partnership with nature into our life and work.

RELATIONSHIP WITH THE GIFTS OF NATURE FOR LIFE AND HEALING

Humankind is called to co-create. With nature's help, humankind can set into creation all that is necessary and life sustaining. God's majesty is glorified in the manifestation of every manner of nature's fruitfulness (Hildegard of Bingen, quoted in Uhlein, 1983, pp. 106–107).

As we become more conscious of our relationship with nature, we begin to see the many ways we can work in co-creative partnership to bring healing and balance to ourselves and our world. We can learn from ancient and contemporary practices that work with nature in a healing partnership—traditions that regard the natural world with respect, appreciation, and awe. People who follow this perspective learn to treat everything in nature with care because they are aware of the wholeness of all life in nature. The bioscientific perspective seeks to distill the "essential" element that affects a particular part of our biological system from a natural substance such as a plant. In contrast are traditions that recognize that the healing qualities of any part of nature derive from the relationship of essential element to the whole—the interconnection with the soil and roots and leaves, and the energy of the whole plant. Rather than seeking the "magic cure" or "quick fix," traditional processes recognize that healing is a sacred process requiring time because it has to do with the whole—with relationships. Rather than viewing natural elements as one more "thing" to be used, we can choose a different approach that recognizes how the life energy of nature invites us into healing relationship.

We easily recognize our reliance on plants and other life forms for food and for healing. What many people have lost, however, is a living relationship with that which nourishes and heals us. Those who grow, harvest, gather, or hunt their own food and healing resources have an opportunity to more consciously connect with the life form offering nourishment or healing. Indigenous peoples again give us the example of conscious relationship in their care, gathering, and preparation of that which nature gives. For example, when hunting, the spirit of the animal or fish is honored and thanked for the life energy it brings to the earth and for being willing to give its life to nourish others. Another example is the traditional use of herbs for healing, which includes a relationship with, not just knowledge about, the plant. Within this relationship, the plant is involved in a conscious way—by asking the plant if it is ready to be harvested, gathering with prayer and ceremony only as much of the plant as is needed, and honoring the plant with prayer and thanksgiving. The plant is acknowledged as an active participant in the healing process, not merely as an object or commodity. Healing within this worldview requires an energetic partnership with the plant as well as with its biochemical properties. Although many traditional uses of herbs are being confirmed by scientific research, and herbs are available to people as commercial preparations, it is worth pondering whether plants that are impersonally grown and harvested for their biochemical properties offer the same healing potential as do those with which we have a living relationship.

Although gardening, fishing, raising livestock for food, and the like offer opportunities for consciously connecting with nature, we are not suggesting that everyone needs to grow or gather their own food and healing herbs to have a living relationship with the natural world. We can appreciate that, whether or not we grow the food, we are being nourished through the gift of nature, and honor and thank the life form, its Creator, and all whose energies bring the nourishment to us. In this way, we acknowledge our interdependence within life's sacred circle.

 ## SELF-NURTURE: Listening to Nature, Being with Nature

- Consciously walk or sit on the earth, feeling her energy, sensing her care and nurture, listening to her needs for healing. Consider how you can participate in healing the earth. Be aware of your elemental and energetic connection with all life forms of the earth. Appreciate that you are a unique note in the cosmic symphony.

- Choose a place in nature—a park, forest, river, meadow, rock cliff, ocean—sit quietly in this place—what do you feel? Listen to the sounds and to the stillness—what do you hear? Attend to one sound, listening carefully to the tone, volume, rhythm, and what it is saying to you. Observe your surroundings—what do you see? Focus on something in the setting that draws your attention noting its color, texture, shape, energy, and other characteristics. Stay with this experience for a few moments. Ask this "something" to reveal itself to you—to teach you about itself, and listen with your heart to its response.

Plants and trees

Plants and trees offer nurture and healing of body, mind, and spirit in numerous ways. The scents and sounds of nature can sooth, calm, enliven, and energize, and open us to the deeper spaces of spirit within us. Consider hearing the birds singing on a fresh spring morning, the pounding of ocean waves as you breath the salt air, the scent of pinon smoke on a crisp winter's night, the smell of flowers, citrus fruit, pine boughs, the crackling of a fire, the rustling of the wind in the trees.

REFLECTION 8–10

- What scents and sounds of nature bring you comfort and feel healing to you?
- How can you include these more in your life?

AROMATHERAPY

Nature's aromatic oils can be used to rejuvenate, balance, and calm body, mind, and spirit through inhalation and sometimes topical application in lotions and compresses (Wheeler Robins, 1999; Stevensen, 1996). These are the essential or concentrated oils extracted from the roots, flowers, bark, stem, or leaf of particular aromatic plants. Buckle (1999) distinguishes between essential oils that are steam distillates derived from aromatic plants, and extracts that are obtained with petrochemical solvents, noting that extracts are not suitable for clinical aromatherapy because it is impossible to remove all of the solvents. Many people derive healing benefit from aromatherapy in many forms, although scientific exploration of the efficacy of these gifts of nature is in its infancy.

FLOWER ESSENCES

Flower and other nature essences reflect another way that nature partners with us for healing. Those who work with nature to develop these essences remind us that the plant kingdom consciously offers these gifts. Each continent and particular areas of the continent has its own specific essences. Machaelle Small Wright (1988), describes flower essences as "liquid, pattern-infused solutions made from individual plant flowers, each containing a specific imprint that responds in a balancing, repairing, and re-building manner to imbalances in humans on their physical, emotional, mental, and spiritual or universal levels" (p. 3). Wright, who established Perelandra Center for Nature Research in Warrenton, Virginia, more than 20 years ago, notes that plants contain within their makeup particular healing and balancing patterns that are vital for humans. From her research, Wright has learned that nature contains a pattern of healing that relates and responds to specific dysfunctions within humankind, noting that flower essences work directly with the electrical and central nervous systems. Nearly 70 years ago in England, Dr. Edward Bach (1996) discovered that flower essences are useful in dealing with the mental and emotional conditions that contribute to or result from illness. Dr. Bach, whose early medical career was both conventional and successful, came to believe that our health depends on being in harmony with our souls. Bach Flower Essences support healing by addressing the anxiety, depression, trauma, and other emotional factors that can impede the healing process (Bach, 1996; Scheffer, 1988). These and other essences can be used preventively as well. Wild and domestic flowers in various bioregions of Alaska are the source of the Alaskan flower essences. Johnson (1996) notes that many of the Alaskan essences can be especially helpful in opening our awareness to spirit because the plants from which they come have had more interaction with other kingdoms of nature and with the cosmos or spiritual realms than they have had with humans. Both Johnson (1996) and Wright (1996) have expanded their research with nature to include essences containing the energetic resources of expressions of nature such as gems, minerals, and environmental events and processes.

As a natural healing modality, flower essences address the whole person rather than solely the disease or symptom. Specific essences are individualized for each person, responding to what the person needs at any given time. Many people use flower essences to promote bioenergetic balance as part of their regular health promotion practice. Flower essences are safe, may be used by people of all ages, and may be taken on their own or used in conjunction with conventional therapies. However, they are not intended as a substitute for conventional medical care when this is indicated.

When we collaborate with nature for healing, whether we ingest, apply topically, inhale, or merely sit in the presence of various elements in nature, there is an energetic connection. Many people experience a special connection with particular places in nature, noting that they feel better just *being* in these settings. One research participant noted,

> when I'm at the ocean, I could sit there all day long. I guess the water just does something to me, it just calms me . . . just the sound, just walking on the sand, or sitting there at the sunset is just beautiful. Because after I come back it's like I'm a new person. I feel alive again.

PLACES AND TREES

Healing places in nature may be anywhere—a particular spot in the garden, a place in the desert, by the river, in the park, or under a favorite tree. Bouchardon (1998) describes how energetic qualities of particular trees interact bioenergetically with humans to promote healing. He notes that when entering a tree's energy field, our energy adapts and reacts to that of the tree, allowing us to absorb or awaken the quality of the tree within ourselves. For example, the qualities of a pine are light and vitality. Thus, when we consciously stand near a pine we can experience personal vitality and connection with life.

SELF-NURTURE: Energetically Connecting with Nature

Consciously approach a plant, a tree, or a rock, paying attention to how you feel in its presence. Feel its energy and how your energies intertwine. With your inner sense, listen to what it might speak to you.

Crystals and Stones

Healing properties of crystals and stones are other gifts of nature. Natural crystals and stones have been used as part of many spiritual and healing traditions for centuries. Crystals and gem stones interact with human energy fields to assist in balancing the human electromagnetic energy. The way that crystals and stones enhance healing includes raising the vibrational frequency of the auric levels, amplifying signals from the intuition, and transmitting light and color (Chase & Pawlik, 1986; Raphael, 1987). Some people, particularly many from indigenous traditions, experience a very personal connection with the "stone people," from whom they receive knowledge, vision, and healing. The energies of certain stones provide them with power, strength, courage, or healing, either directly or when carved into the image of and imbued with the energy of a particular creature of the earth or heavens.

CO-CREATIVE PARTNERSHIPS WITH NATURE

Reconnecting with the sacred healing power of nature requires that we return to the consciousness that all things are connected and that we are all part of a whole. Barbara Marx Hubbard (1998) envisions the birth of a universal humanity that, experiencing the earth as one operational, living system, intuitively feels connected to the whole. As a universal humanity, whatever is going on in each of us is a reflection of the universe evolving in us. The more connected we feel to the whole, the more we are able to appreciate the variety of ways that nature offers to collaborate with us in all areas of our lives. We are fortunate to have visionary models of working in co-creative partnership with nature. Some of these approaches derive from explanatory models that are quite different from biomedicine; thus, considering them to be viable possibilities may be a stretch for the bioscientific mind. In her book, *Co-Creative Science,* Machaelle Wright (1997) describes differences between the approach of contemporary science and the co-creative approach to working with nature that she has learned from her work at the Perelandra Center for Nature Research. Co-creative science involves working with nature in a direct and conscious manner. Wright explains that contemporary science works to "figure out" reality or nature through observation and testing, drawing conclusions based on what the scientist has observed or understood. In contrast, the co-creative scientist

> acknowledges that there is an inherent intelligence within all of nature, builds a communication bridge that allows him to access that intelligence, and then asks nature directly to explain and provide experiential insight so that he may understand "from the horse's mouth" (so to speak) how something works. (p. 1)

Within a co-creative relationship, one works with nature intelligences in a conscious, coordinated, and educational effort, creating a partnership that emphasizes balance and teamwork. Through this process, new ways of approaching health and environmental issues are evolving. One of the healing programs resulting from Wright's (1996) research with nature is a process for co-creatively working with microbes in our environment to support and balance both the microbes and the biosphere (including the human body) of their environment. In Scotland, people in the Findhorn Community (1975) have been working in conscious partnership with nature via communication with nature intelligence for many years. Bouchardon's (1998) process of discovering the healing energies of trees and Bach's (1996) approach to discovering the healing properties of flower essences are yet other approaches to developing conscious connections with nature. Organizations such as the Collective Heritage Institute (CHI) in Santa Fe, New Mexico, offer a more conventional bridge between contemporary science and co-creative partnership with nature. CHI promotes understanding of the human-nature relationship to enhance cultural and spiritual connection with nature. CHI does this partially by bringing together *Bioneers,* scientific and social visionaries working to develop practical solutions for restoring the Earth and for nurturing a dynamic Earth-honoring community that can permeate society.

As nurses and others who recognize the interrelationship between our health and the health of our planet, we appreciate that

> healing ourselves and working to resolve the contradictions in the human-Earth ecology is the same work . . . everything we do transforms and reshapes the world. If our actions can destroy, so can they heal. In this light there is no difference between work and prayer, no distinction between physical activity and the work of the spirit. (Roberts & Amidon, 1991, p. 90)

Our spirits prompt us to honor the sacredness of all life, as we recognize that our well-being and, indeed, our survival is intricately dependent on our relationship with nature. Expanding our own boundaries to engage in more conscious participation with nature enables us to reconnect with our true selves, appreciating the wonder and mystery of our own places in the sacred circle of creation, the universe.

REFERENCES

Bach, E. (1996). *Bach flower essences for the family.* London: Wigemore.

Beinfield, H., & Korngold, E. (1991). *Between Heaven and Earth: A guide to Chinese medicine.* New York: Ballantine Books.

Berry, T. (1998). Earth systems . . . human systems. In B. Webb (Ed). *Fugitive faith: Conversations on spiritual, environmental, and community renewal* (pp. 31–43) Maryknoll, NY: Orbis Books.

Bouchardon, P. (1998). *The healing energies of trees.* London: Gaia Books.

Buckle, J. (1999). Use of aromatherapy as a complementary treatment for chronic pain. *Alternative Therapies in Health and Medicine, 5,* 42–51.

Burkhardt, M. A. (1993). Characteristics of spirituality in the live of women in a rural Appalachian community. *Journal of Transcultural Nursing, 4*(2), 12–18.

Burkhardt, M. A. (1994a). Environmental connections and reawakened spirit. In E. A. Schuster & C. L. Brown (Eds.). *Exploring our environmental connections.* New York: National League for Nursing Press (Pub. No 14–2634).

Burkhardt, M. A. (1994b). Becoming and connecting: Elements of spirituality for women. *Holistic Nursing Practice, 8*(4), *12–21.*

Burkhardt, M. A. (1998). Reintegrating spirituality into health care. *Alternative Therapies in Health and Medicine, 4,* 127–8.

Burkhardt, M. A. (2000). Healing relationships with nature. *Complementary Therapies in Nursing and Midwifery, 6*(1), 35–40.

Burkhardt, M. A., & Nagai-Jacobson, M. G. (1994). Reawakening spirit in clinical practice. *Journal of Holistic Nursing, 12*(1), 9–21.

Burkhardt, M. A. & Nagai-Jacobson, M. G. (1995). *Understandings of spirituality among men.* Presentation at the American Holistic Nurses Association and American

Holistic Medical Association Conference, *The Changing Face of Healing.* Phoenix, AZ, June 21–25, 1995.

Burkhardt, M. A. & Nagai-Jacobson, M. G. (2000). Spirituality and health. In B. M. Dossey, L. Keegan, & C. Guzzetta (Eds.).*Holistic nursing practice: A handbook for practice* (3rd. ed., pp. 91–121). Gaithersburg, MD: Aspen.

Chase, P. & Pawlik, J. (1986). *Healing with crystals.* Farmingdale, NY: Coleman.

DeWitt, C. (1998). The oneness of Biblical and ecological teaching. In B. Webb (Ed). *Fugitive faith: Conversations on spiritual, environmental, and community renewal* (pp. 92–101) Maryknoll, NY: Orbis Books.

Fields, R., Taylor, P., Weyler, R., & Ingrasci, R. (1984). *Chop wood, carry water.* Los Angeles: Jeremy. P. Tarcher.

Findhorn Community (1975). *The Findhorn Garden.* New York: HarperPerennial.

Fox, M. (1991). *Creation Spirituality: Liberating Gifts for the Peoples of the Earth.* San Francisco: Harper San Francisco.

Habito, R. L. (1993). *Healing breath: Zen spirituality for a wounded earth.* Maryknoll, NY: Orbis Books.

Hifler, J. S. (1996). *A Cherokee feast of days, Volume II.* Tulsa, OK: Council Oak Books.

Hubbard, B. M. (1998). *Conscious evolution.* Novato, CA: New World Library.

Jeffers, S. (1991). *Brother Eagle, Sister Sky: A Message from Chief Seattle.* New York: Dial Books.

Johnson, S. (1996). *The essence of healing: A guide to the Alaskan flower, gem, and environmental essences.* Homer, AK: Alaskan Flower Essence Project.

Nattrass, B. & Altomare, M. (1999). *The natural step for business: Wealth, ecology, and the evolutionary corporation.* Gabriola Island, BC, Canada: New Society Publishers.

Niehardt, J. G. (1972). *Black Elk speaks.* New York: Washington Square Press.

Nightingale, F. (1859). *Notes on nursing: What it is, and what it is not.* London: Harrison and Sons. (Commemorative Edition printed by J. B. Lippincott, 1992).

Ornish, D. (1998). *Love and survival.* New York: HarperCollins.

Porritt, J. (1991). *Save the Earth.* London: Dorling Kindersley.

Raphael, K. (1987). *Crystal healing.* New York: Aurora Press.

Roberts, E., & Amidon, E. (1991). *Earth prayers from around the world.* San Francisco: Harper San Francisco.

Rockefeller, S. C. (1998). Reconnecting to what sustains us physically and spiritually. In B. Webb (Ed). *Fugitive faith: Conversations on spiritual, environmental, and community renewal* (pp. 71–82) Maryknoll, NY: Orbis Books.

Seattle, C. (1992). *How can one sell the air?—Chief Seattle's Vision.* Summertown, TN: The Book Publishing Company.

Scheffer, M. (1988). *Bach flower therapy.* Rochester, VT: Healing Arts Press.

Schuster, E. A., & Brown, C. L. (1994). *Exploring our environmental connections.* New York: National League for Nursing Press.

Schuster, E. A., & Keegan, L. (2000). Environment. In B. M. Dossey, L. Keegan, & C. Guzzetta (Eds.).*Holistic nursing practice: A handbook for practice* (3rd. ed., pp. 249–278). Gaithersburg, MD: Aspen.

Shaner, H. (1994). Environmentally responsible clinical practice. In E. Schuster & C. Brown, (Eds.) *Exploring our environmental connections* (pp. 233–254). New York: National League for Nursing Press.

Smith, H. (1991). *The World's Religions.* San Francisco, CA: Harper San Francisco.

Southard, M. (2000). *Love notes to earth, 2000 calendar.* Sisters of St. Joseph, 1515 W. Ogden Ave., LaGrange Park, IL 60526.

Steindl-Rast, D. (1998). Belonging to community: Earth household and God household. In B. Webb (Ed). *Fugitive faith: Conversations on spiritual, environmental, and community renewal* (pp. 102–117) Maryknoll, NY: Orbis Books.

Stevensen, C. J. (1996). Aromatherapy. In M. S. Micozzi (Ed.) *Fundamentals of complementary and alternative medicine* (pp. 137–148). New York: Churchill Livingstone.

Swamp, J. (1995). *Giving thanks: A Native American good morning message.* New York: Lee & Low Books.

Swimme, B. (1998). The universe as sacred story. In B. Webb (Ed). *Fugitive faith: Conversations on spiritual, environmental, and community renewal* (pp. 132–148) Maryknoll, NY: Orbis Books.

Too, L. (1999). *The illustrated encyclopedia of Feng Shui.* Boston: Element Books.

Two Elk, T. (1998, October). *Sacred fire.* Presentation at Belonging to mother earth: Indigenous wisdom and healing. Virginia Beach, VA.

Uhlein, G. (1983). *Meditations with Hildegard of Bingen.* Santa Fe, NM: Bear.

Villoldo, A. (1999). *Shamanism and energy healing.* Paper presented at the Fourth Annual Alternative Therapies Symposium: Creating Integrative Healthcare, New York, NY, March 26, 1999.

Webb, B. (1998). *Fugitive faith: Conversations on spiritual, environmental, and community renewal.* Maryknoll, NY: Orbis Books.

Wheeler Robins, J. L. (1999). The science and art of aromatherapy. *Journal of Holistic Nursing, 17*(1), 5–17.

Wright, M. S. (1988). *Flower essences: Reordering our understanding and approach to health.* Jeffersonton, VA: Perelandra.

Wright, M. S. (1996). *Perelandra microbial balancing program.* Jeffersonton, VA: Perelandra.

Wright, M. S. (1997). *Co-creative science: A revolution in science providing real solutions for today's health and environment.* Jeffersonton, VA: Perelandra.

CHAPTER 9

Connecting Through Ritual

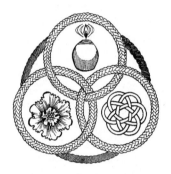

Rituals . . . remind us that we all spring from the center,

the source, the All-That-Is;

that the aliveness of the Great Spirit lives in each of us;

and that we all have an equal place in things

<small>BROOK MEDICINE EAGLE, IN IGLEHART, 1983, P. 122</small>

Rituals help us to connect with our inner core, Sacred Source, other people, nature, and all in our world and universe. Sacred rituals help us to move from *chronos,* or linear time into *kairos,* which is Sacred time, God's time. Rituals help us to remember, to honor, and to change. They involve actions, symbols, and ceremonies that come in many shapes and forms, both secular and sacred. Whether shared with others or highly personalized, rituals are integral to our human experience, and a central part of religious and spiritual traditions and cultures throughout history. Lighting Sabbath candles, routine morning walks, daily prayer time, greeting the rising sun, sharing the day's experiences with family over dinner, or a soothing bath can all be rituals. Basic elements of ritual include actions, meaningful patterns, intention, awareness, and purpose or goal. This is differentiated from ritualistic behaviors, which are repetitive and often empty actions that have little or no meaning. We all have patterned behaviors that we call "daily rituals," related to how we go about the activities of our day. For example, the morning or evening shower, the cup of tea or coffee while reading the morning paper, routine exercise, prayer or meditation, and the hug and kiss as we say goodbye to or greet our children or loved one. Some of these behaviors are so routine that we do them almost unconsciously; yet, if we are unable to do them for whatever reason, our day seems not quite right. Rituals give us an opportunity to pause, to step out of our ordinary routine, to be aware in this moment, to acknowledge and gain perspective on the experiences and events in our lives. In ritual, we have an opportunity to engage our whole selves by using more than words to help us grasp the deeper meanings of our lives. Rituals arise, in part, from our search for connectedness with the Source of our lives, with the meaning of our lives, and with others with whom we experience life. By consciously stepping outside the ordinary flow of our lives, we can attune more to our senses and become more aware of who we are and how we are connected. Pollack (2000) reminds us that doing things the same way helps us to become more aware of the patterns and continuity of our lives.

SACRED AND SECULAR RITUAL

The *intent,* more than the particular actions, differentiates sacred from secular ritual. We have all experienced secular rituals. Consider, for example, July 4th celebrations or graduation ceremonies. Each of these includes patterns of actions. Particular actions vary from family to family, community to community, school to school, but they generally have a basic pattern within each setting such as July 4th fireworks, family picnics, and parades, or graduation robes, processions, speakers, and conferring diplomas. These actions have meaning for those involved—remembrance and celebration of independence or celebration of achievement and passage to another phase of development. Sacred ritual includes a conscious invitation or openness to the presence of the Divine within the ritual. Religious worship and spiritual ceremony within any tradition is sacred ritual. Regular practice of personal prayer or meditation is sacred ritual, as is the family gathered around to bless the food before eating. A daily walk for the purpose of exercise is a secular ritual; when done with awareness of the life energy around us, the intention of sharing love and peace with the earth with each step, or as a body prayer, the walk becomes a sacred ritual.

Rituals help us to connect with the physical and natural world and also link us with that which is unseen, with mystery, and with the energy underlying and flowing through all existence. Ritual provides a process through which we experience the interconnectedness of our physical and spiritual selves. Creating and participating in ritual can bring us into sacred time and sacred space, where our ordinary, every day reality encounters sacred reality. Ritual always begins with our physical selves and provides a doorway for us to experience the more of who we are, our essence that is deeper and more expansive than the body. Perhaps you have had the experience of a special sense of the divine Presence during a religious service, or when gathering with friends for a solstice celebration, or when sharing thanks for a meal with your family. You might experience this as a pervading sense of love, gratitude, or peace, a stillness that seems especially deep, particular insight or sense of knowing or, as Pollack (2000, p. 23) writes, "the sense of awe and wonder that fills us—that tingling all over the body, the hair standing up. The desire to laugh, or cry out, or maybe weep, not from sadness or even joy, but just from so much amazement, and love, filling our small selves." Within ritual, we are simultaneously in the physical and the spiritual worlds with awareness. Sacred rituals open us to direct experiences of the numinous, the sacred, and invite the Divine into our lives.

Rituals reflect who we are and what is important to us in our journeys through life. Through ritual, we both create and express that which is meaningful in our lives. Lighting a candle in remembrance of a loved one who has died expresses our love and sense of connection with that person. At the same time, the act of lighting the candle creates the space within which we can remember the person and reinforces the importance of our remembering. When we regularly gather with others for prayer or meditation, we re-create the energy that makes this practice meaningful as, through our actions, we express the importance of gathering together.

REFLECTION 9–1

- What are your "daily rituals"—the things you "always do"?
- Consider both the sacred and secular rituals in your life. What makes these rituals important for you? What differentiates those that are secular from those that are sacred?
- How have you experienced ritual taking you into sacred time and space?
- How do these rituals help you gain perspective on your life and help you to experience your connections?
- What rituals have the most meaning for you?
- Do some rituals that once had meaning for you no longer have meaning? What contributed to this change?

Many people in contemporary society no longer find meaning in religious and other rituals that once were significant to them or their parents. The hunger for meaning has prompted many to explore spiritual and healing traditions from other cultures, and the rituals that are part of these traditions. Some find greater spiritual sustenance as they fully embrace another tradition. Others borrow and adapt rituals from various traditions to fit in with their own practices. For example, people whose spirituality includes a deep sense of connection with nature might gravitate toward indigenous traditions that are grounded in earth spirituality. Some people fully embrace these traditions, seeking teachers and following all the practices associated with these traditions. Others learn the basics of certain rituals that help them to experience their connectedness with nature, and they integrate these rituals into their personal or communal spiritual practice. These people might, for example, use traditional herbs such as sage and cedar to smudge or cleanse their home, or as part of an opening prayer or ritual for a worship service. They might use a sweat lodge or Medicine Wheel at their homes, or call in the sacred directions as they begin meditation.

Achterberg and colleagues (1994) note that rituals create and reflect individual and cultural values. These rituals store and transmit information about a society's beliefs through the symbols of ritual. When we adapt rituals from another tradition, we need to be aware of the relationship of the actions and symbols to our belief system. Because belief is an important element in healing, Achterberg and colleagues suggest that rituals that are consistent with our belief systems are more likely to be used with faith and hope, noting that trust that a ritual works for its intended purpose is a key factor in healing.

RITUAL AND EMOTION

Rituals involve our whole selves in search for truth. Quoting Jamie Phelps, Morseth (1999, p. 18) writes, "in African-American culture the emotional is not the opposite of the spiritual, nor is there any separation between the emotional and the intellectual. Both the mind and the heart are needed to grasp the truth." We often think of sacred ritual as a solemn event or process that requires us to be serious, devout, and "holy." Ritual, however, relates to and expresses all our emotions. Pollack (2000, p. 19) offers examples of several moods of ritual. Rituals for *celebration* call us to be joyful. These can include singing, dancing, laughter, and feasting. A wedding is a ritual of celebration, as is a May Day observance, a bar mitzvah, a house blessing, and a regular "date" with your life partner. Rituals for *transformation* help us shift old patterns and release us to new ways of being in life. These rituals call us to be with areas of our lives in which we might feel stuck, or overwhelmed, or victimized, or in need of healing in other ways. The Native American purification (sweat) lodge is a transformation ritual, as are the process of the Alcoholics Anonymous Twelve Step Program and processes of forgiveness and atonement found in many traditions. A person who wishes to get on with life after a divorce can create a ritual that acts out leaving the pain behind and crossing a bridge to a new and better path. Rituals for *mourning* allow people to fully enter the pain of their loss so they can begin to open to healing. In Western traditions, people often expect funerals to bring closure, and within a few days or weeks, consider that people should be through the grieving process. In many traditions, however, a year or more is given to mourning, with various rituals and expectations being part of this time. For example, Jewish rituals related to death include the immediate family observing seven days of mourning (sitting *Shiva*) after the funeral, with a memorial candle burning continuously during this time, and recital of the mourner's *Kaddish* for the deceased for eleven months. Rituals of *rest* enable us to honor our need for leisure and relaxation. An afternoon nap on the weekend, routine evening walks, and regular practice of prayer and meditation are but a few examples. Creating and practicing such rituals provide opportunities to set time aside for renewal and rejuvenation.

REFLECTION 9–2

- What rituals of celebration are part of your family tradition? Are there rituals that have been passed on from one generation to another?

- How do you include rituals of celebration into your life? Do your celebrations include ordinary experiences as well as the "special" occasions?

- What rituals of mourning are part of your tradition? How do these rituals help people to deal with the dying and grieving process?

- What are your rituals of rest? How do you incorporate these into your life?

- When have you experienced rituals that have supported processes of personal transformation?

RITUALS AND LIFE TRANSITIONS

Life transitions are acknowledged and honored through ritual in many societies. By helping to mark beginnings and endings, rituals of transition help us focus on and bring closure to old aspects of our lives so we can be more open to new situations and experiences. Rituals can help us through difficult transitions by pointing the way to new possibilities and mobilizing our energy for the new phase in our lives (Iglehart, 1983). Consider the many secular and sacred rituals that people have surrounding birth, death, and the many transitions that come between. For example, rituals surrounding birth include the kind and content of pre-natal care, many elements of the birthing process, baby showers, care and burying of the umbilical cord, naming, and other ceremonies that celebrate the child's identity as a member of a particular family and community. Rituals that mark cycles of growth and development include birthday celebrations; academic, sports, and other achievement awards; puberty rites and initiation ceremonies marking the transition from child to adult; confirmations; bar and bat mitzvahs; graduations, and weddings. Rituals surrounding dying include the ways we care for and support the dying person and family, prayers and ceremonies to support the person through the transition, special clothing, care of the body after death, wakes, obituaries, funerals and memorial services, burials, placing of tombstones or memorial plaques, and days or times of remembrance of those who have died.

SELF-NURTURE: Small Transitional Rituals

In her book, *Woman Spirit,* Hallie Iglehart (1983, p. 130) describes these small transitional rituals that she does within her daily routines:

Frequently I stop and say goodbye to my house when I leave it, sometimes imagining it protected. When I arrive at a gathering, I often spend a few minutes by myself, breathing or resting my eyes, to get centered. When I get together with someone, we may hold hands in silence for a few minutes. This helps us leave behind the busy-ness we have come from, and focuses us so that we can be together more fully.

Using these, and other ideas of your own, incorporate small rituals of transition into your everyday personal and work life.

Achterberg and colleagues (1994) view illness as a rite of passage through which we move from one phase of life or way of being to another. They describe three phases of rites of passage that can be found in individual rituals of healing. The first is the *separation phase,* the symbolic or actual breaking away from everyday busyness in which we make personal time and space away from routine activities so we can focus on the intent of the ritual. Within this phase are two distinct parts: the *trigger* that motivates us to take the time away and the *deliberate activities* of moving from one mode of being and acting to another. The second phase is the *transition phase*, which calls for identifying and focusing on areas of life that need attention. This time between the worlds, in which we have moved into sacred space, is the time spent doing the ritual. The third is the *return phase,* the time of reentry or reincorporation into daily life, bringing the benefits of the ritual practice of the transition phase into every day activities. In essence, ritual gives us time apart so that we may return to our world in a clearer, more centered way.

RITUALS AND HEALING

Nurses can incorporate meaningful rituals into care with patients and help patients create their own healing rituals. Simple rituals for small transitions can help nurses to be present with patients. For example, nurses might take a few minutes to center when entering their workplaces, or they can consciously wash their hands or pause to take a breath between patients to leave the former encounter behind so they can be focused with the next patient. Conscious nursing rounds that include good assessment, caring touch, and verbal acknowledgment of each person can help all concerned stay connected in a context of care. Within each phase of ritual just described are opportunities for nurses to suggest or support actions or processes that facilitate patient healing.

Relating these phases to the experience of illness and healing, Achterberg and colleagues write that illness or crisis prompts the separation phase by forcing us to separate from usual activities or change our ways of doing things so that we can restore harmony or health. With a minor illness this could be as simple as taking a day off from work, going to bed earlier than usual, or taking more time for meditation and using imagery to assist in mobilizing and supporting the immune system. Diagnosis of serious illness is often the trigger that prompts more profound change in behaviors and patterns and the creation of personal rituals of healing. A mixture of activities can be part of the separation phase. This phase might include *going to a sacred or healing place* to think, process, and begin planning for the future and *sacralizing* the healing place through use of symbols or natural elements such as water, candles, incense, flowers, crystals, art, feathers, prayer beads, or music. There could be an actual or symbolic *forming a circle* (of people, stones, string, flowers) that symbolizes both the separation between sacred and secular and wholeness and connection within self and with others. There might also be *symbolic acts of breaking away* that reflect moving from one way of being to another, such as removing shoes or other clothing, washing, untying a knot, and opening or closing a door (Achterberg et al., 1994, pp, 22–25). A simple way of noting the separation is signifying that this time is different by staying in one's pajamas all day. Jean Watson retreated to a healing place for her "time out and time in." Esber Tweel's separation began with his hospitalization and continued with being homebound for several months. He sacralized the room where he spent most of his time with pictures of his family, crystals that brought him rainbows, and treasured art work from special places he had traveled.

When related to healing, the transition phase could be the time of the illness itself as well as the time spent actually doing healing rituals. As with many mythic journeys, the experience of illness brings us face to face with uncertainty, mystery, and seeming darkness through which we can discover the light of more of ourselves, "what is real and worthy and healing in the broadest sense" (Achterberg et al., 1994, p. 26). Within the experience of serious illness, the transition phase is that time spent focused on self and the processes needed for healing. This process can include surgery, therapies, intensive medications, initiating lifestyle changes, or doing more inner work. This could be a time of reflection and life review related to what is important, what changes are needed, what is possible, and envisioning and planning for transformation. Achterberg and colleagues (1994, pp. 25–29) discuss several aspects that are characteristically part of the transition phase: *time alone,* either chosen or forced by the circumstances, provides the space for inner reflection and for recuperation; imagery related to *symbolic death and rebirth* that help us envision letting go of old ways and transitioning to a healthier and better way of living; entering into *unusual states of consciousness,* which enable us to see things from another perspective or open us to our connections with our inner selves and Sacred Source; *rehearsal of activities* through which we mobilize our physical, mental, and spiritual resources to assist us in dealing with whatever is needed to achieve healing; *gathering information* from various sources regarding all aspects of the healing journey. A reflection from Esber's journal illustrates part of his process during his long transition phase:

Life changed moment by moment and day by day. I began to realize how much we take these precious moments for granted. It is not that we have become overly excited about every little thing, but it is how we have become so active in everything, that we have forgotten the little things. For example, how fast we eat a meal with someone who we do not see or hear because we are in such a rush to get to what is next. We don't even taste it or feel the texture of the food. Our minds operate at such a high speed that we see with our eyes briefly, and hear with our ears in a whirlwind of sounds; therefore we have bypassed hearing with our souls. We begin to take for granted the banquet that is placed upon this table of life. There is one thing I will never take for granted, and that is walking, or the ability to use my arms and legs like I did before. Life is precious, and yet we spend considerable energy living in an illusion we have created, distracting us from merging with the façade, and emerging with appreciation into the "grace" that embraces us. (Tweel, 2000)

The return phase is the reincorporation into usual life, including the benefits of the transition phase, after the healing work or ritual is completed. Actions that support this phase might include seeking encouragement for continuing our healing processes and changes in behaviors by connecting with others who have had similar experiences; continuing rituals that nurture our whole being; frequently returning to healing states of consciousness through imagery and other processes; and formally releasing the events of the crisis through action or imagery (Achterberg et al., 1994). This is illustrated in a simple ritual done on the bone marrow transplant unit where my niece, Sheila, was a patient. For several weeks following the transplant, the child remains in the same room in strict isolation. When the child's condition improves to the point of being able to be on a more open unit, the nurses have a "breaking out" ceremony in which they place colorful streamers across the entry to the isolation room and the child literally breaks through them to move out of isolation. Although this ritual did not signify a return to normal activities, it provided encouragement along the path of healing. It symbolized as well to child and parents the transition from the immediate post-transplant crisis to the next phase of the healing process.

We see in stories shared in this book, and know from our own life experiences, that serious illness, whether our own or that of a loved one, can be an incredibly transformative experience that leads us deeper on our spiritual paths. Because transformation requires reassessment of our goals, values, and priorities, and letting go of behaviors and patterns that are not supportive of our growth, it is hardly an easy process! With serious illness, we are confronted with challenges to our whole being—physical, emotional, mental, and spiritual. Experiences of illness can involve pain, suffering, fear, anxiety, uncertainty, feeling helpless, sense of isolation, and dealing with personal mortality—all of which prompt questions of meaning. In the midst of the experience of illness, ritual helps us to connect with the deeper resources within ourselves, with the support of family and community, and with Divine love, strength, and wisdom, all of which contribute to the healing process. Achterberg and colleagues (1994, pp. 13–19) suggest several reasons why rituals work as a healing force:

- Rituals contain steps for recovery—including guidelines and processes that lead to health when they are followed.

- Rituals reduce anxiety and depression—through meaningful and creative activity that is substituted for nonconstructive worrying.

- Rituals reduce feelings of helplessness—through repetitive actions that are life-sustaining and life-enhancing, clear and quiet the mind, and allow us to access our inner wisdom and spiritual grounding.

- Rituals allow for demonstration of family and community support—through presence, love, and bonding during the time of crisis and throughout the healing process.

- Rituals encourage self-acceptance and compassion for ourselves—through loving attention and care focused on ourselves by self and others and by offering an opportunity to renew and reframe beliefs and concepts about ourselves.

- Rituals can directly evoke a Higher Power or Healing Source—through prayer, love, focused energy, inviting and opening to the presence of the Divine.

- Rituals in general offer a welcoming space and comforting rhythm of thoughts and activities, providing structure and boundaries that unclutter our minds; allow us to reflect our values and convey messages to self and others about who we are and what we are experiencing; and enable us to connect with our inner wisdom. The support and presence of others experienced through ritual strengthens us in dealing with issues that are difficult to face alone.

 ## SELF-NURTURE: Connecting with the Inner Healer

Go to a quiet place where you will not be disturbed for 15–20 minutes. Arrange the environment (lighting, temperature, furniture, and the like) so you are comfortable. Play some music quietly in the background if you would like. Sit or lay down in a comfortable position, and close your eyes if this is comfortable for you. Begin to pay attention to your breathing. You do not have to change it, just become aware of your breath as you inhale and exhale. After a few breaths, begin to be aware of the space between the breaths and gently allow this to lead you into your inner being, to a place where you feel a sense of peace, of love, where you feel safe. With the inner senses of your imagination, look around and pay attention to what this place is like, listen to any sounds, be aware of scents. Continue allowing your breath to draw you even deeper into this place where you feel the love and support of your soul, your spirit. Invite your inner healer to be with you in this space. You may begin to sense, or perhaps see with your mind's eye, the presence of a very wise and loving being. Invite this being to sit with you for a little while. Tell this being about an area of your life that needs healing. Describe what is going on, and ask this being what is needed for you to move toward healing in this area. Spend as much time with this wise one as you wish to gain clarity about what is needed for your process of healing, or at least the next step for you along the healing path. When you are ready to take your leave, thank this wise one for all that you have received. Know you can return to this place and meet with your inner healer at any time. Return your awareness to your breathing. After several breaths, gradually return full awareness to your surroundings. You may want to stretch as you slowly open your eyes. Thank yourself for giving you this time of healing.

NURTURING SPIRIT THROUGH RITUAL

*Rituals, mantras, prayers may build nests in our hearts and stay there
to nourish us throughout a busy day. (Adapted from Jones, 1999)*

Rituals provide a rich resource in caring for the spirit. They mark both ordinary and significant life events and experiences. Rituals serve as reminders—calling us to attention and helping us remember to allow sacred time and space in our lives. Both the ritual behavior and the mindfulness that accompanies it are important aspects of ritual. The intent of a ritual focuses our actions and attention, bringing our awareness to the present moment. We find an example of this in Bill Moyers' (1995) conversation with Sekou Sundiata in which they talk of the enthusiasm and passion within many Black churches. When Moyers reflected that, in the churches he visited, "the music rose from some deep vein of inner experience," Sundiata offered this understanding: "Yes, I think the passion has to do with the way people come to those churches to experience God at *that* moment in *that* church. Somehow that experience in itself is a way of knowing. The aim there is to actually create a ritual that allows one to experience God . . ." (p. 393). Experiencing God or the sacred in this way implies a receptive openness of both heart and mind. Rituals help us to bridge the oft-experienced chasm between *head* and *heart,* between our thinking, rational selves and our feeling, sensing selves. In discussing ritual in the Judeo-Christian tradition, Morseth (1999) reflects that to comprehend the richness of heart in ritual, we must appreciate that in the Jewish tradition

> the heart is the center of the whole person, the core of personal character, including thought, emotion, intuition, will, and imagination. Thoughts both good and evil arise from the heart, as well as motives and desires. When the heart is turned toward God, it is filled with grace and truth. When the heart turns away from God it dwells in delusion. Prayerful rituals, then, those done "by heart," have us responding to God with our entire beings. We are moved both in our feelings and in our commitment to a deep relationship with God and all of God's creation. (p. 17)

Because rituals involve us at all levels of our being—our senses, our imaginations, our thinking, our emotions, and our intuitions—they assist us in connecting with all of who we are (our wholeness), with nature, with others, and with Sacred Source.

Engaging the Senses

My senses are the five wide-open windows of my soul. (Shaw, 1999, p. 43)

Vision. The mere act of truly looking at a flower, a sunset, a work of art, or another person can be a ritual for nurturing our spirit. Looking in this way means seeing with our hearts as well as with our eyes, opening our vision to experiencing the energy behind the form. Although we notice color, shape, and characteristics, we are not analyzing, nor even trying to fit the object into a category. Our intent is to be with the object, scene, or person. Many mindfulness processes call us to gaze softly at an object. We also involve our sense of sight in ritual as we shape the space, provide colors and textures, place symbols, create altars, and perform actions.

REFLECTION 9-3

- Consider what is visually appealing in the space where you find spiritual nourishment.

- How do the visual elements in this space help you connect with your spiritual being and your sense of the Sacred?

- What visual reminders would support you spiritually and bring comfort in times of crisis or illness?

- How does your sense of sight help you connect with your spiritual being?

Hearing. Consider how your spirit lifts or is soothed at the sound of a loved one's voice, as you listen to certain music, as you sit quietly taking in the sounds of the ocean, or when you hear the ceremonial drumbeat. Our sense of hearing helps us connect with spirit within ordinary life circumstances and through use of ritual sound. When we think of how sound is used in ritual, we often think about singing, chanting or drumming. However, favorite prayers or hymns, spoken or sung aloud, are also ritual sounds. Music, sounds of drums, bells, chimes, fingers snapping, hands clapping, blowing of conch shells or Shofar, or instruments of many varieties are part of rituals in various traditions. Another way of using hearing in ritual is to enter into, and "listen" to the silence. The "sound of silence" as it were, helps to open us to the sacred, to move us from our ordinary experience to the place of deeper connection with our spirit. Sometimes when we feel scattered, confused, or overwhelmed, just being still for a few moments and listening to the sounds around us, our own breathing, some special music, or a bird singing, is enough to bring us back to center. Listening to an inspiring speaker or poem can touch our hearts. Pollack (2000) writes about the power of the sound of words when spoken as names or as affirmations. Affirmations are short, positive phrases that, through frequent verbal repetition, help us to reprogram areas of our lives we would like to change, or to move toward a particular goal. With an affirmation, we use the kinesthetic sense as we write it, the visual sense as we read it, and the auditory sense as we speak it. Names are often given or chosen because of the sound or energy they express. Brooke Medicine Eagle (1991) reflects that names can call forth aspects of ourselves from the realm of spirit and mystery. She writes that, acknowledging the uniqueness of each person, "our people allowed the Great Spirit to help them attune to the name that would match the essence of the child, thus helping, as the name of the child was called out and spoken again and again, to bring forth the child's true nature and gifts"(p. 173). The Dagara people in West Africa have a similar practice in which the elders of the village select a child's name that reflects the child's life purpose (Somé, 2000).

Our words are the link between the inner experience and the outward clarification of that experience. Because of this, we must take care to choose words "connected to our hearts . . . words not so much to describe data, but to break through the surface to the real truth" (Morseth, 1999, p. 9). Pollack notes that the Creator in both Hindu and Jewish traditions brought the world into being through sound. The tone of certain words in Sanskrit and Hebrew can help to balance our physical and energetic bodies as they move us to deeper levels of consciousness. The Christian scripture says that in the beginning was the Word, the Word was with God and was God. Brown (1986) notes that within indigenous cultures, the potency of words is integral to their specific sounds, and what is named is understood as being literally, not symbolically, present in the name. He writes

> An aspect of the sacred potency latent in words in primal tradition is the presiding understanding that words in their sounds are born in the breath of the being from whom they proceed, and since breath in these traditions is universally identified with the life principle, words are thus sacred and must be used with care and responsibility. Such quality of the spoken word is further enhanced by the understood close proximity of the source of breath, the lungs, with the heart, which is associated with the being's spiritual center. (p. 3)

Within these traditions, words are especially powerful when they are spoken in ritual or ceremonial context. For example, as Brown writes, recounting a myth of creation "is understood to be an actual, not a symbolic, recapitulation or reenactment of that primordial creative process or event, which is not bound by time" (p. 3).

REFLECTION 9–4

- What sounds help you connect with your spirit and the Sacred Source?

(continued)

- How has sound been part of ritual in your own spiritual tradition? Are there particular sounds, such as songs, prayers, instruments, that take you back to particular spiritual experiences?
- What sounds enliven your spirit, or soothe you when you are distressed?
- What sounds are healing for you?

My experience with, and practice of, spiritual discernment
tells me that we really need more than words to assist us
in grasping the intimate relatedness of our humanity and God's
transcendence. (Morseth, 1999, pp. 2–3)

Kinesthetic: Because we are embodied, we always use our physical, kinesthetic senses in ritual, even if we are being still. As noted in Chapter 5, we experience and express our spirituality through our bodies. The body is integral to ritual in all spiritual traditions. Our movements, gestures, and postures bring our physical being into the experience as we pray, sing, dance, sway, clap, or lay-on-hands (Morseth, 1999). The way hands are held for prayer or used during a ceremony, prayer postures, dance, procession, walking, embracing, joining hands, using prayer beads, anointing the body with sacred oil, corn meal, herbs, or water may all be integral to ritual. Our bodies store memories of our life experiences. Pollack (2000) reminds us that whether or not we are conscious of doing so, we are expressing what we are feeling any time we move. She suggests that we can awaken knowledge of ourselves and deepen sacred awareness by including various kinds of movements, particularly dance, in our rituals. Brooke Medicine Eagle (1986, 1991) speaks of the importance of rituals that include physical action in healing and transforming many areas of our lives. She notes that physical acts and movements are the most powerful ways to transform ourselves, to re-program our computers, so to speak. By using a physical metaphor to express the shift or change we wish to make, we make it more real and create energetic shifts within our whole being that support and assist us in moving toward our goal. The ritual actions can be very simple, such as signifying a move from one phase of our life journey to another by going to a bridge and literally crossing it, releasing old hurts by writing them down and burying them so the earth can transform them to nourishing soil, moving into a new and uncertain situation by taking a leap of faith, literally jumping off something high enough to cause some uneasiness without being unsafe, and landing on solid ground.

REFLECTION 9-5

- What postures or physical gestures are integral to rituals in your spiritual tradition?
- How do you connect with your spirit through physical sense and movement?
- How do physical movements or gestures enliven you or help you to become more centered?
- How have you experienced the use of sacred or blessed oil, water, herbs, or other elements, in prayer, ceremony, or rituals for healing?

Scent and Taste: Sacred rituals often engage our senses of taste and smell. Rituals may include burning elements such as incense, tobacco, herbs, or candles. The smoke from burning sage, cedar, or sweet grass is used to smudge or cleanse both people and the space before many Native American ceremonies. Incense and candles are integral parts of many spiritual rituals. Flowers and other plants may be part of the ceremony or be used to help create the sacred space. Food and drink are integral to many rituals. Blessing and sharing of bread and wine are done in different ways within both Jewish and Christian rituals. In some traditions, certain foods, drinks, or herbs are considered sacred, and may be used only in spiritual ritual. In some African traditions, spiritual practice requires that food be left for the spirits of the ancestors. Ritual meals or feasting are part of some celebrations. For example, wedding celebrations in most cultures include food shared with family and friends. Aromas and tastes evoke memories and emotions that help us connect with experiences of the spirit. For example, the smell of incense takes me back to a profound sense of the holy that I experienced within Catholic rituals of my youth, and the scent of burning sage awakens within me the experiences of sharing sacred ceremony within Native American traditions and with close women friends.

REFLECTION 9-6

- How do scents or tastes help you to connect with your spirit or the Sacred?
- What elements, food, or drink are integral to spiritual ritual in your tradition?

Stories and Ritual

Stories often accompany ritual. For many years, stories were shared in the oral tradition, told and re-told for centuries before being written down. The power of these stories is evident in their survival over time. Such stories engage our minds and our hearts, drawing us into the intent of the ritual. We connect with the characters in a story intellectually, imaginatively, and energetically. Stories within ritual help us learn about and connect with the Sacred Source, with healing energy, with cycles and seasons of nature and of our own lives, and with accepted values and behaviors of our tradition. We see this in the story of the escape of the Israelites from Egypt that is recounted as part of the annual Jewish Passover Seder Ritual, or the repetition of the actions and words from Jesus' "Last Supper" during Christian Eucharistic or communion rituals. Navajo healing rituals include the stories of how particular spirit beings sought and received healing. Chanting the story of their history from the time of creation to the present is integral to the Zuni *Shalako* ceremonial. Stories help us remember and imagine possibilities. Using guided imagery as part of ritual incorporates images and senses that become part of a story. For example, when we guide someone to imagine or visualize following a path that leads to a safe place, noting the sounds, sights, textures of that place, possibly meeting a very wise person there, we are helping the person we are guiding to experience and co-create part of the story of their healing process. Words and images of prayers and sacred texts are parts of the greater story of our relationship with the Sacred. Consider how the following words reflect relationship with the Sacred in different traditions: from the psalms, "taste and see that the Lord is good," and "the Lord is my shepherd"; from the *Tao Te Ching*, "being at one with the Tao is eternal. And though the body dies, the Tao will never pass away"; from the Koran, "in the name of God, gracious and merciful. All that is in heavens and earth, exalt the glory of God, he is omnipotent and wise; the kingdom of the heavens and earth is his"; from the Navajo chant, "I walk in beauty before me, I walk in beauty behind me, I walk in beauty below me, I walk in beauty above me, I walk in beauty all around me, in beauty it is finished."

Altars and Shrines

Altars and shrines help create sacred space, connect with the world of Spirit or the Divine, and often serve as a focal point for ritual. We find altars and shrines in homes, in nature, in places set aside for sacred ritual. The family photos displayed in many homes are secular shrines of sorts that help us connect with family and friends both living and dead. The cross, Bible, or statue of the Virgin Mary; the star of David, menorah, or Sabbath candles; the crystals, special herbs, and goddess statue; and the feathers, pipe, and tobacco pouch all help mark the space as sacred and connect us with the spiritual. Crosses, wreaths, or flowers placed along the roadside where someone died in an accident is another type of shrine. Altars serve as reminders of the connection between our spirituality and our everyday life. They can be as simple as a candle on the corner table or a special picture and stone placed in the window of your work place.

In many traditions, people create home altars or shrines that can include a statue or other representation of a saint or deity, sacred or power objects, elements from nature, or whatever represents the presence of or connection with the Sacred. Altars may be located in a particular place, or they may be able to be carried with you. Villoldo and Krippner (1987) describe the shaman's *mesa,* a collection of power objects that is also the place the shaman comes to meet the spirits. The shaman carries the mesa with him, setting the objects in a particular configuration on the ground on a cloth when doing a ritual. The mesa described by these authors was divided into three areas that did not signify either positive or negative forces: the *campo ganadero,* or field of the dark, on the left, the *campo justiciero,* or field of light, on the right, and the *campo medio* or neutral field and place of balance in the middle. In other traditions, altars or shrines might honor one's ancestors or the spirit protector of the family.

In her discussion of creating home altars, Pollack (2000) notes that personal altars reflect who we are, helping us to define and clarify who we are spiritually and emotionally. As we gather and arrange objects that are outside us, yet represent our inner connection with spirit, we both express and learn about ourselves. The act of creating the altar is also a commitment to our own growth. The altar creates a space of sanctuary that reminds and invites us to incorporate those practices and processes that enable us to experience our spiritual connectedness. When we or another needs healing, we might use our altar as part of our healing ritual. As Pollack suggests, creating a healing altar can be as simple as keeping a candle burning in front of a picture of the one needing healing. Such a ritual enables us to be more intentionally present in healing ways with the other, whether we are in the same physical location or at a distance.

Labyrinth

The labyrinth offers a particular kind of spiritual walk or journey that is at once literal and symbolic. Walking the labyrinth is a process that can clear the mind and give insight into the spiritual journey (Artress, 1995). In contrast to a maze, there is no way to get "lost" in a labyrinth; there is one way into the center, and the same path is followed on the return. Artress reflects that, as a tool to deepen self-knowledge, empower creativity, and guide healing, the labyrinth offers a stable and sacred space in which to focus attention and listen to the soul's longing. The act of walking the labyrinth is a ritual, a body prayer through which we take time from ordinary life to journey to our own center and truth. As we return to our routine outer life, we carry with us the sense of energy, grounding, and empowerment that comes from connecting with the inner self. The labyrinth is a sacred pattern based on spirals, which reminds us that the spiritual journey, indeed the life journey, is never a straight line. Although the path at times seems to take us away from our goals, continuing to traverse it ultimately brings us to our center. The labyrinth is a reflective walk that we may enter with a general sense of openness, with a special question or focus, or perhaps with a familiar prayer. Then, without any particular expectations, the process takes us where we need to go and enables us to bring the essence and insights of this journey back into our daily lives.

CONNECTING WITH OTHERS THROUGH RITUAL

Rituals include both personal and communal experience. Rituals have a special power and energy when shared with others. As we connect with others through ritual, we increase our sense of community. The process of sharing the ritual expands the energy to become greater than the sum of each individual's energy. In a very real, though not always tangible way, the energy of shared ritual brings greater presence of the sacred into society as a whole. Larry Dossey provides an example of this in his book, *Meaning & Medicine* (1991). He cites a study that reported the effects of a group doing transcendental meditation (TM) in Jerusalem that demonstrated an inverse correlation between the size of the meditating group and crimes and violence in Israel, and war deaths in Lebanon during the same period (war deaths decreased 70% on days that meditating was high compared with when it was low). Citing a similar study in Washington, D. C., he notes that there was an inverse correlation between the size of the meditating group and the level of violent crimes in that city (pp. 186–187).

Religious services are rituals shared within community. One purpose of religious and other traditional rituals is to bring people into physical harmony with one another to renew and reweave the social fabric of the community (Achterberg et al., 1994). Pollack (2000) gives an example of this in the Dagara society in Africa in which adult participation in communal rituals provides the basis for effectively carrying out family rituals. In turn, family rituals provide the groundwork for individual rituals that must be performed to help maintain and support the family's and community's connections with the gods.

We connect at the level of spirit when we join with others for prayer, meditation, or spiritual ceremony. Ritual connects us with people with whom we might not connect in other ways. Consider how religious worship brings people together who may have little else in common. Have you ever experienced the deep sense of presence with another by sitting in silent prayer or meditation together? I have had this opportunity during silent retreats in which I have experienced a real sense of knowing other participants even though we do not verbally converse with each other. Consider the bonding that comes through simple family rituals such as bedtime stories and prayers, the hug and kiss on parting in the morning and returning in the evening, the special Saturday breakfasts or Sunday dinners. Unlike in Western cultures, where healing is focused on the individual, in many societies, the family and community gather for a healing ritual. Sharing in the ritual provides energy and support to the one who is ill and acknowledges that the whole community is affected by both the illness and the healing process. Healing the one brings healing to the community as well.

SELF-NURTURE: Deepening Connection with Others

Consider how you connect with others through ritual. The following are a few ways to deepen your connection with others through simple ritual. Use these, modify them as needed, or create your own way of connecting soul-to-soul with people in your life through ritual.

- Gather once or twice with family or friends for a period of silent prayer or meditation. Decide together on the length of time and be in silence together for this time. You might want to begin with a short inspirational reading. When the time is finished join hands in a circle for a moment to signify closure.

- Consider a ritual way of sharing a sunset with another. You join with another person and merely sit in silence together watching and enjoying the changes from the time the sun begins to set until all the colors fade. There is no need to discuss or comment on what you are seeing or feeling either during or after the process. After you have enjoyed the sunset together, just thank each other, and return home or to your usual activities.

- At the beginning of your workday or shift, join with your co-workers for a few moments to center for the day. You might join hands and together do several deep, cleansing breaths. You might do a brief "check in," saying something about where you are in the moment, or something you feel good about, or something you feel concerned about. You can also use this process at the beginning of meetings.

CONNECTING WITH NATURE THROUGH RITUAL

Rituals connect us with the world around us enabling us to experience our relatedness with all in our world and universe. Nature provides the basis for seasonal and cyclical rituals. Religious and sacred calendars cycle with the moon, the sun, the stars, the planets, and the seasons. Spiritual traditions that reflect a close connection with nature celebrate seasonal rituals related to the patterns of nature. An example is the Celtic Wheel of the Year, which has eight seasonal rituals (Pollack, 2000). These rituals include the winter solstice (December, 21st), Imbole (February 2nd), spring equinox (March 21st), Beltane (May 1st), summer solstices (June 21st), Lughnasadh (August 1st), fall equinox (September 21st), and Samhain (October 31st). Rituals in this cycle acknowledge dependence on the Divine for sustenance and celebrate the gifts of creation through the cycle of planting, growing, harvesting, and resting. Many people join in secular and spiritual celebrations of the solstice and equinox cycles. Machaelle Small Wright (1993) who has spent more than 20 years learning to work more effectively in partnership with nature, describes how she observes these days as nature holidays: She uses each of these days to take time out, step back, reflect on, and connect with the specific nature processes related to each day and celebrate the partnership between humans and nature.

The cycling of the full moon determines the time of sacred ceremony in many traditions. The moon is used to determine the timing of special religious observances such as Christian Lent and Easter, Jewish High Holy Days and Passover, and Muslim Ramadan. In many Native American traditions, a woman's *moon time* (menstrual period) is considered a sacred time where women step away from routine activities so they can focus inward and listen to Spirit's guidance for themselves and the community. Observing and celebrating the cycles of nature is an especially important way for those who do not live close to the land to nurture connection with nature.

Creating a visual shrine or altar outside using stones, plants, a tree, or other elements of nature helps us remember our connectedness with all life and is a way in which nature facilitates our connection with spirit. The Native American Medicine Wheel is an example of creating a place of prayer and ceremony that incorporates elements of nature and the directions. The Medicine Wheel is a sacred circle built of stones representing the Wheel of Life or the full Circle of Life that is used in ceremonial ways for healing, giving thanks, praying, meditating, seeking guidance for one's journey or life path (Medicine Eagle, 1991; Sun Bear, Mulligan, Nufer, & Wabun, 1989). The Medicine Wheel is divided into various aspects, generally including four quadrants that represent the four directions (north, south, east, west). Each direction is aligned with one of the four seasons of the year and of life and offers gifts and teaching associated with these seasons and cycles. The Medicine Wheel represents any human cycle, whether this is a project, a time of change, or a lifetime. "We travel around and around the wheel in our Earth walk, and if we remember to spend as much time in the releasing and quieting quadrants as in the sprouting and doing quadrants, we find a balanced way of life (Medicine Eagle, 1991, p. 287).

CREATING SACRED RITUAL

Rituals come in all shapes and sizes, and one size does not necessarily fit all. You might be attracted to a ritual from a particular tradition, but a certain part may not fit. How might you change it to make it your own while staying true to the overall intent of the ritual? Whether we participate in ritual within the context of the religious or spiritual tradition we were raised, share spiritual or other rituals with friends, or create our own rituals, we need to be able to personalize the process at some level. In *Rituals of Healing*, Achterberg and colleagues (1994) offer many rituals that incorporate relaxation and imagery to enhance the healing process. In preparation for doing a ritual they encourage us to tend to our basic comfort needs, ensure that the environment will be supportive of the process, alert others to our need for uninterrupted space, have all needed materials handy, and pay attention to our physical needs during the time. The basic format that they suggest for personalizing or creating rituals incorporates the three phases of ritual noted earlier. Begin with the separation phase during which we settle in, begin to relax, create our intention, and enter a healing state of consciousness. During the next phase of transition, we become more attuned to our relaxation and use our imagination to mesh our senses of sight, hearing, taste, touch, and smell with the condition needing healing. This might mean following an imagery script or allowing spontaneous images to emerge. We close this phase with personal and general images of wholeness and healing. The return phase brings us back to a wakeful state in which we notice our deeper sense of relaxation and renewed energy and make note of any insights or images that emerged during the ritual.

The template for ritual described by Pollack (2000) includes similar process of making preparations, gathering what we need, and stating the intent for what we wish to accomplish or create through the ritual. She also suggests purifying self and the space in some way, such as using incense or sprinkling salt water, and creating a sacred circle either physically or energetically. This can be done by imagining a circle or bubble of energy around the space, lighting a candle or placing stones in the north, south, east, and west, or walking around the space with the intention of filling the whole area with love. This process can also involve inviting the spirits, energies, or deities that you wish to assist in or guide the ritual to be in the space. The work of the ritual may involve many processes such as breath work, singing, dancing, drumming, blessings, ritual action, sharing food. As a way to close a ritual, she suggests grounding the energy so that it becomes more real in our lives, expressing thanks, offering a blessing, and returning to our daily life carrying with us the benefits of the ritual.

The ritual of Sabbath in the Jewish tradition is one example of this process within a religious context. Sabbath observance begins with the lighting of candles, signifying the separation from the week of work and moving into the time of sacred rest. The transition phase includes the various activities, including religious services, of the Sabbath day. The Sabbath ends with the *Havdala* ceremony, which signifies the closure of sacred time of Sabbath and moving back into secular time, carrying the blessings of Sabbath into the rest of the week. Indeed, within any religious worship service, we see the basic elements of ritual. The separation comes as we move from our routine life into the place of the service. The transition phase includes the various activities of the service such as prayer, music, reading sacred texts, blessing and sharing bread, wine, other elements, particular movement or actions, interactions with others, and all that is occurring within ourselves. The service often closes with a blessing, which initiates the return to our usual activities with the reminder to carry the sacred more consciously into our daily life.

We can create sacred ritual alone or with others, with prior planning or spontaneously. Any ritual that helps us reconnect with ourselves and with Spirit helps to ground and revitalize us. We see this in Jude Fleming's (personal communication, 2000) experience of creating such a ritual when she "went on an adventure into the Rockies" with her daughter and a friend. Noting that she and her companions were "needing to ground in Earth Mother," she described finding "a slice of heaven," spending time sitting under a big Jeffery Pine, hiking up a trail, and pausing to take in "a truly magnificent canyon with a river running through it." After returning to where the car was parked, she reflected

> I pulled out my pipe, a few candles, some special stones and I set an altar. We all prayed, we wrote on paper what we were willing to give up, and then we ceremonially burned the paper in an abalone shell. We sang a few songs and we cried and we laughed and I could see the spirits uplift. We shared a meal. In exactly the right moment we put the last thing in the car, closed the door and the rain fell. We went off to find the Canyon. We just drove, talked, shared words and silence and we once again came back to what was real. We were revitalized. I keep remembering that all we need to do is stay on our path, focus on our love for Spirit . . . that is it, all that we need. I am sad when I realize how long I go between communications. I would not treat a human that I love the way I treat Spirit and I love Spirit more than life. Well, it was a wonderful, completely self-care day that we all so desperately needed. It serves to remind me of where my roots are, and it also reminds me of just how powerful and real ceremonial acts are when intentions are honest and from the heart.

REFLECTION 9–7

Consider the place of rituals in your life.

- What rituals are currently a part of your life?

- Are there other rituals you would like to make a part of your life, and how might you bring that about?

- When and how have you created sacred ritual, alone or with friends? What was the experience like for you? How did the ceremony revitalize you and help you reconnect with Spirit?

Developing an awareness of the place of ritual in our own lives establishes a basis from which we can facilitate and provide opportunities for patients to consider and experience the place of ritual in their lives. We can explore what rituals are significant for a particular patient and what rituals might support the patient's healing process. These could be rituals that are part of their spiritual traditions or rituals that we help them to create. We need to consider what constitutes sacred space for various patients and to explore with patients the resources that might help them better understand and include supportive rituals in their lives.

CREATIVE EXPRESSION

> *Defining creativity is almost an oxymoron, but I will venture the beginning of a definition. A blessed birthing of newness. We don't have to wait for some spectacular birth. Creativity is an approach to how you use your gifts . . . it is new every morning. Christ's ministry was defined by creative acts, like healing on the Sabbath or creating a new thing from bread and wine. (Weems, 1999)*

Rituals are often born from the soul's longing for that which is beyond words, and from experiences of wholeness and brokenness that are part of life's journey. We often need "visible, tangible, and symbolic vehicles of grace . . . to assist us in grasping the intimate relatedness of our humanity and God's transcendence" (Morseth, 1999, pp. 2–3). Creative expression, whether incorporated into ritual or engaged in for its own sake, can be such a vehicle of grace. "The relationship that we come to understand between our faith and our creativity, is linked to our desire to explore and understand mystery—the unknown—and to achieve personal transformation, as well as interconnectedness" (Morseth, p. 23). By considering the nature of creativity and its place in healing and wholeness, we may better understand the healing process and the spiritual journey as well.

Remembering Madeleine L'Engle's understanding of creativity as a way of living life and reflecting on Weem's "beginning definition" of creativity as birthing of newness, we gain a sense of creativity as that which is present within everyday happenings and routines, as well as what we more frequently might acknowledge as works of art. Nursing literature reflects a growing interest in and exploration of the relationship between the creative arts, creativity, and nursing (Chinn & Watson, 1994; Picard, Sickul & Natale, 1998; Rose, 1999; Wilkstrom, 2000). In both the appreciation and experience of creativity in myriad forms, and the participation in acts of creability, persons find nurture of, and expression for the soul. "Art and healing are sisters. They are tied together by a silver thread," so begins an article in which Picard and colleagues (1998) offer their reflections on the healing power of aesthetics in the experience of suffering and the need for care. As nurses recognize and illuminate that silver thread, creativity can be incorporated into the healing process in forms as numerous and varied as the persons on the healing journey.

Nursing's story is filled with acts of creativity. How many nurses have fashioned different ways of positioning a limb to relieve a person's discomfort, or helped a woman feel more attractive in the aftermath of chemotherapy when her hair is gone? How many times have you stopped to figure out a new way of addressing a problem or phrasing a question? As a hospice nurse, I was always taught many lessons of comfort and care by the families and friends who cared for the patient— ways of preparing food to enhance its taste or attractiveness, comfort measures designed for a particular situation, creative uses of familiar objects such as a coat hanger being fashioned into a tool for reaching objects.

REFLECTION 9–8

- Recall some creativity you have experienced in your professional life.

- What current situations offer an opportunity for the use of your creativity?

- What are your experiences of being refreshed, renewed, challenged, or enlivened by a work of art, whether a song, a painting, an object, a dance, or any form of artistic expression that engages your being?

- How do you seek to incorporate creativity and art into your being and doing in a conscious way?

In her book, *Composing a Life,* Mary Catherine Bateson (1989, p. 1) calls attention to "the act of creation that engages us all—the composers of our lives." The composition of a life requires improvisations. Batson speaks of the need to discover the nature and shape of our creation along the way rather than following a predetermined vision or plan. The notion of improvisation is one that nurses and patients alike experience as they use both the known and the unfamiliar in fashioning a new unity. Sharing with patients the image of "composing a life" might be helpful as they live the new and often unexpected chapter of their lives.

The arts provide us glimpses into not only the souls of the artist but our souls as well. For this reason, painting, music, narratives, poetry, architecture, and sculpture might all evoke strong, sometimes unexplainable, feelings. Simply exploring with patients the place of the arts in their lives, and the forms in which creativity expresses itself in their lives, opens the door to their connections with the healing potential of the aesthetic. Some traditions, particularly the non-Western traditions, incorporate art into healing rituals and ceremony. Dress, body adornment and painting, and music, singing, and dance accompany rituals of healing. Some hospices take special care to make the environment a healing one through placement of works of art (quilts, paintings, sculpture) and use of music.

Thomas Merton said that art attunes the soul to God. Levoy (1997) suggests that perhaps art was the original religion, practiced to put us in sympathy with unseen powers and to invoke the spirits. He quotes the Jungian writer, James Hillman, in saying "When I ask, 'where is my soul, how do I meet it, what does it want now?' the answer is 'Turn to your images'" (p. 126). Picard and colleagues (1998, p. 40) remind us that "a perspective focused exclusively on symptom management and control can be a barrier to understanding the wholeness and uniqueness of the experience." In the challenge of making meaning out of suffering, the arts offer possibilities. Picard and colleagues share this story of a man recovering from cancer treatments, who was unable to sleep at night:

> Listening to music became an activity for my body. I love running most when moving is pervaded by a sense of rhythm, and listening to Bach's music gave me a sensation of movement. The origins of music are inseparable from the dance, and dance is one of the great metaphors for life itself. Until I was ill, I had never heard so clearly the dance in the music, and life in the dance. Illness taught me beyond anything I can do, my body simply is. In the wisdom of my body's being, I can find myself over and over again. (Picard et al., 1998, p. 41)

Art as a means of self-expression may be a part of our health and healing. We might ask, as do some of these authors, "can I change my understanding of something by dancing it?" The artistic creations by children and youth living with cancer reveal their images, not only of illness but also of wholeness and life, as they grace calendars and holiday cards. Poet Laureate of the United States Robert Pinsky's special undertaking was his Favorite Poem Project, in which he invited any and all Americans to write to him about their favorite poem. The resulting book (Pinsky &Dietz, 2000) reflects the power of poetry and its ability to capture and evoke deep human experiences. This is poignantly illustrated in Sandra Melville's poetic expression of how she has come to live with her chronic illness of transverse myelitis.

THIEF IN THE NIGHT

I never asked you in, thief in the night
Slowly, silently you came
Stealing each day a bit more of me
Fingertips then fingers

Hands, wrists, forearms
Like a giant "What's this" game for a child,
You named
And claimed
Parts of me.

Hands which once held a pencil to capture another's image
Held a pen to share a thought
Hands which threw a lightning bolt to start a dying heart
Or stroked the cheek of one I loved
You named
And claimed
Parts of me.

Feet and legs which danced on air
One with music, became the music
Feet and legs which danced with a mountain
Pine and snow and sky unending
Feet and legs which ran with my children
Laughing, racing, catching, cuddling,
You named
And claimed
Parts of me.

Energy and motion
Whirling here and there
Checklists conquered
Activities deftly balanced and moving
Like a juggler tap dancing in the street
Even this you took, uninvited guest
Leaving only bone-drenched fatigue
Where to cross a room is a victory
You named
And claimed
Parts of me

I never asked you in, thief in the night
Or asked for the gifts you brought and left me with
Claiming the stillness of my arms and hands:
Leaving a thrum
Constant buzz,
Rippling like a stone-thrown lake
At any tender touch or gentle breeze.

Freezing burning evening gloves of pain
Sunburn from no friendly sun
And dancing now only with the Earth,
As I fall to greet her.

And yet
Unwelcome guest, thief in the night,
You have not claimed my self, the heart of me
There is a room you cannot enter
A claim you cannot make.
I draw
Though it be shakily
I write
Though it be with my voice
I dance
Though it be in my heart
I touch
Though it be with my cheek.
And I live, and laugh, and love
Though it be with the pain.
I have you, uninvited guest, thief in the night
But you do not have me.

Consider how all the poems and psalms shared throughout this book offer insight into the soul journeys of their authors.

Our friendship and correspondence with prisoners has awakened us to the talents and gifts of persons who are incarcerated, many of whom have recognized and developed those gifts during their prison years. Their artwork enlivens the hallways and waiting rooms of some of the prisons, as well as the letters and cards they send to friends. Spiritual and religious themes are often present in their art. In describing his art, one young man says "It's Jesus that I've come to know who helps me live right in here. I've found that I can draw and share some of what keeps me going."

The act of naming is an affirmation, and by naming the creativity we see in others, we may strengthen its presence and practice in their lives. Persons who are ill might want to journal, draw, knit. A friend who died from liver cancer enjoyed working with wood until a short time before he died. Journaling, art, composing—all can be part of our wellness and wholeness. "For many creators, 'creation' is a misnomer because the creative act does not involve making something new, but linking with a complete and timeless wisdom that already exists, God . . . the Absolute . . . Lazlo's field of information . . . Whatever term is used, this dimension is often considered sacred by the creative individual" (Dossey, 2000, p. 16). Whether it is watching a child engrossed in her watercolors, a teenager absorbed by music, or standing in awe of a work of art, the connection with the soul, the "silver thread" between healing and art is present. Breunig (1994) offers these words for nursing and art:

> The big creativity, the creativity that permeates one's life, that seeps out of artists' studios and into their lives, expresses itself in creative moments and caring moments alike. Sometimes there is a product to look at and touch; sometimes there is not. The creative product may be a new way of seeing, a new way of approaching one's life and challenges. Sometimes it is a more authentic way of living—or of dying . . . Authentic caring is what turns craftsman into the nurse artist (pp. 196–197).

REFERENCES

Achterberg, J., Dossey, B., & Kolkmeier, L. (1994). *Rituals of healing: Using imagery for health and wellness.* New York: Bantam Books.

Artress, L. (1995). *Walking a sacred path: Rediscovering the labyrinth as a spiritual tool.* New York: Riverhead Books.

Bateson, M. C. (1989). *Composing a life.* New York: Atlantic Monthly Press.

Breunig, K. (1994). The art of painting meets the art of nursing. In P. Chinn & J. Watson (Eds.), *Art and aesthetics in nursing.* New York: National League for Nursing Press.

Brown, J. E. (1986). *The Spiritual Legacy of the American Indian.* New York: Crossroad.

Chinn, P., & Watson, J.(Eds.) (1994). *Art and aesthetic sin nursing.* New York: National League for Nursing Press.

Dossey, L. (1991). *Meaning & medicine.* New York: Bantam Books.

Dossey, L. (2000). Creativity: On intelligence, insight, and the cosmic soup. *Alternative Therapies in Health and Medicine, 6*(1), 12–17, 108–117.

Iglehart, H. A. (1983). *Woman spirit.* San Francisco: Harper & Row.

Jones, T. (1999). Which way to God? In C. de Vinck (Ed.), *Personal reflections on Henri NOUWEN THEN.* Grand Rapids, MI: Zondervan.

Levoy, G. (1997). *Callings—Finding and following an authentic life.* New York: Crown.

Medicine Eagle, B. (1986). *Healing through ritual action.* Audiocassette Tape. Sky Lodge, PO Box 121, Ovando, MT.

Medicine Eagle, B. (1991). *Buffalo woman comes singing.* New York: Ballantine Books.

Morseth, E. (1999). *Ritual and the arts in spiritual discernment.* LaVergne, TN: Lightning Print.

Moyers, B. (1995). *The language of life: A festival of poets.* (J. Haba, Ed.). New York: Doubleday.

Picard, C., Sickul, C., & Natale, S. (1998). Healing reflections: The transformative mirror. *International Journal for Human Caring, 2*(3), 40–47.

Pinsky, R., & Dietz, M. (2000). *America's favorite poems.* New York: Norton.

Pollack, R. (2000). *The power of ritual.* New York: Dell.

Rose, B. H. (1999). A basket metaphor for nursing. *Journal of Holistic Nursing, 17*(2) 208–217.

Shaw, L. (1999). Nourishment for the journey. In C. de Vinck (Ed.). *Personal reflections on Henri NOUWEN THEN.* Grand Rapids, MI: Zondervan.

Somé, S. (2000). It takes a village to make a relationship work. *Utne Reader* (Sept-Oct), 64–69.

Sun Bear, Mulligan, C., Nufer, P., & Wabun. (1989). *Walk in balance: A path to healthy, happy, harmonious living.* New York: Prentice Hall.

Tweel, E. N. (2000). Unpublished personal journal of illness experience. Charleston, WV.

Villoldo, A., & Krippner, S. (1987). *Healing states: A journey into the world of spiritual healing and shamanism.* New York: Fireside Books.

Weems, A. (1999). A conversation with Ann Weems. *Alive Now* (May/June), 21–25.

Wilkstrom, B. M. (2000). Nursing education in an art gallery. *Journal for Nursing Scholarship, 32*(2), 197–199.

Wright, M. S. (1993). *Perelandra garden workbook: A complete guide to gardening with nature intelligences* (2nd ed.). Warrenton, VA: Perelandra.

PART
3

Sharing Sacred Journeys

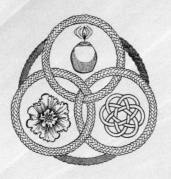

*T*his section focuses on our sharing sacred journeys with others. Spirituality exists not so much in individuals as in the relationships between and among persons and God or Sacred Source. We do not soul-search in isolation; rather, we find nurture and sustenance for ourselves as we share this with others. Appreciating that we are all stories-in-process affirms the spiritual journey for ourselves and others, providing room for both light and darkness, joys and sorrows, questions, pondering, and embracing mystery. Grounded in appreciation of our own spiritual journeys, we enter more consciously into sharing the sacred journeys of others, recognizing that our journeys often follow winding and spiraling paths that take us through rugged as well as peaceful terrains. Spiritual caregiving calls us to develop competence and confidence in our abilities to be with others in ways that enable us to recognize their spiritual questions and issues and to support and assist them in attending to their spiritual natures.

Connecting with Others

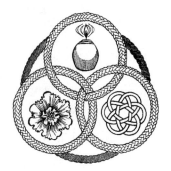

One of the gifts White Buffalo Woman brought to the Lakota people

was the rite of hunkapi, *the making of relatives.*

And today, when we really care about someone and want to be close

to them through our whole lives, we adopt them as relatives—

as sister or brother or grandmother. I think this is what we're doing

in our world right now—becoming relatives.

Becoming family with each other in a whole new way.

<small>BROOKE MEDICINE EAGLE, IN ANDERSON & HOPKINS, 1991, P. 200</small>

The spiritual journey is more a search for right relationships than it is a search for right answers. As humans, we are social beings whose very survival is linked to the ways we connect with others. Our need for belonging is very strong—belonging to a family, to a tribe, to a community, to a culture, a world, a universe. Because human relationships provide the framework and grounding for the way we live and experience our personhood and place in the world, they are a major aspect of our spirituality. Our values and spiritual perspective are shaped by our relationships with family, friends, community, and culture and find expression as we interact within these circles. We first learn of love and experience care within a family. Here, too, we experience conflict and learn that relationships are not always easy. Within this setting, we receive our first impressions of how the world works, our purpose in being, and our place in the cosmos. Family also provides our first sense of how to relate to others, to the earth, and to the Sacred. Our relationships provide sustenance, help us to discover meaning, support us in all areas of our being, and can be the source of our greatest joy. We discover who we are through our relationships, both those that are comfortable and nurturing and those that bring us pain and discomfort. Because the very same relationships that offer love and support also bring us hurt and sorrow, they can provide us with our greatest challenges and opportunities for learning. Feeling disconnected or alienated from others is dispiriting. When we feel isolated or feel a lack of support, we are more prone to physical and emotional health problems. Feeling alienated from that which provides us sustenance can cause us to question our own value and place in the world. Such questions can lead to depression, or they may lead us to explore ourselves more deeply, discovering those deeper and more expansive levels of our own being.

RELATIONSHIPS AS CONTEXT AND CONTENT FOR OUR SPIRITUALITY

> When we attempt to lead our spiritual lives apart from the nurture, support, and accountability of others, we end up distorting our spiritual growth. The presence of fellow travelers is essential for our growth. We need companionship and communion with others. (Hawkins, 1987, p. 117)

The spiritual journey calls us into relationship. Indeed, from the vantage point of our spiritual nature, all life is about sharing sacred journey with those around us. Buber (1958) maintains that spirituality does not exist so much in individuals as it does between and among persons. We see this in the stories people share when they talk about how spirituality manifests in their lives, stories that often focus on the various facets of their relationships with the significant people in their lives. These stories reflect how our relationships with others, both close and intimate connections and those of a more casual nature, provide the context within which we live our spirituality. Our relations with others provide much of the content of our spiritual expression and experience as well. People speak of the joy of holding their new infants, memories of family times on vacation, special things they learned from a grandparent, sharing of important life events with various friends and family, delight at seeing their life partners, pain at the death of a child, the distress of not having spoken with a sibling for many years, and the sense of betrayal when a friendship ended. Within our relationships, we encounter the full gamut of human experience, and this is what our spiritual journey is all about.

Relationships are sources for the growth and change that are naturally part of the spiritual journey. We connect with our spiritual selves through the joys and sorrows, harmony and discord, of our relationships. The teaching of many great spiritual traditions that God is equally in all things helps us appreciate that all aspects of our relationships are important to the unfolding of our spiritual path. Because we expect spirituality to manifest in care and concern for others, we may find it easy to appreciate that being with others in loving and supportive ways is an expression of spirituality. However, we need also to recognize spirituality manifested in our struggle and presence with painful and difficult situations in relationships with family, friends, and acquaintances. Attending to the healing that is needed in relationships that have been frayed is an essential part of the spiritual journey.

HOW RELATIONSHIPS NOURISH OUR SPIRITS

This connectedness with others, and yet beyond self and others,
keeps alive our common humanity. It helps us to stay connected
with the human spirit . . . (Watson, 1999, p. 117)

We are nurtured spiritually, physically, emotionally, and mentally through our connections with others, indeed we need contact with others in all these areas to survive. Joni Walton (1996, p. 240) reflects that "the soul is found in the depths of our relationships," suggesting that our connectedness with self "begins and is nurtured in relationships," and that we cannot soul-search alone. We need to touch and be touched, we need to be able to express and share our thoughts and emotions, and we need to feel a kinship with others at our deeper levels of spirit. When we do not have this interaction, we die at some level of our being. Failure-to-thrive infants suffer developmental delays, and waste away and die when they do not experience sufficient caring touch and interaction, even when basic needs for food and shelter are met. Our spirits impel us to connect with others, recognizing that we ultimately find our sustenance within our relationships.

Our spirits are nourished within our ordinary experiences of daily living as well as in special times shared with others. Consider the joy of watching your child at play, the delight in sharing a meal and conversation with friends, the comfort of having your sister call when you have had a particularly hard day, or the excitement of sharing a holiday with your family. These interactions provide the energy of life that sustains and nourishes us. The daily interactions of greeting and saying goodbye, preparing and sharing meals, attending to our emotional and physical environments, and engaging in our various activities connect us with those around us. The love and care, strain, and struggle that we experience within these relationships provide opportunities for us to know ourselves and others. In the ordinary events of life we often discover that which is most meaningful for our existence, what is truly important for living. A friend who recently lost her job at the same time that she ended a significant relationship reflected how important it was to have a place to come "home" to, where she felt the love and presence of caring friends. She noted how difficult it was for her to develop deeper friendships where she had moved, and how hard it was to feel so alone when she felt lower than she had ever been. A 90-year-old woman who grew up and raised her own family in coal camps reflected that even though life was hard in the camps, everyone looked out for everyone else. She experienced a sense of community and support in the coal camps that she found lacking when moving upward in the socioeconomic sense meant moving out of the camps.

When we are joyful, our joy expands as we share it with others. When we are hurting, our pain is eased when shared with those who care. Another's eyes can help us see beauty we might have missed. Another's ears can help us hear what our hearts are truly saying. Another's touch can help us feel our worth when we have come to doubt it. Another's presence can help us feel safe when we are afraid. Another's belief in us can help us appreciate our own potential. Desmond Tutu's (1995) eloquent words remind us of

> a fundamental truth about us—that we are made to live in a delicate network of interdependence with one another, with God and with the rest of God's creation. We say in our African idiom, "A person is a person through other persons." A solitary human being is a contradiction in terms . . . We are made for complementarity. I have gifts that you do not; you have gifts that I do not. *Voila!* So we need each other to become fully human. (p. xiv)

Our connectedness with ourselves is grounded in and nurtured through our relationships. Indeed, we cannot know ourselves outside of the context of our relationships. We trace our roots through parents and grandparents. Within our families, we are daughter or son, mother or father, sister or brother, aunt or uncle, niece or nephew, cousin. Within our work settings, we might be employer, employee, or co-worker. In school, we might be teacher, student, and friend. Our sense of self comes partly from our experiences within these relationships—how we see ourselves, how others perceive us and treat us, how we perceive and treat them. Hawkins (1987) reflects that our selfhood comes to us as gift "through those means of grace that God's prevenience has always provided: our often flawed and sometimes destructive relationships with friend, family and community" (p. 19). Our sense of self as loved, lovable, and capable is grounded in our experiences within our family and our social interactions. Low self-esteem, sense of worthlessness, or limitations in our abilities derives from these experiences as well. Although some relationships can cause distortions in our lives, Hawkins reminds us that the attention, care, and mutuality of our social relationships is essential to our humanity.

REFLECTION 10–1

- How have your relationships helped to shape who you are?
- What relationships have nurtured that which you like best about yourself?
- What relationships have presented challenges to your becoming your truest self?
- How does your relationship with important people in your life contribute to their self-becoming?
- Which relationships seem to bring out what you consider the worst in you?
- In what relationships do you feel you are your truest and best self? Consider the nature of these relationships. What makes them "work" for you?

RELATIONSHIPS AND OUR SENSE OF THE SACRED

Receptive openness to Love, Light, Life, and Presence of the Sacred Source, experienced directly and through others, is a spiritual stance. Our experiences with others help shape both our sense or image of God and our understanding of our relationships with the Divine or Sacred Source. It is easier to imagine a loving, caring, and merciful God when we have known ourselves as loved by parents and other people who are important to us. Our sense of God as judgmental, impartial, detached, or vengeful is also colored by our human relationships. Images of God or Sacred Source as mother, father, or friend reflect our own experiences or ideals for these relationships. Teilhard de Chardin (1960) reminds us that we cannot love God without loving others and that we cannot love others without in some way moving closer to the Divine. Our relationships can help us to experience more fully the qualities of Sacred Presence. Every relationship is a potential doorway for moving us to deeper connection with the Sacred Source within and beyond our being.

INTIMACY

Only in the intimacy of the timeless present can we awaken. This intimacy connects us to one another, allows us to belong, and in this belonging, we experience love. In this way we move beyond our separateness, our contraction, our limited sense of ourselves. (Kornfield, 1993, p. 333)

Deep and lasting relationships with family, friends, or lovers require intimacy. Our natures prompt us to seek intimacy because intimacy is essential to our health, our wholeness. Understanding that true intimacy goes beyond the physical closeness of sexual relations, we might find that our most intimate relationships are with friends and family rather than with lovers. The path to discovering true intimacy with another is similar to the processes of discovering intimacy with God or the Sacred Source and of becoming intimate with ourselves. Indeed, as Fields and colleagues (1984) remind us, the qualities that help us along our spiritual paths are the same as those that encourage intimacy with others. These qualities include being present in the moment, surrender, honesty, trust, and letting go of judgment. We can only experience intimacy with another in the present moment, being open to the shared experience of the now. In this moment I am aware of my feelings, expectations, fears, vulnerability, and sense of safety and am willing to be seen by another as I am. At the same time, I am open to receiving the other person as she or he is.

This openness and willingness to receive another is the essence of surrender (Ray, 1980). We generally think of surrender as giving up our power to another. In the context of the spiritual journey and developing intimacy, however, surrender means releasing the barriers to and letting go of defenses against closeness or union with another, whether this is another person or the Divine. In surrender, we allow ourselves to be authentic. Surrender in this understanding increases our power, as, through our openness, we take in more love, more freedom, and ultimately, more God or the Divine. Honesty means letting ourselves be seen and known as we are and receiving another's truth with loving generosity. We are willing to face the truth of ourselves and to share this truth with the other. Although at times fear may tempt us to withhold or hide something about ourselves or our behavior, honesty guides us to trust instead the Love that grounds our relationships and receives all things without judgment. Trust in our own truth and inner knowing and in the love and compassion of the other are essential for intimacy. True intimacy is possible and liberating only if we feel safe, requiring a level of trust within the relationship. Part of this trust is knowing that we are valued by another who does not make judgments about our worth based on his or her needs, expectations, or shoulds. Russell (1998) reminds us that when we judge others, our view of them is being filtered through our concerns for the future or through eyes of the past, and this keeps us from seeing them as they really are in the present moment. The inability to see someone in the present moment impedes the process of developing intimacy.

Feelings of vulnerability and fear limit our willingness to move toward intimacy and the relationships for which we long. The loneliness and isolation that result are associated with suffering and decreased well-being. Experiencing trust and a sense of safety in a relationship increases our willingness to risk vulnerability that can lead to the joy and healing that can come from intimacy. Dean Ornish (1998) notes that communication is essential in the process of choosing in each moment either to keep our hearts open to possibilities of love and intimacy or to close them in the fear that leads to isolation. He discusses the importance of paying attention to what we are feeling and reminds us that expressing our feelings leads to deeper connections than speaking only our thoughts. Thoughts, processed and filtered in the head and largely an intellectual endeavor focusing on the past, offer a different perspective from feelings. Flowing from a deeper heart connection, feelings tend to reflect what is going on with us in the present and reflect our own truth. Recognizing our own feelings and learning to disclose them clearly and directly when appropriate can open the door to communication in which we are able to listen carefully to another's feelings, acknowledging the shared intimacy with compassion, empathy, and caring.

To know and be known as we are means that we do not have to use our energy to erect and protect the masks that keep our essence hidden. Intimacy helps us to remember and experience who we are. A very dear friend once sent me a card with a verse that says, " A friend is one who knows your song, and sings it to you when you forget." I keep this card in a place where I see it daily, to remind me of how important it is to have people in our lives who know us so well that they can call forth our essence even when we have lost sight of it. We see this reflected in a beautiful story told by Jack Kornfield about a way of life within a tribe in Africa that promotes a sense of deep intimacy and belonging:

There is a tribe in east Africa in which the art of true intimacy is fostered even before birth. In this tribe, the birth date of a child is not counted from the day of its physical birth nor even the day of conception, as in other village cultures. For this tribe the birth date comes the first time the child is a thought in its mother's mind. Aware of her intention to conceive a child with a particular father, the mother then goes off to sit alone under a tree. There she sits and listens until she can hear the song of the child that she hopes to conceive. Once she has heard it, she returns to her village and teaches it to the father so that they can sing it together as they make love, inviting the child to join them. After the child is conceived, she sings it to the baby in her womb. Then she teaches it to the old women and midwives of the village, so that throughout the labor and at the miraculous moment of birth itself, the child is greeted with this song. After the birth all the villagers learn the song of their new member and sing it to the child when it falls or hurts itself. It is sung in times of triumph, or in rituals and initiations. This song becomes a part of the marriage ceremony when the child is grown, and at the end of life, his or her loved ones will gather around the deathbed and sing this song for the last time. (Kornfield, 1993, p. 334)

REFLECTION 10–2

- Consider how it would feel to be known and loved from before you were born and throughout your life through the expression of your unique song.

- Who in your life knows your unique "song"?

- When have you experienced the deep intimacy that is more than physical closeness with another? What enabled or supported your process of opening to intimacy?

- What discoveries have you made about yourself through intimacy with others?

- When have your fears kept you from sharing intimacy with another?

- How do you provide a safe space for others to open in intimacy to you?

RELATIONSHIPS AND HEALTH

Exclusion from meaningful relationships renders human life impossible. (Hawkins, 1987, p. 16)

Love, intimacy, and a sense of belonging are manifestations of Spirit; they are also, as Dean Ornish (1998) writes, essential to our health and survival. Close ties with others nourish us spiritually and emotionally, and ultimately support our physical well-being. Ornish discusses a wide range of research regarding the impact of relationships and social support on health. He cites community-based studies conducted in various parts of the United States and Europe suggesting that loving relationships, intimacy with another; social support from family, friends, and other groups; and community ties help us stay healthy and have better outcomes when we do become ill. He cites research indicating that support groups may be particularly beneficial for cancer patients and that people with more developed social ties tend to have less heart disease. Married people tend to live longer than those who are single, separated, divorced, or widowed do. People who are, or perceive themselves to be, socially isolated have an increased risk of dying prematurely. Loving and supportive relationships can help protect against infectious diseases, whereas conflict in relationships can cause the immune system to be less effective. One thing that helps women in abusive relationships find the courage to leave is forming other relationships. Even kindness from strangers is important. The totality of the relationships that touch our lives provide our safety net when we are faced with any crisis or major decision. One woman who finally left a very controlling and abusive marriage of many years stated that the kindness and encouragement of a teacher at her children's school gave her the courage to leave. Connecting with her own inner resources through the support and help that she experienced at the local domestic violence shelter, she has been able to keep from going back to that relationship and to move forward with her life through scary and uncertain times.

When researchers explore the impact of love and support on health, they look at the impact of both the quality and the number of our relationships with others on our health and well-being. To elicit information about the number of social contacts or relationships, researchers ask questions such as "How many people do you meet in an ordinary week?" "How many people do you share common interests with?" "With how many friends and family members can you talk openly? When measuring the quality of relationships, researchers ask people questions about such things as whether they have someone special they can lean on, who feels close to them, who would hold and comfort them, and who they can share feelings with and confide in. Researchers also explore whether there is someone at home who really appreciates what the person does for him or her, or if there is a friend who would drive them to the clinic or hospital if they were ill, someone who would loan them money if they needed it, or who would help care for their children if they were sick (Ornish, 1998). Ornish notes that of ultimate importance is having someone who really cares for us, who loves us and wants to help when needed, and in whom we can confide. He comments that people who feel loved and cared for are more likely to choose life-enhancing rather than self-destructive behaviors, and that those without such relationships have three to five times higher risk of premature death and disease from all causes (p. 28).

REFLECTION 10–3

- Use the questions just described to reflect on the quantity and quality of your own social relationships. *(continued)*

- How do you experience love and care in your relationships? How do you share love and care in relationships?
- How have you experienced the interplay between health and relationships?
- What areas of your relationships might have a negative impact on your health?

Religious Participation and Health

Spiritual and religious communities offer both spiritual and social fellowship and support. Levin's (1994) research suggests that religious participation provides people with a sense of belonging, social support, and fellowship that can buffer adverse effects of stress and anger, and support biological processes that enhance health. Koenig (1999) and Benson (1997) address the influence on health of religious faith and social support experienced within the faith community. Research indicates that religious participation contributes to overall healthier lifestyles and life satisfaction and improves the ability to cope with stress. Religious faith can also contribute to stronger and healthier relationships within families. Religious faith is at the same time personal and communal. Sharing this faith with others is a source of comfort and support and can provide a means of connecting with others at deeper levels of intimacy. Through religious ritual and celebration and through social gatherings people connect with each other at many levels—physically, emotionally, mentally, and spiritually. The interpersonal relationships of religious congregations can extend to other aspects of a person's life as well. Congregations often offer support to people in need, both those within their circles and others in the community.

Perhaps . . . our resources come to us from beyond our lives. They come quietly into our lives through the social relationships, the mutuality and sociality hat constitute the fabric of our lives. Perhaps such sociality and mutuality are in fact the means of God's prevenient grace. (Hawkins, 1987, p. 18)

 SELF-NURTURE: Supporting Your Health Through Relationship

- Make a date to spend some quality time with someone with whom you feel you can be truly who you are, with whom you share love and care.

- Make a conscious effort to express your feelings in communication with others and listen carefully and with compassion to the feelings expressed by others.

- When you are feeling lonely or isolated, contact someone who will be present with you—in person or by phone. This might be a family member, friend, spiritual advisor, counselor, or other caring professional.

- Participate in a group where you experience fellowship, support, and sharing of common values and important areas of your life. This could be a faith community or another group or organization in which you feel your Spirit comes alive.

CREATING COMMUNITY—ALL RELATIONSHIPS ARE SPIRITUAL

. . . we learn from one another how to be human, by identifying ourselves with others or by finding their dilemma in ourselves, and by connecting with the universal human experience. (Watson, 1999, p. 117)

We live our lives within any number of groups or communities, each of which provides a context for our relationships. These groups include family, schoolmates, co-workers, religious or spiritual communities, social and service organizations, clubs and self-help affiliations, health-care settings. Although we tend to think of having our spirituality addressed primarily within religious or spiritual communities, any of these social structures can be a place where spiritual aspirations are mediated. Many people experience spiritual nurture and growth through participation in groups such as Alcoholics or Narcotics Anonymous, support groups focused on particular health concerns, circles of friends who share life concerns, organizations focused on social and ecological issues. For some people, these groups are their spiritual homes. Whether or not they are active in or belong to a particular religious tradition, their connection with others in the group provides a sense of belonging and an opportunity to share their own experiences, struggles, joys, and gifts. Indeed, some people reflect that they experience more of God's presence and connect more with their spiritual nature when involved in groups such as these than they do in traditional religious settings. Even groups that include people whom we do not know, feel little in common with, or perhaps dislike, provide a milieu in which we can deepen our experience of our common humanity. Such groups offer opportunities for us to discover what we have in common with others as we appreciate as well our diversity. When such groups call us to and provide a safe place for deeper levels of sharing from the heart as well as from the head, we have the opportunity to connect with others at the level of spirit.

Spiritual nurture comes both from people with whom we connect on an intermittent basis and from individuals and groups who are part of our daily lives. Some people have a particular gift for maintaining close connections with others over time and distance. I recently had a visit from a friend who maintains ties with people with whom he has lived and worked in several countries across the globe. Although he has not lived here for more than 10 years, and we see each other only every couple of years, there is a sense of continuing closeness. His visits also prompt gatherings of mutual friends whom I see only occasionally, even though we live closer. His regular communications about his life and work with a small community in Central America help keep us connected with him and connect us as well with the people in his village. I feel grateful for people like him in my life who remind me that love and care transcend time and distance and who help me to appreciate the joys and struggles that we share in similar and diverse ways with all people. People like him truly do help connect the world.

Any of our relationships can be spiritually instructive, whether they are with family, friends, neighbors, teachers, students, patients, co-workers, professional colleagues, members of groups to which we belong, or casual acquaintances. We recognize that "we cannot approach God without also approaching our very human brothers and sisters . . . not . . . just a few, carefully selected brothers and sisters who are close spiritual friends . . . [but] the mixed multitude of friends and acquaintances and strangers that we encounter daily" (Hawkins, 1987, p. 39). Relationships provide the milieu in which we live our spirituality, sort of like a laboratory for developing our spiritual awareness and attuning to our deepest values. In our various settings and circumstances we have the opportunity to share times of joy and sorrow, when things are going well and when there is struggle. Spirituality expresses in our experiences of love, anger, patience, frustration, the whole gamut of moods and emotions that come with our relationships. Through these relationships we learn about those times when it is easy to love and what challenges our abilities to be with others in a loving way, what prompts anger and where we respond with patience. We recognize and experience patterns of behavior that we like and those we would prefer to change. In the midst of the many dynamics of our relationships, Spirit prompts us to foster caring connections, even though this is not an easy task. We often find that this "making of relatives," is slow work requiring "not just caring, but the courage to face misunderstandings and emotional struggles—along with whatever else needs to be worked through—in order to grow together over the long term" (Anderson & Hopkins, 1991, p. 222). Whatever the challenges of our relationships, they also are the source of great blessing. Jude Fleming (personal communication, 2000) illustrates this with a personal experience of her transition into a new work setting:

> I left my position in a small rural hospital, a place of comfort and encouragement, took a position in a large city hospital, working in an Emergency

Department/Level II Trauma Center, a very different environment. I did my best to present myself as a holistic nurse, actively taking a role of love, care, and acceptance towards all with whom I practice, but this choice came with a great challenge and a valuable lesson. As my period of orientation was short, I knew I would have to learn much, fast. My new nurse colleagues, the antithesis of those I had left behind, became my very active critics, especially regarding my attempts to calm and soothe terrified patients. Although it was difficult to go to work each day under this scrutiny and criticism, I believed that if I chose to engage in activities of counter assault, I would bring shame to my role. As a holistic nurse, I am called to higher, more gentle ways of being. Thus, I chose to go to work each day filled with the light and focus of Spirit, engaging my gifts and intellect to learn, returning a loving spirit to injustice, and trusting Spirit to handle the details. I knew that I had a choice of how "to be" and a knowing that makes it possible to love. Whenever possible, I suggested that we work to unite the staff with an attitude and energy of mutual caring, support and nurture. Although I believed my choice was right, I would often go home at night saddened, cry and ask for the strength to do it again the next day. Over time there has been a significant change of attitude in our unit. We have identified that this work is very difficult and highly stressful, and that we need to count on and care for each other. New nurses beginning their practice are held and nurtured by many of us who do not want a hostile workplace. I do not see myself as the only change agent, but I do see myself as one who was able to take a challenging situation and turn it to a very positive and powerful lesson for me first and then the department as a whole.

REFLECTION 10–4

Consider how you live your connectedness, your spirituality, within the various contexts or circumstances of your life.

- How do each of your relationships reflect your spiritual self?
- How do you deal with someone who is different from you, or whose personality really irritates you?
- How do you express your care and concern for people in your life?
- In what areas of your life do you feel most spiritually nourished?
- In what settings or situations do you feel you are most able to live the fullest expression of yourself? What supports this in the setting or situation?

(continued)

- In what settings or situations do you feel your spirituality is stifled? What needs to change so you can express your spiritual self more fully there?

Belonging to the Family of Humanity

> *To love is to discover and complete one's self in someone other than oneself, an act impossible of general realization on earth so long as each man [person] can see in his neighbor no more than a closed fragment following its own course through the world. It is precisely this state of isolation that will end if we begin to discover in each other not merely the elements of one and the same thing, but of a single Spirit in search of itself.* (Teilhard de Chardin, 1964, p. 92)

Spirituality is evident in our appreciation of the common bonding we share with all humanity, the sense that we are all connected. There is a sense, as one participant in our research stated, that the "process of us being connected to one another . . . that is spiritual . . . the emphasis on cooperation, connecting ourselves with other people, our common humanity, we all have to take care of ourselves and help each other try to do that." The spirituality that flows from our innermost being is interactive in its manifestation. Spirituality calls us to appreciate the gift of diversity within our common humanity. Recognizing our relationships within a common human family prompts our concern for the well-being of people distant from us, who we do not know personally, as well as for those in our closer circle of relationships. We express spirituality through our loving appreciation and acceptance of others for who they are, regardless of race, religion, nationality, ethnic heritage, sexual orientation, or other things that artificially divide us. In contrast, religious, social, and political structures sometimes emphasize that which separates us, cautioning us to avoid contact with those who are different, and even denouncing certain groups of people and defining them as enemies. Lisa's Story illustrates one person's process of discovering the deeper connection with others members of our common human family.

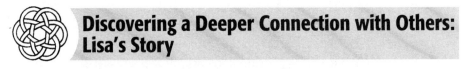

Discovering a Deeper Connection with Others: Lisa's Story

I used to see patients as totally separate from myself. They were people who had problems, and I was the nurse who had answers. Now though, the more I investigate philosophy, the less sense that attitude makes. If we are truly part of a larger whole (the *body of Christ* of the Catholic Church, *collective unconscious* of Jung, *Mind* of Dossey, and *Self* of Wilber), then the dualistic approach doesn't work. I am still my self (to use Wilber's distinction self with a small "s"), and all the boundaries of self apply. Yet at the same time I am part of the Self, the Self which includes all of creation. (A small digression here—Do you think perhaps creation is God's way of self examination? Let us splinter into all these wonderful things so we can look at ourself better?)

So here I am the nurse. I know who I am, I know what I am supposed to do (at least part of the time), yet I am not totally distinct from the patient. A part of me knows that I am part of the Self which this other person is also part of. So I cannot maintain distance, or not care. It would be as if my hand did not care about my foot. In this way I am open to compassion. I used to have pity. "Oh that poor person." Which is actually a condescending attitude. Now I think "so this is what the part of the Self which suffers this way looks like." I wonder what particular fear led this patient to alcoholism, and know that I have fear in me too. I don't condone destructive behavior, I just don't condemn it. I wonder if environmental pollution or some error in genetics led to this person's cancer, and I know that I also live in this environment, I also share the human gene pool. It is not as safe to stand with someone in their suffering, yet that is what compassion calls for. It is much safer to list the ways we are different, and why whatever happened to them could not happen to me. I can no longer maintain this duality. I must stand in compassion, for what happens to my patient, in a very real way happens to me. So much harder, and so much better. How much more so do I feel the being of the human family of which I am a part. So the success of others does not take from my success. I am also in their success. The sorrows of others are part of me, rather than "not my problem." It becomes important to help others be as whole as they may, so we all may be whole. It is also important for me to be as whole as I may be, to do my part well, for me, and for the whole Self. (Lisa Wayman, personal communication, July, 2000).

NURTURING SPIRIT THROUGH SERVICE

> *When people are blessed they discover that their lives matter, that there is something in them worthy of blessing. And when you bless others, you may discover this same thing is true about you. (Remen, 2000, p. 7)*

Many people express their spirituality in service to others. Indeed, connecting with others through altruistic service is an important precept and teaching among spiritual traditions world wide. Within many traditions, we are told to "bear one another's burdens," to care for the widow and orphan, the poor and the sick. We are instructed to honor our parents and elders and to receive the stranger. To "act as if one has no relatives," implying a lack of concern for or assistance to those in need, is a serious breech of traditional Navajo norms. Jesus taught that we serve God by giving food to the hungry, drink to the thirsty, clothes to the naked, and by visiting the prisoner. We hear this same sentiment in the Dalai Lama's address in absentia to the Millennium World Peace Summit (August 20, 2000), reminding us that there can be no world peace as long as poverty, oppression, injustice, and inequality persist. To inspire us to continually reach out to others in need he shared one of his daily prayers, composed by an 11th-century Indian Buddhist master: "for as long as space endures, and for as long as sentient beings remain, until then may I, too, abide to dispel the misery of the world."

Benson (1997) notes that people who help others often report better health and generally feel better than do peers who do not engage in some kind of service to others. In this sense, he suggests that altruism can be a significant way of caring for ourselves. Such service may be to family, friends, or strangers. Walton (1999) discovered that giving of oneself, one's time, energy, and resources to others was an essential component of spirituality among people recovering from a myocardial infarction. We express and nurture our spirituality as we care for the daily needs of family members or when we assist them in times of illness or other special need, when we help a friend pack to move or take time to listen to their joys or concerns, when we volunteer at the local school or serve meals at the homeless shelter, when we offer a kind word to the harried grocery clerk or visit residents of the local nursing home. We pass this heritage of service on to our children by letting them help others with us so that they experience the personal service that connects us person-to-person. When we share genuine presence with another, with its implicit loving honesty and intimacy, we are manifesting our spirituality (McKivergin, 2000; Walton, 1999). Connecting with others through service is a blessing for both of us. Rachel Remen (2000) reminds us that we serve not the weak or the broken but, rather, the wholeness in each other and in life, and in this way, we strengthen the life around us. Noting that we serve through kindness, generosity, compassion, and acceptance, she writes, "the part in you that I serve is the same part that is strengthened in me when I serve. Unlike helping and fixing and rescuing, service is mutual . . . when we offer our blessings generously, the light in the world is strengthened around and in us" (p. 7). Each time we connect with another in a conscious and meaningful way, we share in the life energy that blesses and sustains, the Divine Light expressing in and through us. When we connect with another or others from our spirit, we share in communion, foster community, and help to make Love more manifest in our world.

Linda Noble Topf lives with the illness of multiple sclerosis. In her wonderful book, *You Are Not Your Illness* (1995), she discusses how, for someone who depends on others for many activities of daily living, it is easy to forget the many ways of giving that do not require physical strength and mobility. Her suggestions for giving are worth incorporating into our lives, whether or not we are physically challenged. She writes that we give in the following ways:

- Through caring, sharing, loving; through being a good listener when others close to us want to share their thoughts and feelings.

- By offering little intimacies with those we care about, such as a foot massage, a back rub, telling a joke.

- From the heart by sharing our vulnerabilities and expressing our emotions, through forgiveness of ourselves and others.

- By discovering our own qualities, such as compassion, understanding, courage, perseverance, humor, enthusiasm, gratitude, and joy, and finding ways they can make a positive difference in someone else's life.

- By learning the joy of giving without conditions or attachment, and even the joy of anonymously doing random acts of kindness such as sending flowers to someone who rarely receives acknowledgment (pp. 168–169).

 ## SELF-NURTURE: Serving Others, Serving Life

Choose a way of serving others that reflects the mutuality and blessing of service. You might apply this to situations in which you are already offering the gift of yourself to others, or you might put your time and energy into a new area of service.

- Include at least one area of service in your life, other than your family or work setting, in which you act on the precepts that urge us to care for those in need.

- Cultivate the practice of daily listening to at least one person through your heart to her or his heart.

THE SPIRIT OF RECEIVING

Although we often think of spirituality in terms of what we do for another, we also express our spirituality when we are able to receive from others. Our spirits call us to seek a balance in the give and take of relationships. Loving sexuality is a good example of the mutuality of receiving as we also give; we must open to the other in a receptive way to give of ourselves. We might feel more vulnerable when we are the receivers, yet the willingness to entrust another with our vulnerability is also a gift.

True intimacy with another calls us to receive the wholeness of who the other is, and allow the other to receive our wholeness, warts and all! How often do we hesitate to ask a friend for help or support for fear of being bothersome? Yet inviting friends to assist us or to share our pain, struggles, and concerns gives them the opportunity to share the gift of themselves. Topf (1995) reflects that as we open ourselves to receive, we might consider what we want the giver to experience, such as joy, gratitude, appreciation, and expression of what we are experiencing. She also suggests that we allow ourselves some time to just receive, paying attention to the many ways people gift us, and giving nothing but a thank you in return. During this time, pay attention to how we feel when we receive. Consider how you feel when someone does something nice for you for no particular reason, or when a friend recognizes your need for support and is there for you. As your spirit is nurtured, so is your friend's spirit nourished. Experiencing someone else receiving us helps us open to and receive ourselves. As we receive from another, we acknowledge our interconnectedness, that we are not self-sufficient. We see this in Esber's experience of receiving the prayers of others during his illness:

> Today I want to express a few thoughts about prayer and how much it meant to me during the time of those very critical first three or four months of this illness. When you know people are praying for you, you feel a bit embarrassed and have a feeling of unworthiness. It is like you don't want to impose yourself upon anyone or feel like you have to depend on anyone. But on the other hand, when you hear people are praying for you, it is a very humbling experience. At that time you just don't have the energy or desire to do anything. At first when I heard people saying "we pray for you," I thought it was some cliché. But now in reflection, I see it as one of the greatest sources of energy and empowerment that came to me as a gift between Heaven and earth. The knowledge that all these words and thoughts were offered up on my behalf became overwhelming in a good sense. You recognize your humanity and acknowledge the divine spirit that became a living presence. All those words from the heart from all the people became a gift of blessing and a vital source in recovery and in my "coming back." This coming back is a state of mind that projects a sense of hope. Gracious prayers offered by many people revitalize that feeling of hope. It gives one a perspective of a new tomorrow, while being very much aware of the present. (Tweel, 2000)

REFLECTION 10–5

- How do you connect with others through both giving and receiving? Which feels more clearly a reflection of your spirituality?

(continued)

- In what ways do you feel drawn to give of yourself to others?
- How have you experienced the mutual blessing in giving and in receiving?
- Where do you need better balance in giving and receiving in the many relationships in your life? How can you move toward this balance?

RELATIONSHIPS—OUR MIRROR AND OUR PLAY

All the world's a stage, and all the men and women merely players.
(Shakespeare, As You Like It)

Spirituality is reflected in a recognition that relationships are a source of growth and change. In their own ways, relationships are a path to our self-becoming. Noting that the Sanskrit word *yoga* means union, Russell (1998) speaks of relationships as the yoga of the west. The broadest understanding of a *yoga* is a path to spiritual awakening, any path that leads to union with the cosmos and with one's inner essence. Our relationships become a mirror in which we see ourselves reflected and a play in which we act out the various facets of who we are—both our light and our shadow. Relationships provide an opportunity for us to see our unloving as well as our loving behavior—our shortcomings and limitations in our thinking and behavior as well as our caring and openness. Unloving behaviors often stem from our own fears and insecurities. Cruel words, blame, anger, and resentment can arise particularly when we feel someone is not meeting our needs or expectations. Behaviors that might not be as obviously unloving include hiding thoughts, feelings, and past actions, trying to prove we are better than another, insisting on a particular belief or point of view, manipulating others so they will behave as we wish, saying or agreeing to things we do not believe to win another's approval, or being the way another would like us to be rather than being ourselves (Russell, 1998, p. 100). When we are willing to pay attention to our behaviors and reactions within relationships we can become more aware of our inner fears and vulnerabilities, and see where we continue to be caught in old attachments, patterns, models, and identities. Relationships offer an opportunity to develop mindfulness through which we can use even painful situations as an opportunity for growth.

CONNECTING WITH OUR LINEAGE

Relationships through which we express and experience our spirituality are not limited to those who are living, but extend as well to people no longer embodied on this earth. Maintaining connection with spirits of Ancestors who have died is an essential element of spiritual practice in some cultures. Remembering our lineage need not be limited to those with whom we are related through blood lines. Wise ones and teachers, spiritual guides and mentors, and special friends, all help to shape our lives, and thus become part of our personal lineage. Through acknowledging with gratitude our connection with those who have gone before us, we place ourselves within a vast community extending through time (Anderson & Hopkins, 1991). Brooke Medicine Eagle (1991) reflects that when we experience ourselves as a strong part of community, we recognize that we receive energy and love even from those who do not know us personally. Spiritual elders support and pray for us across generations. The understanding of the communion of saints within the Christian tradition reflects our connection with those who have gone before us. Photographs and things that belonged to loved ones who have died help us continue to feel connected to them. Memories of their presence and how they were with us in life can help to inspire, support, and guide us when we have questions, struggles, and concerns. We see this illustrated in a story of a young boy who had a very special relationship with his grandfather. The two of them enjoyed not only doing things together but also simply being together. This grandfather was a listener as well as a great teller of stories, and in his presence, this young boy felt both listened to and well loved. The boy was as happy as could be when his grandfather would sit in his favorite chair, holding the boy on his knee, and listening to the boy's adventures or telling him stories about the animals and the people who once lived on the land around their farm. These two comrades learned a lot from each other and grew to know each other's hearts in a way beyond words. And so, when the grandfather died, the young boy was quite lonely and sad, for he had lost the person he considered to be his best friend in all the world. Then one day, as he was walking through the house, he passed his grandfather's chair, and a wave of loneliness and missing his grandfather swept over him. But then, he paused and rubbed the wood of the rocker's arm, and then he slipped into the chair and pushed himself back with his feet, settling into the chair. As he sat in that chair, he could feel his grandfather's arms around him. And ever after, he would go to sit in that chair when he needed to know his grandfather's presence . . . to be listened to . . . to hear wisdom . . . to be welcomed. Perhaps even now, as a grown man, he sits in that chair and, like his grandfather before him, holds a child on his knee and listens, and learns, and shares . . . and feels his grandfather's presence still.

FOSTERING CONNECTEDNESS

Being conscious in our relationships is a primary way we integrate spirituality into our lives with people. The very nature of our work as nurses brings us into relationship with people in times of suffering, struggle, and uncertainty, times when people often feel vulnerable and afraid. We also accompany people in times of joy, accomplishments, and through everyday events of life. As noted in Chapter 4, the presence we bring to any of these situations is an important way we express our spirituality. Being fully present and listening with our whole beings helps to create a sacred space in which patients can feel safe in expressing and discussing spiritual matters. Our verbal encouragement can help patients share spiritual concerns. Reflections such as "You said that it is hard to understand why all of this is happening," says that we are willing to hear their deep concerns. Remain present in the silence, if needed, while waiting for the patient's response. Noting observations and recognizing that the person has deep concerns often facilitates sharing.

Cricket Rose (1999) reflects how her roles as nurse and artist have engendered a deeper way of connecting with people. Using baskets as a metaphor for nursing, she illustrated the totality and the simultaneity paradigms of nursing through patterns, colors, and shapes of different baskets. She writes that she has witnessed a transcendence of her practices in both weaving and nursing through her reflection on her beliefs about nursing roles and baskets that represent these roles. "I weave now with more consciousness of the emerging relationships and more questions of their usefulness and meaning to myself and others. I nurse now with the same awareness in consciousness, mindful of the space between my caring and the needs of my patients" (p. 215). In a personal communication (September, 2000) she commented that she finds spiritual expression in her weaving, which, for her, is very much a desire to communicate God's grace and mystery. However, "like putting our words down to try to describe a sunset, weaving only gives a hint of the feelings. If I weave with a purpose or an event or a person in mind, I am inspired to think of all the patterns in our lives and how they interplay. Events, purposes, and people all have revealing sides, like patterns. Weaving to represent someone's life force or gifts means holding their actions in thought while allowing patterns and shapes to emerge from the weaving. Some images are so strong they can only be explained by inspiration, others are intuitive and more representative of the forms and functions the recipients demonstrate to the weaver." We need not be weavers to apply Rose's insights to our relationships with others. Recognizing and affirming the patterns and textures of another's life and how they help to create the uniqueness of this individual fosters our connecting at the deeper levels of spirit.

Attending to spiritual concerns requires a willingness to be present with mystery, uncertainty, pain, or suffering, seeking not to "fix" or to "answer," but to be in the mystery with another. Saying with our whole being and intention that we are willing to stay the course through times of difficulty, pain, and mystery provides encouragement when, ultimately, we can only say, "I don't understand this either." Our presence might help family, friends, and the patient to understand that their presence and expressions of love and care are essential and valuable components of their healing support, even when they feel that there is nothing they can do.

Physical contact or touch in its myriad forms is essential for our survival and an important factor in developing and maintaining relationships. In using touch therapeutically, however, we must be sensitive to the meaning of touch for each person. When used appropriately, gentle touch can establish connection, a handclasp can convey understanding and presence, a hand on the shoulder can provide support, an arm around the waist can literally and figuratively give a lift! One patient described a nurse's supportive touch and presence in saying "When the doctor came in to give me the news, she (the nurse) was standing beside me and I could feel her hand on my arm the whole time he was talking . . . I was so glad that she was just there with me." Esber offers us a very poignant reflection in this regard:

> Over the years I have come across many women from our cancer support group who have stated that at the beginning of their illness there was a feeling of fear from family members and friends to touch them or hug them, as if they had some form of leprosy. The patient, in many cases, feels they are unclean to begin with because of the medication, the taste in their mouth all the time, they even begin to perspire in such a way that the odor and taste seem to exude from their pores. This can leave one in a state of dissociation from themselves as well as others. I have experienced this feeling, not because of people not touching or hugging me, but because of the feeling within myself. Your body identity changes with an illness; you break out in rashes, you begin to feel disgusted with your own appearance, and you become conscious of how other people see you, or what they may be experiencing with odors, looks, and so on. You feel that you become an extension and an expression of "gross anatomy"! This feeling came to me the other day when I was at my massage therapist, and how good it felt having someone massaging my muscles, and having that touch for a brief moment. How important it is to have that touch from another human being who does not have a fear about touching. Being able to overcome our inhibitions to touch those who are sick, to embrace each other, has a healing effect that gives one a sense of acceptability, balance, and compassion . . . St. Francis embraced the leper! Jesus healed the lepers. Did He heal them physically, or did he heal, by his embrace, the emotional, unclean feeling that the leper has for him or herself? (Tweel, 2000)

REFLECTION 10–6

- Consider how you touch patients and others who are sick. What messages do you communicate through your touch?

- How can you incorporate more conscious use of caring touch into your care with patients and families? *(continued)*

> • List three ways you can become more aware of relationships
>   that are important for your patients, and begin to include
>   these more consciously into your care.

Along with being attentive to our relationships with our patients, we address spiritual needs through the ways we acknowledge our awareness and appreciation of important relationships in the patient's life and by integrating these relationships into care. The presence of parents is especially important for children who are hospitalized. For example, four-year-old Sheila clearly stated that her mom and dad being with her when she was in the hospital for her leukemia helped her through the scary treatments such as "the IV's and spinals." Awareness of a patient's significant connections enables us to encourage and seek ways of strengthening meaningful and supportive bonds with these important people. Recently, when a very dear friend was in the hospital for coronary by-pass surgery, I was with her both before and the day of the surgery. When I stopped to see her in the coronary care unit the day after the surgery, the nurse asked if I was family (as only family were allowed to visit). When I hesitated and then said I was a very close friend, he interrupted me, saying, "you are family." This nurse saw beyond the rules to the importance of our relationship and encouraged my visit. We can remind patients of their network of care and support by recognizing and affirming the presence of significant others. "You seem especially close to Marta," might provide an opportunity for sharing about a special relationship and bringing Marta close in thought. Acknowledgments such as "You always seem brighter after a visit from your artist friends," "Your daughter seems like a big help to you," and "I can see you have a very special relationship with your grandson" affirm the value of important relationships and provide an opening for further exploration of these relationships. When people talk about these relationships, they bring the whole power of the relationship to the present; that is, the very act of sharing and affirming the relationship brings the power and meaning of the relationship into the moment. We see this, for example, when faces light up when they mention a favorite grandchild, their spouse of many years, or the dog who has been their constant companion. The thought and mention of the person or pet brings the Presence of the person into that space in a very real way. In healthcare settings, we sometimes find that relationships developed with the receptionist, the cleaning person, and the dietary person become very significant. When considering important relationships we need to be aware of the total web of connections that are supportive.

When we become aware of discordant relationships, we can explore with patients or others how the discord came about and consider both readiness for and ways of beginning the process of healing or reconciliation. We need not try to "fix" the relationship. Rather, when we note that a particular relationship appears troubled and provide an opportunity for the person to process factors contributing to the discord, the person will often come up with his or her own insights or plans. Patients might have difficulty expressing their deeper concerns, even when they very much want to let others know what is going on with them. We can offer our assistance as they seek to share some aspects of their situation. Questions such as "What would you like to say to her?" or "How much information or detail about your condition do you think he can handle?" or "How do you think you would feel or respond if she walked into the room right now?" can help them find and rehearse the words they want to say. Offering to be with them as a resource and support is another way of fostering their important connections. For some people, visits from pets might be as spiritually uplifting as those from human companions! Have you ever included pets as visitors officially or unofficially? Recognizing the healing benefits of animals, many long-term care facilities and pediatric units are beginning to include pet therapy as routine practices.

Photos, artwork, and other memorabilia of loved ones, including pets, provide reminders of connections beyond the confines of illness or injury. We can help people connect with important places, people, and experiences through imagery, pictures, and stories. Asking about the people in a photo or the story behind a picture or special object acknowledges and provides the chance to learn more about the significance of particular relationships. "What was it like on your first date?" provides an opening for a woman to share happy memories about her dying husband. "Describe your favorite place on your farm" allows a man to speak of how his spirit is nurtured through his life in nature. As we learn to understand the relationships and connections that frame a patient's life, we begin to be more aware of recurring themes and concerns. When such themes are noted, we can reflect on and validate them with the patient. Statements such as "It seems I have often heard you speak of. . . . with great concern," give the patient the opportunity to know our perceptions and to validate or correct them. Most often, it is reassuring to the patient to know that we are indeed listening and responding to their deep concerns.

Family members sometimes feel awkward and uncertain about how to be with a loved one who is sick or hospitalized. They might need our encouragement and guidance in visiting and calling. We might need to encourage families and friends to share physical expressions of care and concern in the sometimes-intimidating environments of our health care institutions. We can guide and encourage them with statements such as "It's okay to hold her hand, you won't interfere with the tubes." "He mentioned that you give a wonderful back rub, would you like to give him one today?" "She seems to know when you are here and holding her hand." "I can show you how to massage her feet." "Would you like to brush her hair?" We need to recognize differences in our comfort with touch and the conditions in which we may want to share touch. Awareness of our own feelings about and comfort with touch help in assessing the place and potential use of touch in the patient's situation. When words cannot be found, or in circumstances where persons are more comfortable with physical expression than with words, touch can be a powerful expression of spirit and an instrument of healing.

Whether sick or well, people are part of family, society, and world. When we are ill, contact with persons from religious, social, business, neighborhood, school, hobby or interest groups remind us of our connections with and participation in the larger community and world. If our participation in these groups is a source of stress, reminders of these connections might not be particularly healing, however! The atmosphere of some health-care settings, such as intensive care, long-term care, chemotherapy, and dialysis units, potentiates the development of bonds of mutual caring among various patients, families, and caregivers. I recently observed and felt the bonds that developed among people in the coronary-care unit waiting area at a large urban hospital. People would reach out to others in many ways. When someone would get news, others shared their happiness or concern. Food served as a way to connect. One man brought donuts to share, saying that he remembered being hungry as he waited during a similar experience. The networks of support that arise can become very significant in the lives of all those involved. Recognizing the healing potential in such relationships, nurses can actively foster their development through actions such as introducing patients and family members to each other, asking someone who has been in the setting longer to help the newer person find their way around, and facilitating sharing of experiences among patients who are undergoing a particular procedure. Whatever ways we can help patients and families to feel connected rather than isolated supports the health, healing, and spirituality of all concerned.

REFERENCES

Anderson, S. R., & Hopkins, P. (1991). *The feminine face of God.* New York: Bantam Books.

Benson, H. (1997). *Timeless healing: The power and biology of belief.* New York: Simon & Schuster.

Buber, M. (1958). *I and Thou.* (R. G. Smith, Trans). New York: Charles Scribner's Sons.

Fields, R., Taylor, P., Weyler, R., & Ingrasci, R. (1984). *Chop wood, carry water.* Los Angeles, CA: Jeremy P. Tarcher.

Hawkins, T. R. (1987). *Sharing the search: A theology of Christian hospitality.* Nashville, TN: Upper Room.

Koenig, H. G. (1999). *The healing power of faith.* New York: Simon & Schuster.

Kornfield, L. (1993). *A path with heart.* New York: Bantam Books.

Levin, J. S. (1994). Religion and health: Is there an association, is it valid, and is it causal? *Social Science and Medicine, 38,* 1475–1482.

McKivergin, M. (2000). The nurse as an instrument of healing. In B. M. Dossey, L. Keegan, & C. E. Guzzetta (Eds.). *Holistic nursing: A handbook for practice* (pp. 207–228). Gaithersburg, MD: Aspen.

Medicine Eagle, B. (1991). *Buffalo woman comes singing.* New York: Ballantine Books.

Ornish, D. (1998). *Love & Survival.* New York: Harper Perennial.

Ray, S. (1980). *Loving relationships.* Berkeley, CA: Celestial Arts.

Remen, R. N. (2000). *My grandfather's blessings.* New York: Riverhead Books.

Rose, B. H. (1999). A basket metaphor for nursing. *Journal of Holistic Nursing, 17*(2), 208–217.

Russell, P. (1998). *Waking up in time.* Novato, CA: Origin Press.

Teilhard de Chardin, P. (1960). *The Divine milieu.* New York: Harper & Brothers.

Teilhard de Chardin, P. (1964). *The future of man.* New York: Harper & Row.

Topf, L. N. (1995). *You are not your illness.* New York: Simon & Schuster.

Tutu, D. (1995). *An African prayer book.* New York: Doubleday.

Tweel, E. N. (2000). *Unpublished personal journal of illness experience.* Charleston, WV.

Walton, J. (1996). Spiritual relationships: A Concept Analysis. *Journal of Holistic Nursing, 14* (3), 237–250.

Walton, J. (1999). Spirituality of patients recovering from an acute myocardial infarction, *Journal of Holistic Nursing, 17*(1), 34–53.

Watson, J. (1999). *Postmodern nursing and beyond.* Edinburgh, Scotland: Churchill Livingstone.

Sandra Melville's Story

Sandra Melville, who lives in the Boston area, is no longer able to practice as a nurse because of her *Uninvited Guest*. She shares her experience of living with a chronic and debilitating illness, reflecting the prime importance of the caring and support from others in this journey. In a personal communication, she spoke of the identity change required as the disease has become part of her and her family, and how she has had to learn to give herself permission to make the needed changes, and to take care of herself without feeling guilty. As she daily embraces the mystery of living with this *Uninvited Guest*, she reflects that it is not the ending of one's path that is important, but how you make the journey that is the issue. She says, "The Journey is All." (Story copyright Sandra Bauer Melville, MSN, RN-C, reprinted with permission of the author.)

THE UNINVITED GUEST

One never plans to be a patient. One takes care of patients. Throughout a long and varied nursing career, I'd never planned to be on the other end of the stethoscope. But here I am, and the irony is not lost on me. I now pour more pills for myself to take in a day than I used to for 6 patients in the CCU. I'm on a first-name basis with the pharmacist, and I have the longest medication list of any of my primary care physician's patients. I use the skill and experience that used to enable me to find veins in the critically ill to enable the home health care nurses to find veins in me. When I'm admitted to the hospital for one of my periodic visits, I bring my medications from home and a medication list. Yes, I'm one of those patients, the one who comes complete with charts and graphs because we're trying to figure out how to live with this illness that has entered our lives, this Uninvited Guest that has come to stay.

I have a disorder called transverse myelitis (TM). You might think of it as "single sclerosis," or MS of the spinal cord, for it is a demyelinating disorder similar to multiple sclerosis, only usually occurring in a single lesion somewhere along the spinal cord. It is a rare disorder, occurring in three to five per million of the population. I suppose if one has to be ill, one might as well have a rare disorder. It crept upon me slowly, starting with some numbness of the fingertips, progressing over a period of days to weeks up the arm, gradually becoming bilateral. As a busy nurse practitioner, wife, and mother, I didn't pay too much attention to it. When it persisted, I consulted with a friend neurologist, and as it was unilateral at the time, we thought it might be a brachial plexus injury. When it became bilateral, and more severe, I was ultimately diagnosed with TM. (The story of reaching that diagnosis, and the need to become an educated consumer, I may tell another time.) One spinal tap, two MRI's, three grams of SoluMedrol later, and I was home to begin to negotiate what my relationship would be with this new entity in my life.

You may have heard the expression "a person living with AIDS." I now became a person living with transverse myelitis, and it almost seemed to be a person itself. There were several facets to it. One was the pain and sensory changes. These varied on a day-to-day and sometimes hour-to-hour basis. The freezing, numb, deep-sunburn type discomfort came and went, worse with increased activity, fatigue, stress, and weather changes. I woke in the morning, almost pain free, just a little drumming in the hands, and would wonder what the day would be like. Would this new entity be kind and quiet today, so that I might accomplish a day's work? Or would it be hateful and mean, driving me to take medications and lie still, waiting for it to settle?

Another aspect was the fatigue. Stress, heat, lack of sleep, all would bring on this bone-wrenching tiredness. I had no choice but to become horizontal, and be grateful that my children were no longer toddlers but now able to amuse themselves. A morning of driving my children to swimming lessons, picking up the groceries and fixing lunch now exhausted me. I applied to myself those things I had used with my patients. I had taught my cardiac rehabilitation patients pacing of activities. Now I used those principles myself. I had only so many "coins of energy" to spend, and I would spend them wisely. Still, some days I might feel almost normal. What would the Uninvited Guest bring today?

In many ways, it was like the relationship one has with a new lover. One is very focused on the moods and changes of the other one. One learns how to bring out the best in the mutual relationship. One learns as much as one can about the other. I had no old yearbooks, but medical texts and the Internet provided information. One might chat up the other's friends to get a more rounded view; I found an Internet chat group of fellow TMers. I found myself wanting to tell my friends about this new entity in my life, thinking it might be as important to them as it was to me.

Through this, I was always the nurse. Isn't it interesting, I'd think, how the nervous system reacts? Anti-convulsants and anti-depressants for the pain—how fascinating that they work this way. Medication schedules adjusting to give me the "best" times during family hours. Balancing fluid intake to maintain blood pressure and avoid incontinence during social events. Consulting with the neurologist to determine how to treat this Guest that not only was staying, but that refused to settle into a routine.

The Guest invited another guest—sympathotonic orthostatic hypotension. An even rarer disorder, also in the autoimmune family. (I had a passing thought about what other members from that family might come, but didn't stay there). Now I had no choice, I had to go to the hospital.

Nurses there were busy, short staffed with critically ill patients on the floor. I wasn't ill—as long as I was flat, I was cheerful, looked normal. It was only when I stood up, and my blood pressure became unobtainable, that I looked as if I belonged. So I stayed in bed, and mostly saw aides except at pill times. Still, some of the nurses, even though busy, took a moment to chat, came in my room to chart. I felt less alone, distracted for a time from the ever-present Guest.

In the work-up, it was discovered that I had an unstable C-spine, requiring immediate surgery. Bear in mind, my hands don't work well; and surgery aggravates the condition. I awoke in considerable pain, and a nurse bustled up. "Now dear, you have this PCA pump. Just press this button and it'll give you some pain medicine." "I'm sorry," I croaked, hoarse from the intubation and extubation. "My hands don't work, I had this surgery, I can't press the button." "Oh," she said, "well, we'll just put it in the other hand." "No, I'm sorry," I rasped, barely able to manage a whisper. "The other hand doesn't work either." "Oh," she said temporarily defeated. Then she brightened. "Well," she beamed, gesturing to the nurses' station, surrounded by a cacophony of critical care noises. "You just yell out, and one of us will come push the button!"

I was soon out of critical care, and had IV's out; but the pain and that Guest acting up prevented me from getting enough oral fluids. I was dry, and I knew it. I told the surgeon I needed an IV, and he agreed. He left to write for it, then popped his head around the corner. "What do they usually give you, and how fast?"

That night the IV was feeling funny, and I asked the nurse to check it. "I don't know what you're worried about; you don't need the IV anyway." It was too much. The Uninvited Guest had been niggling and naggling all this time; and I'd rarely given in . . . but this was too much. I started to cry.

Another nurse came in to look at the IV. She flipped on the light, took in the tears leaking from my eyes, and sniffed, "I don't know what you're so upset about. You have nothing to cry about!" Nothing to cry about! The Guest laughed. I cried.

I escaped the mercies of that pair, and eventually went home. I was encased in that medieval torture instrument, the cervical collar. The home-care nurses were nice, professional, generally young. We worked together well. The one who stands out, though, was a little older. She plumped my pillow, got a cloth for my brow, opened the collar to cool my neck, gently touched my shoulder with one hand while taking my pulse with the other. It didn't take any longer. She did all the high tech things the others did, with a practiced hand. She also remembered high touch, the nonspoken but essential part of nursing.

The Guest is still here, uninvited, moved in. We have our routine. I like to think I have things in balance. The Guest goes with me though, always with me, and always has to be dealt with, always tugging on my elbow. As a nurse, I was confident of my ability to provide quality compassionate care for individuals with chronic illnesses, individuals who struggle with uninvited guests for control over their lives. As a patient, I realize how much more there is to understand.

CHAPTER 11

The Power of Story

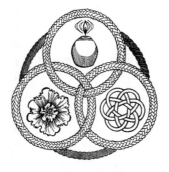

The people who come to see us bring us their stories.

They hope they tell them well enough

so that we understand the truth of their lives.

They hope we know how to interpret their stories correctly.

We have to remember that what we hear is their story.

COLES, 1989, P. 7

Story is defined as a narrative, either true or fictitious, in prose or verse, designed to interest, amuse, or instruct the hearer or reader, a tale (*The Random House Dictionary,* 1987, p. 1879). And, as Lawlis (1995, p. 40) reminds us "storytelling, an art founded in the beginning of human history, has been a central feature in the transfer of important and critical forms of information from one generation to the next." Consideration of story's place in the art and science of nursing is reflected in nursing and health-care literature (Boykin & Schoenhofer, 1991; Kiser-Larson, 2000; Lawlis, 1995; Liehr & Smith, 2000; Martin, 1999; Nagai-Jacobson & Burkhardt, 1996; Sandelowski, 1991, 1994; Sherwood,

295

2000a; Wagner, 1999, 2000; Wilson, 2000). Sherwood (2000b) addresses the significance of story by calling attention to the presence of story in all cultures as a way to exchange knowledge and information, as well as to entertain. She states,

> Story is comprised of experiences that are significant to the person, that define who one is. People connect through shared story in a powerful interaction that communicates relationships, transmits culture, socializes a new generation, and communicates expectations. Reflections on story help us understand how to live and discover meaning. The use of story is consistent with the quest for quality of experience and healing in health care institutions to offer balance to high technology.

STORY AS VESSEL FOR THE SPIRITUAL

Nurses often feel the conflict inherent in being asked to give "personalized" care while fitting patients into various systems of coding and grouping that seem designed to decrease the individuality and uniqueness of each patient. Sherwood's comments alert us to the potential power of recognizing each person as a story in progress and thereby gaining an appreciation for the other's uniqueness as well as a clearer understanding of the context for the present experience that we share. Sandelowski (1994, p. 25) asserts that story enables the listener to discover "critical sources of information about etiology, diagnosis, treatment and prognosis from the patient's point of view." In the process of telling and hearing stories, persons often come to new insights and deeper understandings of themselves because stories include not only events in our lives but also the meanings and interpretations that define the significance of the events for particular lives.

Sachs (1987) reminds us that what makes us unique is not so much biological makeup as our narrative or story, which is always and often unconsciously evolving. As nurses well know, five women with the diagnosis of breast cancer will have five different stories about the meaning of the illness in their lives, five different narratives unfolding. In breast cancer survivor groups, the participants share stories that contain both threads of their common experience and reactions as well as highly individual responses and experiences. In our research studies regarding spirituality and health, we found that participants very often told stories and shared anecdotes from their lives to convey their understandings and experiences of spirituality. Stories are a natural way to communicate and nurses in any health-care arena are presented with stories. Kindig (1997, p. 12) quotes novelist James Carroll as saying, "We tell stories because we can't help it." One frustration for health-care providers who are seeking answers to questions on an information form is that persons often respond to such questions as "What brings you to the hospital?" by telling a longer-than-time-allows story of all that led up to this hospitalization. As one novice nurse said, "Where do I put all that other information she gave me. . . . I know it's really important, but I'm not sure for what."

Persons tell us these stories and anecdotes in the hope that we will better understand their particular life situations, they want us to see "the whole story." Hearing the story, the nurse might indeed gain a clearer understanding of the answer to the particular question and, perhaps more significantly, a richer understanding of the person who is answering the question. A sometimes-quoted bit of advice for medical and nursing students urges them to get to know not only the disease the patient has but also the patient who has the disease. As patients tell their stories they sometimes begin to understand themselves in a new way in the context of their larger story and are able to move into the future in ways that are congruent with and affirming of their wholeness. Stories thus become instruments of healing and wholeness. In sharing her experience of breast cancer and its impact on her life, Penny described herself as coming into her own authentic relationship with God, contrasted with "the one I had grown up with that really belonged to my family and was kind of passed on to me." This authentic relationship involved expressions of anger and rage, hurt and frustration as she literally shook her fist at God and sometimes used language that "wasn't pretty." Along the way, she experienced "a white light . . . the peace that passes all understanding . . . that is with me to this day." Hearing her story gives us a glimpse into her wholeness, her healing journey.

Part of the art of human caring is recognizing and facilitating the opportunity for encountering story, recognizing the potential for healing that is a part of sharing stories. Understanding all persons, including ourselves, as ongoing and unfolding stories offers nurses a valuable perspective from which to approach spiritual caregiving. Spirituality is multidimensional, reflecting the depth, breadth, and complexity of a person's being, and embracing that person's connections with God or Sacred Source, the earth, other persons, and the self. Story and metaphor often provide a language and form for conveying the richness of our spirituality when factual statements of experience fail to do so. Hearing Floyd describe his "wrestling with God on my couch . . . we really wrestle with this thing. I mean real *contact*" offers insight into his "up close and personal" relationship with God. Wrestling, unlike boxing, is a form of struggle that means being engaged with our whole body in a way that does not allow much "backing off." In the midst of his life with cancer, Floyd's language tells us that he is in a relationship with God that is "real tight." Stories give us insight, bring us enjoyment, teach us to solve problems, help us understand and form identity, and are wonderful teachers. Stories can be heard when a lecture falls on deaf ears.

Bruchac (1997, p. xi) states, "Few things have helped me understand the world better than a good story." As nurses, we might say that few things have helped us understand patients better than their stories. Few things help us understand ourselves as well as reflection on our own stories. Through the vehicle of story, we learn to know others and ourselves from many perspectives as human beings who experience relationships, emotions, conflicts, and struggles and whose responses are at once both personal and universal. From such a vantage point, we listen in new ways, being open to that which the patient wants to share as well as that which is requested on the information form. As nurses we, too, are formed and informed by our life stories. An awareness of our own life stories deepens the awareness with which we listen to another's story, for we are aware of the influence of the listener on the receiving of the story. For a time, however brief, nurses become a part of the stories of their patients. As Kindig reflects,

> Storytelling is a monumental act. In its finest hour, it becomes a psalm of praise and thanksgiving for the love and connection of family. No one else can tell your stories. . . . The stories you tell bind you close to one another, yet they give you wings to fly out confidently into the larger world. They teach you how the world works and where you belong in it. But most of all, they open the door to that holy and magnificent place where heaven and earth converge and time hangs in sweet suspension, if only for a moment . . . (1997, p. 2)

REFLECTION 11–1

- What are your memories of story in your life? Was yours a story-telling family? When did you hear stories? Are there family stories that are shared among family and passed down through generations?

- What is the place of story in your life today? When did you last hear or share a story? What was the story? Recall it again.

- Remember stories you have shared in your professional life. With whom did you share and what prompted the sharing? What was the experience like?

LISTENING FOR AND BEING WITH SACRED STORY

Sherwood (2000a, p. 159) observes that although there is a growing recognition of the positive influence of a strong, well-based spirituality on health and well-being, health-care systems often challenge rather than support or reinforce the personal connections that are the basis of holistic care that embraces the whole person as spiritual being. From her study of the experience of spirituality in nurse-client interactions, Sherwood relates the essential truth for caring practice, in the words of study participants: "When caregivers are willing to listen, clients share their innermost selves" (Sherwood, 2000a, p. 170).

Story brings us face to face with quandaries, insights, struggles, joy, suffering, pain, and healing moments. Stories may make us feel helpless in the face of perceived hopeless situations. Stories may also help us recognize the hope that lies in such a situation. Stories challenge nurses to understand the wholeness of a person, to listen for the meaning of a life. One nurse commented, "I used to think that people who told me stories about their lives were just wasting my time and theirs, but now I realize that they are telling me about what is really important. I've learned to listen and to use what they say to help them see who they really are, what they can really do. Even when they tell me things that are really hard to hear, or even to understand, it seems like they just want me to know that it is part of their life too." Stories are a way of helping nursing process fit the patient rather than requiring that the patient fit the process. As we listen to stories, we seek to be able to hear, to hold that which we hear in awareness without drawing premature conclusions, and to remember that the meanings of stories evolve over time and can change with reflection and retelling.

Kindig (1997) defines sacred stories as any story that redeems and affirms us. Affirmation and redemption are found not only in the extraordinary but in the ordinary as well. For the nurse who is able to see and hear the sacred in every person, extraordinary moments fill the days as she recognizes courage, love, perseverance, faith, mercy, kindness, and grace in the lives of persons around her. She hears with compassion the bitterness of a woman twisted by arthritis who says, "You nurses are always talking about how brave that lady with cancer is, but, to you I'm just a crabby old woman with arthritis. I don't think you know what it's like to hurt all the time and know you probably won't die!" And, listening to the words beneath the words, the nurse hears an invitation into the story of the woman whose angry accusation might turn another away.

> *Answer, if you hear the words under the words—*
> *otherwise it is just a world with a lot of rough edges,*
> *difficult to get through, and our pockets full of stones. (Nye, 1995, p. 37)*

THE *PERSON* OF THE STORY

The whole-person to whole-person relationship expands the horizons of the nurse-patient relationship beyond the immediate health problem to include the meaning and impact of these events in a person's life. The nurse is with the patient as troublesome questions surface: Will I be stuck here all my life? What if I can never walk again? Should I call my son who hasn't talked to me for years? Coker (1998) addresses the concept of personhood saying, "within the heart of every individual lives the most desired of needs—to be recognized as a person" (p. 435). She describes personhood as a process rather than as a product and differentiates between *person* and *personhood.* Coker describes person as the incorporation of body, mind and spirit of an individual that defines one's essence. Personhood, in this understanding, refers to the continuing development toward self-actualization by our total being in spiritual, sociological, psychological, and physical dimensions. Although Coker's research focused on older persons in a residential-care unit, the factors that she identifies as influencing personhood apply to all persons: historical perspective, the culture, value system, education, family and life experiences, relationships, and movement toward self-concept and self-esteem. Story is a valuable means of understanding and relating to our personhood, this multidimensional, whole-person ever becoming.

 ## SELF-NURTURE: Attending to a Special Story

Is there a story (it may be in the form of a poem, movie, painting, or memory) that is for you a sacred story, one that affirms or illuminates your life? Take time with that story and reflect on its meaning for you in this time of your life. What is the message of this story for you?

Bruchac (1997) says that stories can help us find our way home. Madeleine L'Engle (1993), in her book *The Rock That Is Higher—Story As Truth,* titles her first chapter "Story As Homecoming" and shares the experience of finding that familiar Biblical stories sustained her in the long and difficult recuperation after a serious automobile accident. She describes her discovery that the stories of Samuel, David, and Jesus the Christ offered "life-giving, life-saving . . . story that transcends facts" (p. 20).

Going to my first meeting as a facilitator for a Parents Anonymous meeting, I was anxious and wondered if anyone was going to show up, what they would be like, and whether "facilitating the meeting," which had sounded so simple when I had agreed to take on this responsibility, was going to be something I could do in any helpful way. My memory of that night and what followed have become one of my stories of redemption and affirmation. That night two young women came and shared their fears and pain, trusting, perhaps in desperation, that somehow they would be heard. They shared their fears of coming to a meeting that so openly acknowledged a part of themselves that they feared, even hated, this sometimes uncontrollable anger directed at their young children. Somehow, as they shared their painful stories, what I heard was courage. I found myself moved by the courage of these young women, walking into this unknown place, with unknown people, to share what one woman called "such an awful, ugly part of me."

In the months to come, I witnessed the power of relationships in the lives of these women as slowly, but surely, they involved more people in the stories of their lives, sought help and made difficult but necessary changes. They told and retold stories of their journey and listened well to one another. By the manner of their sharing, their honesty, and their open-hearted listening, they created sacred space from which to live and grow. And, I experienced the power of shared story to affirm and redeem and to help people move into the future in new ways as they envisioned a better future for themselves. There were no "perfect endings" but, rather, the ongoing choice to make the future better than the past. In describing her experience in Parents Anonymous, one of the women said, "Because some of you could hear my story and not turn away I thought that maybe God wasn't going to turn me away either." And, today, when I receive a photo of this woman's first grandchild, held in the arms of smiling parents (my friend's daughter and son-in-law) and a letter expressing her delight in this child and her deep gratitude that the cycle of abuse and fear are broken, I share my friend's joy. And, because we have shared much of her journey from that first Parents Anonymous meeting, through many seasons of challenge and change as she continues her healing and yet is ever whole, my mind and heart have been stretched and challenged and I, too, am forever changed. As Sherwood (2000a, p. 160) reminds us, caregiving encounters affect both nurse and client, especially the nurse's own spirituality.

JOURNEYING WITH MYSTERY

The world is very mysterious. It is full of paradoxes and unfinished stories. Many of us try to avoid these paradoxes and finish the stories. Only a few step deliberately into this mystery. . . . (Sullivan, 1991, p. 5).

As nurses seeking to care for persons as whole beings, spiritual beings, we are often called to step into the mystery and the unknown with our patients. Although our natural inclination is often to try to "make things better" or "fix" the problematic situation, the spiritual journey by definition leads into the unknown. A story told in the present, in the "eternal now," brings to its telling influences from the past in hopes of understanding more deeply the present moment. The word "mystery" has been described as truth that we do not yet understand. In the mystery of the present moment we seek to find the truth of our lives.

Being willing to hear stories of pain and mystery when the nurse can offer only her presence is an important part of holistic care. Bearing witness to stories in which pain and suffering are dominant themes is aided by a sense of our own connection to the Mystery beyond all mysteries. Nursing gives us the opportunity to explore that terrain, the terrain of mystery beyond human understanding and the One who holds even that. The need to articulate, to give voice and meaning to those happenings which batter our souls and psyches, numb our bodies, and break our hearts, is what sends us to a trusted friend, a therapist, a minister, a mentor, or prayer. It is as though at some basic level we understand that to begin healing we need that listener who will help us begin the process of healing. In some situations, the nurse is that first listener, the first to hear the halting words of pain and confusion, anger and hurt in an experience that is becoming a part of one's life story. Some stories will need to be told over and over again, and in the process they might become not only the patient's story, but the family's story and the staff's story as well.

Jean Watson (1999) shared some of the mystery and the meaning of her story at the American Holistic Nurses Association conference. These reflections are hers as she journeys with mystery through a time of tragedy, anguish, and deep physical, psychological, and spiritual pain. As you read some of the words she spoke, take time to take them into yourself . . . hear her story and let it touch your own. Listen for your story in her story, which she offers as a gift. " . . . I live in darkness, yet I experience light; I know fear, yet I dwell in love; I know terror and life's horrors, yet I glimpse joy; I know despair, yet I live in hope; I know doubt, but I reside in faith; I live with and witness suffering for myself and my loved ones, and I learn about deep healing from the inside out; I lose my balance, yet I dance; I have been asked to bear the unbearable as one of my life's journeys."

REFLECTION 11–2

- Slowly re-read Jean Watson's words, taking time to hear each word and feel the emotion behind the word. Describe your connection or disconnection with these words—what is the experience of taking in her words like for you?

- Think about what the word *mystery* means to you—what thoughts, feelings, and images do you associate with *mystery*?

- How is mystery present in your life today? Paradoxes? Questions? Wonderings?

- Reflect on a time when you "stepped into the mystery."

LISTENING FOR AND HEARING OUR OWN STORIES

Remember, what you are hearing (from the patients) is to some considerable extent a function of you, hearing. (Coles, 1989, p. 15)

Just as caring for another's spirit requires caring for our own spirits, so does hearing another's story require grounding in our own stories. As our own lives and stories evolve, so does our hearing of the stories of others change. Picard (1991) notes that as nurses we bring both personal and professional experiences into each encounter. The person-nurse we are today brings a wealth of personal and professional experience to each encounter today; and, the experiences of today will be a part of tomorrow's person. As we are changed by internal and external experience, so does the way we listen to and hear others change.

REFLECTION 11-3

- What are your first memories of yourself? Your family? What stands out for you?

- What led you to become a nurse? What were your feelings about being a nurse?

- What are some of your roles in life other than that of nurse?

- Think about your first days as a practicing nurse. What words or phrases would you use to describe yourself at that time?

- Do you remember particular patients and families from your early days as a nurse? If so, what made them memorable for you?

- Think of experiences that brought you satisfaction. Why were those particular experiences satisfying to you?

- Can you recall an experience that troubled or still troubles you? What was the nature of the experience and why did it or does it trouble you?

- Now take time to think about yourself today. If you draw a timeline of your life, what are some of the major events and how have they influenced you? How would you describe the growth and changes in yourself over the course of your story? Who have been, and are, the major players in your life story? What are your major satisfactions? Disappointments? Plans and hopes for the future? Fears? What words and phrases describe you today?

As we grow in appreciation of ourselves as those who will be hearing stories, we are better able to listen with an awareness of how the person who is hearing the story influences its telling and the way it is received An awareness of ourselves as listeners is an important part of the process of sharing story. How ready am I to listen at this time? What obstacles to my being fully present and listening exist? Am I in a hurry? Distracted? Annoyed? Is my previous contact with this patient and family a hindrance to my listening with an open mind and heart? Have I categorized this patient or family in a way that limits my hearing? What can I do to be fully present with this person at this time?

Understanding our own story is surely the work of a lifetime. Some exercises that can facilitate this process are included in Figure 11–1. Bruchac (1997) refers to our storytelling roots and says that each of us has four roots that tell us who we are, where we came from, and how our lives came to be as they are: *our ancestry, our families, our homes, our own lives.* He urges us to identify and nurture these roots so that our storytelling tree will grow stronger. Each of these four roots is a

---

Exercises to Facilitate Awareness of Story

1. Take a few moments to become quiet, perhaps using some breath awareness. In this quiet space, allow yourself to remember, in as much detail as possible, something about yourself, some event or incident that comes to mind. How has this experience or event become a part of who you are? What meaning does it have for your life at this moment?

2. Keep a journal in which you record events, feelings, experiences, insights, and questions in your life. Periodically review your writings, noting themes flowing through your story. Reflect on your story as it is evolving.

3. Think about books, stories, songs, fairy tales, movies, plays, or works of art that have special meaning for you. Take time to consider why and how they hold that meaning for you. Think about the images, characters, colors, and sounds that are found in each of these and how they are reflective of your own story. What meanings do you find that provide insight into your own unfolding journey?

4. Write an autobiography for your eyes only. Take your time. Re-read and reflect on it. Are there parts you want to share? With whom would you share? What new awarenesses and learnings have come to you?

5. Look at some old family photos or photos of friends. What story do they tell? What memories and feelings come with these pictures? Do you want to tell someone else about them? What do you want to say? Would you like to hear someone else's story about these same photos?

Source: M. Burkhardt and M. G. Nagai-Jacobson, copyright 1997.

Figure 11–1

fertile field of potential information. As Bruchac reminds us, we all have ancestors and each ancestry we have is a source of stories and cultural traditions (pp. 6–9). What are some of the songs, proverbs, and folk tales from your ancestry? For one of us, Japanese fairytales give a glimpse into our ancestry. For the other, marrying a man of Jewish heritage has been an opportunity to hear and learn from stories in the Jewish tradition.

Our families have many configurations—biological, adopted, step-families, and blended families. Lost in the more mobile society where families less often share households or even neighborhoods are some of the day-in-day-out opportunities to hear stories from aunts, uncles, grandparents, and family friends. Bruchac (1997) points out that names have special meanings in every culture and that name stories are one example of family story. Some names are given and others are earned. People tell stories about the meaning of their names, the names' influence on their self-concepts, and about choosing to change a name or be called by a different name. "When I went to college I decided I wasn't going to be Cathy, which made me feel like a little girl; but I would be Catherine, which sounded grown up. Somehow, just being called Catherine made me feel older, more capable. I grew into that name and it really helped me, a small town girl, make the transition from high school to college," is how one friend expressed the power of choosing to be called by another name.

REFLECTION 11–4

- Consider your family, its history, your place in it, the connections and disconnections, its place in the community, its struggles, and its triumphs.

- What might your family motto be?

- What are some of the values, attitudes, skills, and traditions that have shaped you? How do you see them influence your every day life? Your practice of nursing?

- How did your family get its name and what does it mean?

- What name stories are in your family?

- Who are the story bearers in your family and when have you last listened to or told a family story?

- Think about your name. How did you get your name and what does it mean? How do you feel about your name? What is its significance to you?

SELF-NURTURE: My Story and its Messages

- Give yourself some time to reflect again on your story. Write about those persons who have encouraged you, whose presence has brought affirmation, joy, courage, strength, wisdom. Listen again to their messages for your life. You might want to write or call these people and share your reflections.
- Expand your awareness of your own story through the exercises included in Figure 11–1.

HOME STORIES

Our homes have special significance in our lives, and many stories are connected to them. Our city, town, community, and house are all potential sources of stories to inform us about ourselves and where we are in the world. West Virginians hear and tell the stories of John Henry, the Hatfields and McCoys, and the uncertain life of working in the coal mines, as a part of their story. When we bought a home in West Virginia, our feelings about our home were influenced by the stories of the people who had lived there before us, adding to the good feelings we had about our home. And when we tell stories of our life in West Virginia, our home in the hollow beside the creek is a part of those stories.

REFLECTION 11–5

- Reflect on your home at this time. What stories come to mind? What stories are important to the way you feel about your home and the community around you?
- Where is home for you?

SELF-NURTURE: Being Home

Allow yourself some time and space to really come home and truly be present at home. Describe the feelings associated with coming home and with being at home. How do you draw on these feelings to nurture yourself when you need those connections but cannot physically be at home?

Your own life, as you live it moment by moment, contains much food for story. Sometimes it's a difficult story, sometimes a happy one, often a complex tale—but a rich and unique, one-of-a-kind story. It is woven of threads from the universal story and contains strands uniquely yours. We can learn more about our own stories by remembering and reflecting on memories, dreams, feelings, themes of life, seasons of life, significant relationships past and present, and the stories that are a part of our stories. By seeking out persons who are and have been a part of our lives and hearing their stories, we understand our story in the context of other stories and appreciate our many connections over time and space. By learning how we best come to know our own stories we are able to integrate those activities into our lives on a regular basis. Journaling, reading, seeking our family trees, creating (in its many forms from cooking ethnic or family dishes to art and poetry), and studying traditions and cultures are a few of the ways we come to appreciate our stories. Reflecting on our memories, feelings, themes in our lives, experiences of the seasons of our lives, connections past and present, what gives us meaning and purpose, and other questions of the soul deepens our understanding of our story.

REFLECTION 11–6

Think of yourself as a storykeeper for someone else.

- Who is this person?
- What story are you keeping for this person, and why is it important to you and to him or her?
- How and when will you pass it on to them?

STORY AS CARRIER OF WISDOM

In the introduction to his book *Tell Me A Tale,* Joseph Bruchac (1997) recalls how stories from various traditions influenced him throughout his life. He relates how his grandmother told him stories from the Bible about love casting out fear to help him deal with being bullied by larger boys, and how a story from the American Indian Iroquois nation about the importance of peacemaking taught him a similar lesson. He tells us that one of the best things about telling stories to our children is that often we will find them useful to us in our adult lives as well. Bruchac believes that stories have been his friends and guides.

Kurtz and Ketcham (1992), in their book *The Spirituality of Imperfection—Storytelling and the Journey to Wholeness,* address "the continuing story of a spirituality that speaks to both the inevitability of pain and the possibility of healing *within* the pain" (p. 3). These authors share more than one hundred stories from a variety of traditions that offer food for reflection, learning, questioning, mulling over, dwelling with, and enjoying. The first story in the book says simply:

Rabbi Zusya said, "In the coming world, they will not ask me: "Why were you not Moses." They will ask me: "Why were you not Zusya?" (Kurtz & Ketcham, 1992, p. 2)

REFLECTION 11–7

- What does this story say to you?
- What relevance does it have for your life today?
- Can you think of a situation in which it would be helpful to share this story?

Stories that are passed down through the ages have timeless lessons and truths to share. L'Engle (1993) sees story as homecoming, a family affair, an affirmation of God's love, the search for truth, scripture, the Lord's Prayer, community, joy, Good News, redemptive act, creative act, and resurrection. She reminds us that stories can have many interpretations, any or all of which may be right. "Story helps us with questions that have no answers" (p. 103), she says, reminding us that people through the years have told stories as they searched for truth. Jesus used stories to teach, and his parables remain oft-told stories by people of many traditions.

A perusal of bookstore and library shelves reveals books with stories from many cultures and religious traditions. Children's stories from China, Japan, India, Mexico, Zaire, Kenya, Egypt, and many countries and cultures around the world are increasingly common on bookshelves in our shrinking world. Children are often delighted with stories from far away lands in which they hear tales and truths that are at once strange and familiar. In the research for this book, one of the unexpected pleasures was finding the abundance of stories that enlightened and entertained and some that we are reflecting on and pondering even today.

Martin (1999) shares a story about watering watermelons in a drought she has created "in the practice of the story telling tradition to encourage people to make links to their wit and wisdom to survive tough life situations" (p. 8). She explains that one of the functions of stories is letting our instinctual (or primal) natures align with our rational natures to teach us "that growth might exist in a drought, and that there can be abundance and plenty in times of scarcity"(p. 8). She shares some of her spiritual journey in nursing by sharing the questions that she asked herself along the way: Was I able to converse wisely? Was I able to be silent and listen? Was I able to understand this person's situation? At the time, she was forced to answer "no" when she faced the questions honestly. As she reflects back on her journey she offers this understanding: "I would blame it less on the availability of time and more on my lack of awareness of how soul talk happens in conjunction with conversations about physical and technical care. I had to make a commitment to want to consider what might be possible in the moment" (p. 9).

As Martin continued her journey in nursing, she found that through their conversations and stories persons were sharing their ideas on love with her. She quotes a patient as saying, "Love matters to me, Marg," and shares her own recognition that, in the world of nursing, dealing with life-threatening illness did not usually include the need to consider love as a factor. When asked what she thought love was she responded that she did not know, but would let the listener know when she had figured it out. Although she noted to patients that many people have addressed the meaning of love, she discovered that rather than wanting to know what others thought, people would begin to share their own ideas and memories. When she began to ask people who were sharing in this way if this was the first time these thoughts had crossed their minds, they often replied, "No, but it is the first time that I have had anyone to talk to about it" (p. 9). In reflecting on Martin's experience, we were reminded that participants in our research on spirituality shared their appreciation for the opportunity to talk about spiritual things that occupy their thoughts but are seldom shared.

Martin describes her process of finding the courage (heart) and will to move her feet (soul) to be in a new position where she could hear a whole story in the fragments people speak. She tentatively names this process as contemplation. She describes this place of contemplation, this experience of "storying" and conversing as "being in the place of wide open awareness . . . a natural form in nursing . . . it is something akin to making us human." She finds "love stories" that give life and hope to the future when her conversations are based in reflection, consideration, and contemplation. Such stories call attention to the specialness of sharing the present and to possibilities for a better tomorrow. Because Martin's professional work, like that of many nurses, does not allow for being present continuously, she explored ways of providing encouragement for patients to continue reflection and consideration in her absence. Through the process of thinking aloud with questions such as "How does it feel when you're off course?" or "What does being on course feel like?" (p. 11), she began a story process that they could continue in her absence.

In her experience, she has found that talking about nature and the weather is "a soul thing" for the inspiration it brings. "When I began to talk less about myself and more about my love of the land, I could explain the gentle strength that is in water to help find a way for a person not to panic in the face of extreme fatigue" (pp. 10–11). She grew to recognize the healing power in attending to both the physical problem at hand and the soul's needs for soul talk. And, she found that healing and hope for the future called for the development of a lineage with the capacity to transform the worst nightmare into the best that can be done with it. She shares the comment, "while not wishing tough times on anyone else, that this time of change or transition is like no other and we would not have missed this for anything" (p. 11). Martin's story and reflection confirm the understanding shared by many, that stories and storytelling are powerful ways to share our spiritual journeys, the journeys of the soul.

Lawlis (1995) discusses telling stories as "an integral part of the health-care delivery process" because he sees "embedded in the skill of telling stories . . . the essence of health attitudes, education and love" (p. 40). He presents a thought-provoking and convincing discussion on the use of storytelling to provide a coping technique in the "generalized context of a person's experience, not in a situation-specific event" (p. 41). He cites examples of his use of storytelling as part of the medical plan of care for persons such as a 6-year-old awaiting a spinal tap, adult surgical patients, and a 14-year-old facing paraplegia because of a spinal tumor. Lawlis describes the power in presenting "a hero who first captures the patient's reactive stance toward the illness, and then gradually adopts a proactive stance that fits within the patient's actual or potential skill set." This enables the patient to vicariously process the hero's reactions to the situation and learn coping behaviors for the challenge at hand. Lawlis cites the example of presenting coping strategies such as exercise, imagery, and deep breathing techniques within the context of the story in which the hero becomes a model for the listener (pp. 41–42). A saying in Alcoholics Anonymous is "Fake it 'til you make it," suggesting that people can choose to behave in ways they might not want to or feel like in the moment. However, in the long run, modifying their behavior will also change their being. In other words, we can change ourselves and the situation by behaving as though we were, in fact, the people we want to be, our best selves.

REFLECTION 11–8

- Recall a hero or heroine who was a source of inspiration or enjoyment for you.
- What are some of your favorite stories, and why are they your favorites?
- What stories from traditions and cultures other than your own have you enjoyed?

(continued)

- How have stories imparted wisdom, encouragement, and inspiration to you? Which stories did that for you?

- At this time in your life, how do you most often encounter stories, perhaps through books, other people, television, movies, songs, or other means?

SELF-NURTURE: Story for Now

Treat yourself to a story just because . . . Enjoy it.

SHARING AND LIVING LIFE STORIES

As nurses, patients, families, and other care providers find themselves in the midst of busy, often even chaotic, health care systems, how do we make space within ourselves and the system for persons to have their stories heard? Considerations for consciously incorporating story into practice include the following:

- Recognizing each person, including ourselves, as an ongoing, unfinished story

- Understanding our own stories and their influence on the hearing of another's story

- Appreciating the breadth and depth of another's story, even though we can know only a brief part of the story that has brought another to this particular time and place

- Recognizing connections and relationships that enhance the understanding of story

- Developing a growing understanding of theory and research on story as related to nursing practice

- Consistently eliciting, listening for and to the stories of others, especially for the meanings and the "words under the words"

- Strengthening our grounding in our own stories

Sandelowski (1991) cites studies that illustrate "how lives can be understood, revealed and transformed *in stories* and *by the very act of storytelling*" (p. 163). When patients relate the stories of their lives, they often provide a context for explaining events of their lives. Patients' stories also say something about their pictures of themselves, whether positive or negative. Stories in their telling and retelling help people come to terms with life, its challenges, and its mysteries. Nurses have many opportunities for sharing stories, from the many questions they ask as a matter of gathering information, to the time spent in the presence of patients and families for other reasons. As we have been reminded, telling stories is often a natural response as people try to convey that which matters most to them, who they are and what events and experiences mean in their lives. Yes, as Coles (1989) says, patients bring us their stories and hope we understand. Too often today, patients and families relate stories of having nurses and other care providers gather, categorize, classify, and distribute information only to miss the person, and the person's story, which goes unheard and unrecognized. Have you ever looked through a patient's chart and been aware that the patient has been lost amid the professional jargon and laboratory data? Or have you read a chart and felt that it revealed so little of the essence of a person that it might belong to any number of other people? When nurses acknowledge that the data gathered to make an appropriate medical diagnosis is only part of the story, they honor the depth, breadth, and complexity of the person before them.

Sandelowski (1994) identifies several functions of the expert nurse-healer in relation to patients and story: (a) to create an environment in which patients feel free to tell stories, (b) to work with patients to make the structure and meaning of their narratives apparent to them, (c) to construct a unifying narrative for their lives, or (d) to reconstruct a more useful or coherent interpretation of past events and future projects. She states, "the overall objective of narrative intervention is to transform disabling or incomplete, incoherent, or overly restrictive narratives to enabling narratives that permit movement toward an integrated sense of self with future possibilities" (p. 29). Creating an environment that is conducive to the sharing of stories may be a challenge in sometimes busy, noisy, and crowded situations. The presence of the nurse is, however, a potentially powerful instrument in creating a safe place for the sharing of self through story. By both verbal ("I'm so glad we have this time to get acquainted.") and nonverbal (eye contact, appropriate touch, sitting rather than standing with one foot out of the door) behaviors, she is able to convey her desire to understand what life is like for this particular person at this time. We convey our presence by sharing observations ("You seem a little hesitant about that . . .") and gently exploring their meanings ("I wondered if you were worried. . . ."). We invite further sharing of a person's story by asking, "What is that like for you . . . ?" Acknowledging the limitations of the situation and expressing our desire to hear another's story facilitates further sharing. "I know it's a bit noisy in here and this is a busy place, but I want to spend some time with you and hear about . . ."

Working with patients to make the structure and meaning of their lives apparent to them involves listening well, validating what we believe we are hearing, and reflecting with the patient on what we have heard and experienced in the hearing. By listening with our whole beings for not only events and facts, but for the meaning of these happenings in the lives of the patient for whom we care, we establish a relationship based on our appreciation of the wholeness of another, a unique life story in process. Sharing our perceptions of the meaning and structure of their lives often provides them with an opportunity to look at their lives in new ways. "I'd never thought about myself as a strong person, but when I look at myself as you've described me I get a different picture of myself." Often the telling and retelling of stories will in itself bring new clarity and understandings for teller and hearer.

To construct a unifying narrative with patients or to reconstruct a more helpful interpretation of their lives enables them to move toward healing if not curing. "You know, now that I think about it, I've always been the kind of person who took care of his responsibilities. That's why it's so important that I finish this up before my surgery. It's not that I am trying to be stubborn or don't trust them to do it. I need to do it for myself." "I've been thinking about being in a wheelchair. I'm still the same person and I've always enjoyed figuring things out, so I guess I can figure out how to live like I want in this chair." As noted earlier, Lawlis (1995) uses story (in this case, fictitious stories with imaginary heroes) to enable persons to imagine, construct and move into a future in which they are able to cope in new and healing ways with challenges to their well-being.

Kiser-Larson (2000) asserts that "story and caring are inextricably connected concepts in nursing" (p. 31). She describes caring as "a science that guides the nurse in facilitating a healing environment in which the client may express his or her wholeness." She further describes the relationship of caring and story: "The patient's story is often the initial connection between the nurse and the patient. As the nurse manifests caring for the patient, the patient is free to share more of who he or she is. Thus, caring and story become reciprocal as caring invites story and story enhances caring" (p. 28).

Kiser-Larson (2000) cites three nursing paradigms: the *particulate-deterministic,* the *interactive-integrative* and the *unitary-transformative.* She quotes Newman in explaining that the first of the paired words describes the view of the entity under consideration and the second refers to the notion of how change occurs (p. 29). In the particulate-deterministic paradigm, caring is viewed as too "fuzzy," a concept so narrowly defined as to lose its very meaning. Story is difficult to use in this view because story is not easily broken down into individual units to be measured and studied. In the interactive-integrative paradigm, caring may be seen as actions to meet the needs of persons unable to do so for themselves. Caring actions are seen as based in adequate knowledge and skill, and the nurse's actions are congruent with the patient's perception of needs. Story, like caring, receives more recognition in the interactive-integrative paradigm than in the particulate-deterministic paradigm. Kiser-Larson states that in this view, the context and setting of the patient's story are of interest, but the story is broken down into parts to be analyzed and perhaps compared with parts of the stories of others. Kiser-Larson finds the concepts of caring and story of most value in the unitary-transformative paradigm. This paradigm is much more inclusive of the varied understandings of caring, which includes caring as "the adherence to the commitment of maintaining the individual's dignity or integrity" (p. 30). In this paradigm, story is often seen as a way of understanding the patient's life, including the health issues in the immediate story. In the unitary-transformative paradigm, the whole of a person's story provides a means of understanding the uniqueness of a particular person and a basis for appropriate nursing care. Story and caring are recognized as both content and process. "Story is a vehicle to develop the characteristics of mutuality, presence and trust in a nurse-patient caring relationship"(p. 31).

The unitary-transformative paradigm most closely resembles the perspective of holistic nursing in which the whole is unitary in nature, and persons, including patients and nurses, are viewed within the perspective of wholeness. The nurse-patient relationship is one within which both persons are influenced and changed and the emphasis in the nurse's role is on *presence, being with* the patient. In this paradigm, as in the perspective of holistic nursing, the nurse shares the patient's story and "story and caring are melded into a transformative experience where both patient and nurse are changed" (p. 31).

Liehr and Smith (2000) present a theory of attentively embracing story as a guide for nursing practice. They suggest that this theory can help us use story to guide our spiritual care. Their theory embodies holistic nursing's emphasis on purposeful engagement with the whole person for purposes of moving to greater wholeness, the essence of spiritual caregiving. Using this theory, the nurse intentionally engages with the patient to facilitate the sharing of the patient's story. The essence of the nurse's being, the *Self,* is fully present to hear the other's story. The nurse is present as an active listener who is with the patient as the story evolves and as the patient reflects on the story, paying special attention to meanings and themes. Attentively embracing story also facilitates the patient's awareness of self-in-relation to both himself or herself and important others who share in the creation of the present moment. Personal history (which incorporates both the story of the past and the future as experienced in the present) and reflective awareness (which involves reflecting on the present moment) are aspects of connecting with self-in-relation.

Liehr and Smith (2000, p. 15) discuss the nurse's role in "creating ease . . . an experience of relief surfacing," as the patient recognizes the meanings in the coming together of the parts of his story into a whole. As she listens to the story, the nurse guides dialogue to support the linking of happenings that might appear unrelated at first telling and remains aware of the themes that are emerging in the unfolding. In what Liehr and Smith refer to as "the flowing/anchoring paradox," the nurse facilitates the use of story as instrument of healing and caring by staying connected to the deep meanings and themes that emerge (anchoring) as the sharing is encouraged and supported.

Story path is one way of applying story theory to the practice setting (Liehr & Smith, 2000, pp. 15–16). Helping the teller of the story to step back from the story may support the engagement of the teller in sharing the story. Story path is represented by a line on a single, blank page. The current health care event is placed on the line as a marking wherever the patient chooses. "Imagine that this line represents your life's story path and then make a mark where you are at this time." The line can be extended on either end and can represent any span of the patient's life experience that he or she chooses. The patient is then encouraged to use the story-line to record markings that represent significant happenings that could have contributed to the current health concern or happening. In this process, patients are presented with the concept of stepping stones as markings that are important in the reconstruction of events to provide meaning that goes beyond chronological time. Markings and stepping stones are ways of looking at points of significance along a life's story path as well as clues to the uniqueness of each story teller. Liehr and Smith (2000, p. 16) remind us that "although nursing practice guided by theory assures gathering the story, one can never be certain about the way the storyteller will embrace story. The purpose of practice is to create an environment which supports the healing potential of embracing story, knowing that clients choose their own story path."

REFLECTION 11–9

- Draw your own story path in relation to your present experience of nursing. What are the markings or stepping stones on the way to your experience of nursing today?

OTHER FORMS OF NARRATIVE IN HEALING

Life review, psychotherapy, support groups, music therapy, art therapy, psychodrama (a form of psychotherapy), bibliotherapy (involving prose and poetry), and other experiences that incorporate consideration of and reflection on story are examples of the potential use of story in the healing process. In some situations, the patient is in the presence of a listener or listeners and shares story. In some cases, persons are in the presence of a story outside themselves, but which involves their *being* at a spiritual level and has the potential of providing spiritual care and comfort. In some arenas, persons are engaged in physically shaping or expressing story, as through art, dance, or music. In support groups, the power of story is present in the willingness of persons to share authentically and to be listened to by others who are truly *with* the one who tells the story. When a person shares her story in an Alcoholics Anonymous or breast cancer survivors group, she experiences not only the healing in the telling and retelling of story, the benefits of catharsis in situations of pain, but also the soul-to-soul presence of other listeners who want to share her journey.

> *Any work of art makes one very simple demand on anyone who wants to get in touch with it. And that is to stop. You've got to stop what you are doing, what you are thinking, and what you're expecting and just be there for the poem for however long it takes. (Merwin, in Moyers, 1995, p. 2)*

Wagner (1999, 2000) provides moving and vivid examples of the power of story as shared in poetry. Wagner (1999) had the privilege of hearing nurses' stories as they reflected on their experiences of being part of the stories of persons who were dying and their families. More specifically, Wagner asked her nurse-subjects to share their reflections on the family's impact on the dying person's experience. The intent of her study was "to provide deeper insight into the human experience around dying." By recording nurses' stories and then transforming them into poetry, Wagner makes the nurses' knowing more accessible and, for some, more vivid and clear. Wagner (2000) shows the reader that "poetry, infused with a concentration and intensity of image and feeling, brings another dimension to the objective scientific lens." She uses poetry, which "has a magic that is honest, probing, mysterious, and revealing . . . and often captures the inexplicable," (p. 8) to increase self-awareness and connections to others and to move toward understanding the uniqueness in universal human experiences.

STORIES IN THE CIRCLES OF OUR LIVES

Bruchac (1997) talks about moving around the never-ending circle of life and says, "there are certain things we must do if we are to learn and grow and live a good life. The first step is to listen. If we do not listen then we will hear nothing. The second step is to observe. If we do not look carefully at things, then we will not really see them. The third step is to remember. If we do not remember those things we have learned, then we have learned nothing. The fourth step is to share. If we do not share then the circle does not continue . . . And, sharing is what stories are all about" (pp. xiii–xiv). His words have relevance for nurses who are seeking to use the power of story to enhance their care for all persons as spiritual beings. When the understanding of persons as ongoing and unfinished stories is a part of the nurse's being and presence, she or he will be listening for story and facilitate its sharing. Her very being and bearing, his nonverbal and verbal communications, will be a part of their invitation to another for sharing story.

"The human story is a health story in the broadest sense. It is a recounting of one's current life situation to clarify present meaning in the context of the past with an eye toward the future all in the present moment" (Liehr & Smith, 2000, p. 14). The vision of holistic nursing calls for nurse-patient relationships in which the whole being of nurse and patient share part of a healing journey that transforms nurse as well as patient. Each person is recognized to be a story always in progress, always evolving and unfolding. For this time the nurse and patient enter each other's stories. Listening for the story within, between and under the spoken words as well as carried in the physical presence of another, enables the nurse to hear, with the patient, the deeper meanings of this experience for life's story. And, in the sharing and hearing of story, persons are often able to find meaning and purpose in the challenging events of their lives and move into the future in ways that are affirming and congruent with healing and wholeness.

Rachel Remen in her book *Kitchen Table Wisdom,* offers this reflection:

> Everybody is a story. When I was a child, people sat around kitchen tables and told their stories. We don't do that much anymore. Sitting around the table telling stories is not just a way of passing time. It is the way the wisdom gets passed along. The stuff that helps us to live a life worth remembering. Despite the awesome powers of technology many of us still do not live very well. We may need to listen to each other's stories once again (1996, p. xxv).

In our search for ways to offer spiritual caregiving, we need to recognize the opportunities to invite people to the table to share their stories.

REFERENCES

Boykin, A., & Schoenhofer, S. O. (1991). Story as link between nursing practice, ontology, epistemology. *Image, 23*(4), 245–248.

Bruchac, J. (1997). *Tell me a tale.* New York: Harcourt, Brace.

Coker, E. (1998). Does your care plan tell my story? Documenting aspects of personhood in long-term care. *Journal of Holistic Nursing, 16*(4), 435–452.

Coles, R. (1989). *The call of stories.* Boston: Houghton Mifflin.

Kindig, E. S. (1997). *Remember the time.* Downers Grove, IL: InterVarsity Press.

Kiser-Larson, N. (2000). The concept of caring and story viewed from three nursing paradigms. *International Journal for Human Caring, 4*(2), 26–32.

Kurtz, E., & Ketcham, K. (1992). *The spirituality of imperfection—Storytelling and the journey to wholeness.* New York: Bantam Books.

Lawlis, G. F. (1995). Storytelling as therapy: Implications for medicine. *Alternative Therapies, 1*(2), 40–45.

L'Engle, M. (1993). *The rock that is higher—Story as truth.* Wheaton, IL: Harold Shaw.

Liehr, P., & Smith, M. J. (2000). Using story theory to guide nursing practice. *International Journal for Human Caring, 4*(2), 13–18.

Martin, M. (1999). Emerging innovations: A fragment about love from practice. *International Journal for Human Caring, 3*(2), 8–14.

Moyers, B. (1995). *The language of life: A festival of poets.* J. Haba (Ed.). New York: Bantam, Doubleday.

Nagai-Jacobson, M. G., & Burkhardt, M. A. (1996). Viewing persons as stories: A perspective for holistic care. *Alternative Therapies, 2*(4), 54–58.

Nye, N. S. (1995). *Words under the words.* Portland, OR: Eighth Mountain Press.

Picard, C. (1991). Caring and story: The compelling nature of what must be told and understood in the human dimensions of suffering. In D. A. Gaut and M. M. Leininger (Eds.). *Caring: The compassionate healer,* pp. 89–98. New York: National League for Nurses Press.

Random House dictionary of the English language (2nd ed.) (1987). New York: Random House.

Remen, R. N. (1996). *Kitchen table wisdom.* New York: Riverhead Books.

Sachs, O. W. (1987). *The man who mistook his wife for a hat.* New York: Harper & Row.

Sandelowski, M. (1991). Telling stories: Narrative approaches in qualitative research. *Image, 23*(3), 161–166.

Sandelowski, M. (1994). We are the stories we tell. *Journal of Holistic Nursing, 12*(1), 23–31.

Sherwood, G. (2000a). The power of nurse-client encounters. *Journal of Holistic Nursing, 18*(2), 159–175.

Sherwood, G. (2000b). Story: Informing caring nursing practice (editorial commentary). *International Journal for Human Caring, 4*(2), 5.

Sullivan, P. F. (1991). *The mystery of my story.* New York: Paulist Press.

Wagner, A. L. (1999). Within the circle of death: Transpersonal poetic reflections on nurses' stories about the quality of the dying process. *International Journal for Human Caring, 3*(2), 21–30.

Wagner, A. L. (2000). Connecting to nurse-self through reflective poetic story. *International Journal for Human Caring, 4*(2), 7–12.

Watson, J. (1999). *A meta-reflection on nursing's present.* Presented at the 19th Annual American Holistic Nurses' Association Conference: Holistic Healing—Heritage to Vision, Scottsdale, AZ, June 16–20, 1999.

Wilson, C. B. (2000). Caring connections: Self-disclosure of student to teachers in nursing. *International Journal for Human Caring, 4*(2), 19–25.

CHAPTER
12

Attending to Spirit

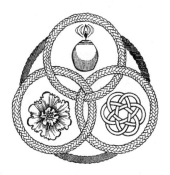

Today, many people are trying to reach the point which intersects

and connects with deeper meanings

and truths created in the path of our time.

We see a search for the spirit and the spiritual at every turn . . .

JEAN WATSON, 1999, P. 80

The previous chapters of this book provide a grounding for attending to spirit and spirituality for ourselves and with others. We attend to spirit through attention to the whole of who we are as body-mind-spirit beings. Basic to integrating spirituality into nursing and health care is an understanding that all people are spiritual and particular awareness of ourselves as spiritual beings. Awareness and clarity about our own spiritual perspective is prerequisite to and grounds our ability to engage in the soul-to-soul encounter that infuses spiritual caregiving. We must recognize the many ways that people express and experience spirituality and remember that, although we respond from our own spiritual perspective, it is inappropriate to impose our perspectives on another. We recognize that religious beliefs and practices are a very important expression of

319

spirituality for many people, but that spirituality is the broader concept and transcends religion.

ASSESSING AND EXPLORING SPIRITUALITY

Recent years have seen a renewed appreciation of the role of spirituality in health and healing within nursing and other health-care disciplines (Burkhardt & Nagai-Jacobson, 2000). Research and scholarly exploration of spirituality is much more evident in the literature today than it was even 10 years ago. The number of professional conferences that list spirituality as a major theme or that include spirituality on the program has increased considerably. Specific courses on spirituality in health are more prevalent in health professions education programs (Barnard, Dayringer, & Cassel, 1995; Carr, 1994; Larson, Lu, & Swyers, 1996; Shelly, 1993; Silverman, 1997). The literature reflects attempts by both clinicians and researchers to make some sense of spirituality within a scientific frame of reference. Although more clinicians and researchers recognize the importance of integrating spirituality into care, they continue to struggle with difficulties surrounding how to assess and measure a phenomenon that defies definition. Part of the difficulty is that professionals are uncertain about how to approach spirituality with others. Like sexuality, spirituality has been treated as a very personal matter that we do not discuss except within intimate relationships. Yet, when we take the time to ask, we find that people are not only willing to talk about this important part of their beings, but also appreciate the opportunity to do so.

We incorporate spirituality assessment into care for ourselves and others, not so much to figure out what is wrong, as to facilitate the process of taking stock and becoming more aware. Spirituality assessment helps us and our patients gain insight into who we are at our deepest cores. Through this assessment we learn what our patients would like to pay attention to, what is really important, and what are the deeper issues of life for them. Our holistic understanding of persons recognizes that all people are spiritual. Spirituality assessment then is not a question of judgment regarding whether or how spiritual people are, or what needs fixing; rather, it is an opportunity to gain insight into their awareness of their spirituality and how it is experienced and expressed in their lives. As we explore experiences and meanings associated with the spiritual journey, we assist patients in recognizing and appreciating the various facets of their unfolding journey.

Although spirituality often seems intangible because it has to do with our inner core or essence, it is not inaccessible. We do, however, need to have a basic understanding of what spirituality is and how it manifests to assess it in clinical settings or explore it through research. Because our essence or soul defies quantification, clinicians and researchers have tended to define spirituality in terms of religiosity and to assess or measure the expression of spirituality that is associated with religious beliefs and practices (Fehring, Miller, & Shaw, 1997; Hatch,

Burg, Naberhaus, & Hellmich, 1998; King, Speck, & Thomas, 1994; Larson, Pattison, Blazer, Omran, & Kaplan, 1986; Larson, 1998; Levin, Larson, & Puchalski, 1997; Taylor, Amenta, & Highfield, 1995; Zorn & Johnson, 1997). A significant problem with this approach, however, is that many people do not express their spirituality within a religious tradition, and conversely, religious practices do not necessarily indicate a person's true spirituality. Thus, seeking to assess and measure spirituality by looking primarily at religious practices might not provide a full understanding of a person's spiritual well-being and concerns. Another factor affecting the measurement and assessment of spirituality is the bias of assessment scales. Many of the scales or instruments that have been used to assess or measure spirituality reflect a grounding in Judeo-Christian beliefs and practices. Although these instruments can provide helpful insights into the spirituality of people from Judeo-Christian traditions, using such scales with persons who do not ascribe to these traditions could lead to inaccurate conclusions about the person's spirituality.

Even when we use assessment scales that are less biased toward a particular tradition and reflect a more inclusive or comprehensive understanding of spirituality, we must view attempts to quantify spirituality with some caution. We need to question what the resulting numbers really tell us about a person's spirituality and how using such instruments enables us to more effectively integrate spirituality into care with people. Hatch and colleagues (1998) suggest that we can facilitate the integration of spirituality into health care by having credible, objective, quantitative instruments for spiritual inquiry. They feel that such instruments would provide a mode of assessment similar to that of the mental status exam, enabling the clinician to infer a patient's spiritual status from his or her response to the questions. Hall (1997) cautions us to look carefully at whether we can truly capture an allusive concept within such scales. She writes that "allusive spiritual phenomena have been operationalized into constructs that have been developed as scales that measure such concepts as spiritual dimension, spiritual well-being and spiritual needs that are supposed to stand for spirituality and are taken by researchers to be spirituality" (p. 86). She notes that when this occurs both the concepts and their measurements can obscure understanding rather than enlighten us about the individual meanings associated with the spiritual journey. Ultimately, relying solely on such instruments to provide a true picture of a person's spirituality and spiritual journey is an inadequate substitute for a holistic understanding of the person.

The differing perspectives reflected by Hall (1997) and Hatch and colleagues (1998) represent an ongoing question surrounding how best to approach spirituality assessment in clinical practice and research. Coming to know a person in the fullness and complexity of her or his wholeness is a goal of holistic nursing. Particularly in the area of spirituality assessment, we need to take care not to substitute knowledge about the concepts for insight regarding the experience. Obtaining *knowledge about* a person through any process of assessment is not an end in itself. Such knowledge is useful only in as much as it contributes to understanding and knowing more of the essence of the person. Any understanding of who the person is must be supported by that person's perspective of the meaning of such knowledge. Although quantitative instruments may more readily capture the attention of the scientific and medical community, an important risk of relying on quantitative measurements is that clinicians may use diagnostic reasoning and structured interview formats as a substitute for the intentional presence and attentive listening that are so basic to soul-to-soul encounter.

INTENTIONAL LISTENING AND PRESENCE

> *I want to write about the great and powerful thing that listening is. And how we forget it. And how we don't listen to our children, or those we love. And, least of all—which is so important, too—to those we do not love. But we should. Because listening is a magnetic and strange thing, a creative force. Think how the friends that really listen to us are the ones we move toward, and we want to sit in their radius as though it did us good . . . This is the reason: When we are listened to, it creates us, makes us unfold and expand. Ideas actually begin to grow within us and expand. (Ueland, 1992, p. 105)*

Attentive listening and focused presence are the heart of caring for the spirit, both for ourselves and others. The core of active listening and presence that is essential in any approach to spirituality assessment lies in our intention and attention as we recognize all persons as spiritual beings. As with many things related to matters of the spirit, although this sounds simple it is not always easy. Good therapeutic communication skills facilitate the exploration of spiritual issues. These skills include the ability to notice nonverbal as well as verbal cues and a trust in our own intuition. As we receive and ascribe meaning and value to what we hear, we need to validate our interpretations with the patient. What we communicate through body posture and physical expressions conveys much about our presence and attention.

Intentional listening and focused presence foster authenticity in the nursing process because we are truly engaged *with* the patient more than doing to or for her or him. Figure 12–1 offers considerations to keep in mind as we incorporate listening as a fundamental process of spirituality assessment. As we listen to another, we need to allow the conversation to flow according to the person's needs and pace. While encouraging persons to tell their stories, we interrupt as little as possible, recognizing that what is not said at a particular moment also has meaning. We recognize that the way the story is told and its sequence are expressions of the person and part of the story. Conversation styles, including the amount of space between words when people talk and the place of silence, vary in different cultures (*Georgetown Magazine*, 2000; Tafoya, 1996). For example, Jewish con-

---

Listening in Healing Ways

- Be intentionally present.
- Maintain focus on the patient/client as a whole person.
- Set aside the need to "fix," "answer," or "correct."
- Learn to be with another in silence.
- Interrupt as little as possible, recognizing that even what is not said at a particular time has meaning and that the way and sequence in which a story is told are part of the story.
- View the other as embodied spirit, ongoing and unfinished story.
- Hear the journey, the relationships, the meanings in the story.
- Listen with all your senses.
- Do not prematurely diagnose.
- Let the conversation flow, noting the pace and tones, being with silence as well as words.
- Breathe!

Source: M. G. Nagai-Jacobson and M. Burkhardt. Copyright 1997.

Figure 12–1

versational style reflects high involvement in which speech is fast-paced, laden with expression, talking simultaneously is a given, and silence indicates a lack of rapport (*Georgetown Magazine,* 2000). In contrast, Navajo conversation style includes a relatively long pause time between words resulting in a slower pace of speech. When one person finishes talking, the listener waits before responding to be sure the speaker is finished. To respond without the space of silence would be considered disrespectful. Appreciating differences in conversation style helps us to pay attention to such things as meanings of language, pauses, pace of speech, and physical expressiveness of the speaker. Sensitivity to the space between the words and being comfortable with silence are important ingredients of listening.

How We Listen and What We Listen For

We listen to another with our whole being, with all of our senses, including the body sense. This is illustrated well in the Chinese calligraphy for "to listen" which is made up of the Chinese characters for ears, eyes, heart, and undivided attention. In listening, we pay attention to congruence or incongruities between words spoken and the energy and expressions surrounding the word. For example, whenever I sense sadness even when the person's words say all is well, I consider the need to explore further. When listening, our focus is on the other in his or her wholeness as embodied soul. Through our listening we receive and honor who they are. As persons share various facets of who they are, we recognize that they, like ourselves, are ongoing and unfinished stories. For this moment, we are part of each other's story, participating in the unfolding of each other's life. It is gift and blessing to receive and be received in this way. Such attentive listening helps us to be aware of the spiritual, the presence of God or the Sacred in the encounter.

REFLECTION 12-1

- When have you been intentionally present for another, listening with your whole being and with an open heart?
- What factors, internal and external, make that difficult for you?
- When have you experienced another as fully present for you?
- How did you recognize that full presence? How did that affect you?

Bruchac (1997, p. 1) reminds us that "it all begins with listening. There are stories all around us, but many people don't notice those stories because they don't take the time to listen." As noted in Chapter 11, people often express their spirituality through story and metaphor; thus, using broad, open-ended questions that encourage people to share their stories is often helpful. Questions and statements such as "What helped you to see things in that light?" "Tell me more about . . . ," "What was that time like for you?" and "I feel like I didn't understand what you were trying to say, help me to understand what you need," assist in developing a deeper understanding of our patients. One of the gifts of intentional listening is that the patient, in sharing with an open hearted and fully present listener, often hears herself or himself with greater clarity and understanding. When we listen to another in this way, we provide a safe space for expression of negative as well as positive feelings and experiences. Within this space, we allow the contradictions, pains, questions, and struggles to be heard without judgment or advice. The opportunity to express, and thereby to hear and better understand her or his situation in all of its richness and complexity, enables the person to move toward the future with more awareness. Expressing an interest in another's spiritual journey acknowledges the value and significance of this journey. Listening with genuine interest to what is shared encourages the person to pay attention to particular nuances, meanings, questions, and experiences related to their spiritual unfolding. We trust that our listening helps them honor this part of themselves more. For example, when we listen to Floyd tell us of his experience of life with cancer and "wrestling with God on my couch . . . we really wrestle with this thing . . . I mean real *contact*" we understand more clearly his relationship to his very real God who is in the struggle with him. When we listen to Penny speak of her journey "through the terrors of breast cancer" we share her anger, fear, rage, and frustration as she struggles and shakes "my fist at God." We also hear that her journey includes experiencing an abiding sense of "light and peace that passes all understanding." As we listen for the story behind the words, we hear the authenticity of the spiritual journey and each person's experience of the Holy.

Listening to another at this deeper level is part of the process of spirituality assessment. Truly hearing and receiving another in this way is a spiritual caring intervention as well. A hospice patient illustrated an experience of intentional listening and presence in describing his relationship with one of the hospice workers on his team. "It just makes me feel good to see him come in. One day he and I both fell asleep, kind of took a nap for a bit. He probably knows as much about me as anyone—because he's the kind of guy who's interested in everything I talk about, my family, my worries, my sickness. Sometimes he asks a question, but mostly he just listens—but I mean really listens, like he wants to know about whatever is on my mind." Our own practice of various spiritual disciplines such as prayer, meditation, and mindfulness enhances our ability to be fully present, available to be with and listen to another.

Spirituality may call to mind our relationship with the Sacred. Thus, spirituality assessment includes listening for mention of God, Spirit, or some other indication of connectedness with the Sacred Source. What words are used to name or describe the Sacred or the Divine and what is the sense of connection with the Sacred that comes through this expression? Persons have different, unique, and personal understandings and experiences of the sacred, and language can pose a problem when talking about this aspect of spirituality. Persons comfortable with the Judeo-Christian tradition of God or Lord, or the Islamic, Allah, might find themselves less comfortable with understandings expressed as Higher Power, Tao, Universal Light, or Absolute. The reverse might also be true. For some people "new age" is a relevant term that connotes spiritual growth and expansion, but for others, anything "new age" is considered suspect and can be spiritually distressing. We address the spiritual when we listen beyond specific words to hear what is most sacred for this person and how that relationship with the sacred can be nurtured.

Spirituality assessment includes exploring particular religious affiliation and any customs, practices, and needs associated with the patient's religious practice. What is the place of formal religion and one's own rabbi, priest, shaman, imam, minister, or spiritual leader? Does the patient want to make contact with someone from his or her religious or spiritual community? If patients attend a place of worship, how often do they go? When someone is sick, what kind of things do they do from a religious perspective? Are particular words of importance to this person? How do their beliefs make it easier or harder to deal with difficult situations? What is the place of music, prayer, sacred texts, books, particular objects, foods, or rituals in nurturing spirit for this person? We must listen for the many and varied ways spirituality is expressed. We listen for their trust and fear, love and support, important persons and experiences along their journey, and relationships that need healing. What is meaningful for people? What is their sense of belonging or place in the world, the cosmos? What is their sense of purpose in life, what do they live for? What brings joy, peace, hope, and sense of worth? Where do they feel alienated, lonely, estranged, and disappointed in themselves? Where do they find their strength in the midst of difficulties and trials? What are important relationships in their lives? What names are spoken with joy and excitement? What memories are shared with wistful longing, or with a sense of regret, or with grateful animation? For example, 15-year-old Elmo, who was in the hospital for treatment of advanced cancer, often spoke of his love of going fishing on the river with his dog. The longing in his voice and the spark in his eye when he spoke of going fishing were indications that fishing was one of the things that nourished his spirit. His parents recognized this, even if the staff did not, when, despite his deteriorating physical condition, they took him out of the hospital (against medical advice) to go fishing!

With people who profess atheism, which is disbelief in the existence of a supreme being, or agnosticism, which is doubt surrounding the existence of God or ultimate knowledge, our understanding that all persons are spiritual directs us to move beyond what is not believed. When people hold these perspectives we listen carefully for what gives meaning and purpose to their lives. What brings joy and satisfaction? What is the nature of their hopes and fears? How do they experience love, support, and connection to others, nature, the world, or cosmos? What are the important relationships in their lives? How does this particular health crisis fit into the patient's understanding of her or his life, and how is he or she dealing with it? Let us again share the example of an astronomer featured on a television program who noted that she was not religious and did not believe in God. Her spirituality was evident as she described her awe and understanding related to the evolution of the universe. She expressed deep wonder in realizing and appreciating that all that had gone before led to her experiences at this particular time, noting that this sense gave her a feeling "that I belong." Although the words voiced were not traditional religious language, her expressions of appreciation, awe, wonder, and meaning reflect her spiritual being.

Barriers to Intentional Listening

Our commitment to incorporating spirituality as part of holistic care implies the ability to assess our own facility as a listener, including any barriers to intentional listening that are part of our own personalities and perspectives. Our discomfort with certain topics can be a barrier to our listening and receiving the other. For example, strong views regarding the morality of certain lifestyles or choices, such as homosexuality or abortion, might interfere with our ability to listen openly to a patient expressing concerns about his gay relationship, or to a young girl who is struggling with a decision about having an abortion. Discomfort in and of itself, however, need not make us an unsuitable listener. Provided we are conscious of being uncomfortable, what is causing or contributing to this discomfort, and how it is manifesting in our being, we can make choices to stay with the listening despite our discomfort, or acknowledge our discomfort to the other and clarify the perspective from which we are listening. Ultimately, becoming more conscious of the various facets of our discomfort deepens our self-awareness and calls us to address the growth edges of our own spiritual unfolding.

External distractions can impede our ability to listen carefully. Consider the impact of a noisy, busy, or energetically frenetic environment on your ability to be present with another. Given distractions from within and without, the ability to focus on the relationship with a particular person in a particular moment is an aspect of healing presence that greatly enhances spiritual care. Feeling the pressure of time can affect our abilities to fully listen by taking us out of the present moment into thoughts about all that we have to do. Nurses often note that the pressure of time and having many responsibilities are factors that interfere with their ability to address spiritual concerns.

SACRED SPACE

Creating a sacred space in which spirituality can be expressed is an important element of attending to spirit. The concept of *sacred space* applies to our inner being as well as to places in our environment. The presence that we bring to the encounter is an essential factor in creating this sacred space. Although to "create" sacred space suggests *doing* something, inner sacred space is often recognized by *being* in awareness and stillness even in the midst of activity. Sacred spaces are home for the spirit, providing rest, stillness, nurture, and opportunities for opening to our various connections. We can transform any environment into sacred space by intentionally bringing awareness of the spirit into the setting. Family surrounding a loved one in a hospital room, a special plant in a sunlit space, the garden, the artist's studio or workshop, a room for prayer or meditation, the porch swing, a favorite rocking chair—each space touched by the intention of those who arrange it—are examples of sacred spaces. We shape such spaces through words such as prayer, poetry, expressions of love and concern; through actions such as helping another with personal care, dance, ritual, or preparing a meal; through use of sounds such as music, chant, drumming, or flowing water; through scents such as flowers, incense, candles, or herbs; through use of colors that reflect particular energy or mood; and through objects such as sacred or religious articles, elements of nature, crystals, pictures, or art. Most people acknowledge buildings such as religious edifices or places such as chapels or shrines as sacred spaces. Many feel the sacredness of places that remind us of acts that call us beyond ourselves, such as monuments to people who inspire us or to ideals that we hold. The Vietnam Memorial in Washington, D.C., is one such example. Places in nature are sacred for many people, especially for indigenous peoples and those who live close to the earth. Within health-care institutions that allow little room for nature, we have to be especially sensitive to people whose spiritual expression is strongly connected with nature. Incorporating pictures or objects from nature may be important elements of creating sacred space. We might also need to arrange times for the person to be outside in contact with the sacred earth and fresh air.

USING GUIDES AND INSTRUMENTS IN SPIRITUALITY ASSESSMENT

A number of guides and instruments for assessing spirituality are available. There are also numerous scales that assess religious belief, participation, and practice (Hill & Hood, 1999). The approaches we include here are examples of assessment processes that are based on a broad understanding of spirituality that can be applied to people from various religious and spiritual perspectives. They are also examples of different approaches to facilitating the integration of spirituality into holistic care. Most assessment guides base their concept of spirituality on literature review and input from content experts. Some instruments for spirituality assessment are grounded in qualitative research as well. Examples of both follow.

Spirituality Assessment Scale

Howden's (1992) *Spirituality Assessment Scale* (SAS) is a 28 item instrument designed to measure spirituality understood as the integrating or unifying dimension of our being (Figure 12–2). Based on literature review and input from content experts, spirituality is conceptualized as a phenomenon that is manifested through unifying interconnectedness, purpose and meaning in life, innerness or inner resources, and transcendence. The four critical attributes that represent spirituality with their corresponding items on the scale are

- Purpose and meaning in life—the process of searching for or discovering events or relationships that provide a sense of worth, hope, or reason for existence (Items: 18, 20, 22, 28).

- Innerness or inner resources—the process of striving for or discovering wholeness, identity, and a sense of empowerment, manifested in feelings of strength in times of crisis, calmness or serenity in dealing with uncertainty in life, guidance in living, being at peace with oneself and the world, and feelings of ability (Items: 8, 10, 12, 14, 16, 17, 23, 24, 27).

- Unifying interconnectedness—the feeling of relatedness or attachment to others, a sense of relationship to all of life, a feeling of harmony with self and others, and a feeling of oneness with the universe or Universal Being (Items: 1, 2, 4, 6, 7, 9, 19, 25, 26).

- Transcendence—the ability to reach or go beyond the limits of usual experience, the capacity, willingness, or experience of rising above or overcoming bodily or psychic conditions, or the capacity for achieving wellness or self-healing (Items: 3, 5, 11, 13, 15, 21).

The SAS is a summated rating scale that uses a 6-point response format ranging from strongly agree to strongly disagree, with no neutral option. The score is obtained by summing the responses to all 28 items; subscale scores are obtained by summing the responses to subscale items using the following numerical rating: strongly disagree (SD) = 1; disagree (D) = 2; disagree more than agree (DM) = 3; agree more than disagree (AM) = 4; agree (A) = 5; strongly agree (SA) = 6. Psychometric evaluation of the scale reveals a high internal consistency (Alpha = 0.9164) for the SAS, indicating that the instrument appears to be a valid and reliable measure of spirituality.

Spirituality Assessment Scale

DIRECTIONS: Please indicate your response by circling the appropriate letters indicating how you respond to the statements.

MARK:

"SA" if you STRONGLY AGREE

"A" if you AGREE

"AM" if you AGREE MORE than DISAGREE

"DM" if you DISAGREE MORE than AGREE

"D" if you DISAGREE

"SD" if you STRONGLY DISAGREE

There is no "right" or "wrong" answer. Please respond to what you think or how you feel at this point in time.

1. I have a general sense of belonging   SA A AM DM S SD

2. I am able to forgive people who have done me wrong.   SA A AM DM S SD

3. I have the ability to rise above or go
   beyond a physical or psychological condition.   SA A AM DM S SD

(continued)

Figure 12–2

4. I am concerned about destruction of the environment. SA A AM DM S SD

5. I have experienced moments of peace in a devastating SA A AM DM S SD
event.

6. I feel a kinship to other people. SA A AM DM S SD

7. I feel a connection to all of life. SA A AM DM S SD

8. I rely on an inner strength in hard times. SA A AM DM S SD

9. I enjoy being of service to others. SA A AM DM S SD

10. I can go to a spiritual dimension within myself for SA A AM DM S SD
guidance.

11. I have the ability to rise above or go beyond a body SA A AM DM S SD
change or body loss.

12. I have a sense of harmony or inner peace. SA A AM DM S SD

13. I have the ability for self healing. SA A AM DM S SD

14. I have an inner strength. SA A AM DM S SD

15. The boundaries of my universe extend beyond usual SA A AM DM S SD
ideas of what space and time are thought to be.

16. I feel good about myself. SA A AM DM S SD

17. I have a sense of balance in my life. SA A AM DM S SD

18. There is fulfillment in my life. SA A AM DM S SD

19. I feel a responsibility to preserve the planet. SA A AM DM S SD

20. The meaning I have found for my life provides a SA A AM DM S SD
sense of peace.

21. Even when I feel discouraged, I trust that life is good. SA A AM DM S SD

22. My life has meaning and purpose. SA A AM DM S SD

23. My innerness or an inner resource helps me deal with SA A AM DM S SD
uncertainty in life.

24. I have discovered my own strength in times of struggle. SA A AM DM S SD

25. Reconciling relationships is important to me. SA A AM DM S SD

26. I feel a part of the community in which I live. SA A AM DM S SD

27. My inner strength is related to belief in a SA A AM DM S SD
Higher Power or Supreme Being.

28. I have goals and aims for my life. SA A AM DM S SD

Figure 12–2 continued

Spiritual Involvement and Beliefs Scale

The *Spiritual Involvement and Beliefs Scale* (SIBS) developed by Hatch and colleagues (1998) was designed to be widely applicable across spiritual and religious traditions, to assess action as well as beliefs, and to be easily administered and scored. The conceptualization of spirituality that grounds this scale was derived from review of the literature and input from people from diverse perspectives of Christianity, Judaism, Islam, Hinduism, and groups whose spirituality does not derive from traditional religious perspective such as the Twelve-Step program. Based on this information, the authors developed a list of underlying principles of spirituality shared by diverse spiritual approaches that include relationship with or belief in a power greater than oneself, purpose in life, faith, trust, fulfillment from nonmaterial things, prayer, meditation, ability to find meaning in suffering, appreciation for mystery in life, ability to forgive, gratitude for life experiences, identity, spiritual activities with others, spiritual belief involvement, and ability to apologize. The 26 items of the scale are designed to assess belief or action embodied by these principles. This summated scale uses a 5-point response format. The scale includes items such as "I can find meaning in times of hardship," "My life has a purpose," "Prayers do not really change what happens," and "Spiritual activities help me draw closer to a power greater than myself." Three items elicit information about the frequency with which the respondent prays or meditates or participates in spiritual activities with at least one other person. Factor analysis of this scale identified four factors around which items sharing similar content clustered: external/ritual, internal/fluid, existential/meditative, and humility/personal application.

Although initial testing of both the SAS and the SIBS indicate that they appear to be valid and reliable, the authors do not address how they would see the scales being used in clinical settings, particularly how numerical scores from the scales would assist health care practitioners in addressing spirituality and spiritual concerns.

Spiritual Assessment Tool

The *Spiritual Assessment Tool* (Figure 12–3) was developed by Guzzetta and Dossey (Dossey, Keegan, & Guzzetta, 2000) based on Burkhardt's critical review of the literature and resulting concept analysis of spirituality (1989). This assessment guide seeks a narrative response rather than levels of agreement with particular items. The open-ended, reflective questions in this instrument assist nurses in developing more awareness of spirituality for themselves and others. These questions are designed to be used as prompts that enable nurses to focus on pertinent spiritual concerns. Similar open-ended questions can be equally appropriate and effective. We need not go through every question with a person at one sitting—doing so might seem tedious and overwhelming. Instead, we follow the person's lead, realizing that some areas might be addressed more fully than others are, depending on particular needs and concerns at this time. The same questions could be explored every day with different nuances arising each time. Instruments such as this are guides that support and enhance the practitioner's comfort and skills with spirituality assessment. These instruments are designed to be interactive rather than given to patients as a self-administered survey.

Spiritual Assessment Tool

To facilitate the healing process in clients/patients, families, significant others, and yourself, the following reflective questions assist in assessing, evaluating, and increasing awareness of the spiritual process in yourself and others.

MEANING AND PURPOSE These questions assess a person's ability to seek meaning and fulfillment in life, manifest hope, and accept ambiguity and uncertainty.

- What gives your life meaning?
- Do you have a sense of purpose in life?
- Does your illness interfere with your life goals?
- Why do you want to get well?
- How hopeful are you about obtaining a better degree of health?
- Do you feel that you have a responsibility in maintaining your health?
- Will you be able to make changes in your life to maintain your health?
- Are you motivated to get well?
- What is the most important or powerful thing in your life?

INNER STRENGTHS These questions assess a person's ability to manifest joy and recognize strengths, choices, goals, and faith.

- What brings you joy and peace in your life?
- What can you do to feel alive and full of spirit?
- What traits do you like about yourself?
- What are your personal strengths?
- What choices are available to you to enhance your healing?
- What life goals have you set for yourself?
- Do you think that stress in any way caused your illness?
- How aware were you of your body before you became sick?
- What do you believe in?
- Is faith important in your life?
- How has your illness influenced your faith?
- Does faith play a role in regaining your health?

INTERCONNECTIONS These questions assess a person's positive self-concept, self-esteem, and sense of self; sense of belonging in the world with others; capacity to pursue personal interests; and ability to demonstrate love of self and self-forgiveness.

- How do you feel about yourself right now?
- How do you feel when you have a true sense of yourself?
- Do you pursue things of personal interest?

(continued)

Figure 12–3

- What do you do to show love for yourself?
- Can you forgive yourself?
- What do you do to heal your spirit?

These questions assess a person's ability to connect in life-giving ways with family, friends, and social groups and to engage in the forgiveness of others.

- Who are the significant people in your life?
- Do you have friends or family in town who are available to help you?
- Who are the people to whom you are closest?
- Do you belong to any groups?
- Can you ask people for help when you need it?
- Can you share your feelings with others?
- What are some of the most loving things that others have done for you?
- What are the loving things that you do for other people?
- Are you able to forgive others?

These questions assess a person's capacity for finding meaning in worship or religious activities and a connectedness with a divinity or universe.

- Is worship important to you?
- What do you consider the most significant act of worship in your life?
- Do you participate in any religious activities?
- Do you believe in God or a higher power?
- Do you think that prayer is powerful?
- Have you ever tried to empty your mind of all thoughts to see what the experience might be like?
- Do you use relaxation or imagery skills?
- Do you meditate?
- Do you pray?
- What is your prayer?
- How are your prayers answered?
- Do you have a sense of belonging in this world?

These questions assess a person's ability to experience a sense of connection with all of life and nature, an awareness of the effects of the environment on life and well-being, and a capacity or concern for the health of the environment.

- Do you ever feel at some level a connection with the world or universe?
- How does your environment have an impact on your state of well-being?
- What are your environmental stressors at work and at home?

(continued)

Figure 12–3

- Do you incorporate strategies to reduce your environmental stressors?
- Do you have any concerns for the state of your immediate environment?
- Are you involved with environmental issues such as recycling environmental resources at home, work, or in your community?
- Are you concerned about the survival of the planet?

Reprinted with permission from B. M. Dossey, L. Keegan, & C. E. Guzzetta, (2000) *Holistic Nursing: A Handbook for Practice*, 3rd ed., pp. 106–107. Aspen Publishers. (Based on M. A. Burkhardt: Spirituality: an analysis of the concept, *Holistic Nursing Practice* 3(3), 69, 1989.)

Figure 12–3 continued

FICA—Spiritual Assessment

In discussing the significance of the spiritual domain to health care, Puchalski and Romer (2000) advocate including spiritual assessment in any patient assessment. They offer the acronym FICA as a guide for spiritual assessment that can elicit significant information within a short time in any patient encounter. Areas for assessment and useful questions for each are:

F: faith or beliefs—what is your faith?
    Do you consider yourself spiritual or religious?
    What things do you believe in that give meaning to your life?

I: importance and influence of faith or beliefs—how important is faith in your life?
    What influence does it have on how you care for yourself? Your behavior during this illness? Your regaining health?

C: community of which you are a part—are you part of a religious or spiritual community?
    Is your religious or spiritual community a support and how?
    Is there a person or group of persons that are especially important to you?

A: address—how would you like me to address these issues with you?
    How would you like me to be involved in the spiritual aspects of your care?

Personal Spiritual Well-Being Assessment

Barker's (1996, 1998) *Personal Spiritual Well-Being Assessment* (PSWBA) and *Spiritual Well-Being Assessment* (SWBA), offer another approach to spirituality assessment (Figure 12–4). Derived from her research (1989) and clinical experiences, these instruments were originally developed in response to a need for a concise and workable method to assess spiritual well-being in primary-care patients. The SWBA is designed as a process for clinicians to help elicit information about the patient's place in the spiritual walk. Spiritual well-being is as important for the clinician as for the patient. Thus, the PSWBA was developed by Barker to assist clinicians in identifying and clarifying personal spiritual well-being so that their interventions in this area with patients would be more effective. The PSWBA is also useful for patients' self-assessment as part of a treatment plan.

Each instrument addresses four broad facets of spiritual well-being discovered through qualitative research. These facets are relationship to self, relationship to God or Creative Source, relationship to others, and relationship to nature. The instruments provide key guide questions for each facet of spiritual well-being. There is no quantitative scale. The participant is asked to verbalize thoughts in each area. The clinician can explore these responses further if the content or patient's affect indicate that it is important to do so. These instruments can be self-administered; however, a greater depth of information and insight is gained through interactive exploration of responses.

Personal Spiritual Well-Being Assessment

Relationship to Self

Overall, in the last month, I feel _____ about myself.

Overall, this feeling is _____ .

Overall, my "well" feels _____ .

Relationship to God/Creative Source

Overall, in the last month, my sense of connection to God/my Creative Source is _____ .

Overall, I feel a purpose to being where I am today _____ .

Overall, I feel _____ about my place in the world.

Relationship to Others

I feel most connected to _____ .

This connection feels _____ .

Overall, my relationships are _____ .

I have one intimate relationship _____ .

This relationship brings me _____ .

Relationship to Nature

My favorite part of creation is _____ .

The last time I was able to experience this part of creation was _____ .

When I experienced this part of creation, I felt _____ .

(continued)

Figure 12–4

Spiritual Well-Being Assessment

What is *(the illness or other concern)* like for you?

What do you do to cope with *(the illness or other concern)*?

What makes you smile?

If you could be anywhere, where would you be?

What relationships are most important to you?

How can I help?

Figure 12–4 continued

The SWBA has also been useful in the restorative care setting. It has been used with hospitalized cancer patients at all stages. An advantage of the SWBA for clinicians was that it was easy to use, did not require calculations or a score to be meaningful, and gave the clinicians a way of exploring what can often be an uncomfortable area as the patient and the clinician deal with questions of mortality and unfinished business. The PSWBA was also helpful for the staff members in oncology to ensure that their spiritual "batteries" were "charged."

JAREL Spiritual Well-Being Scale

The *JAREL Spiritual Well-Being Scale* (Hunglemann, Kenkel-Ross, Klassen, & Stollenwerk, 1996), was developed as an assessment for nurses based on a grounded theory study of spiritual well-being in older adults. Findings from this study reflected the multidimensional nature of spiritual well-being, which includes relationships with self, others/nature, and Ultimate Other existing in the past, present, and future, throughout and beyond time and space. Perceived sense of spiritual well-being results from the harmonious interconnectedness of these various components within the person. The 21-item, Likert-type scale includes items related to prayer, meaning and purpose, personal goals, satisfaction, belief in a supreme being, forgiveness, ability to give and receive love, self-concept, and relationships with others. The three factors identified through factor analysis of this scale are faith/belief dimension, life/self-responsibility, and life satisfaction-/self-actualization.

CLINICAL USE OF SPIRITUALITY ASSESSMENT GUIDES

Using scales such as the SAS, the SIBS, or the JAREL Scale in the clinical setting can assist in gaining an overall sense of a person's spirituality. The assessment potential of such scales is greater when they are administered by a nurse in interaction with a patient, or when given as a self-reporting instrument that is then discussed with the patient. We must be alert for any problems with the patient's vision, reading ability, or comprehension when using a self-reporting instrument. The pattern of responses to individual or groups of items, more than the numerical score, provides us with insights into areas of spiritual strengths and concerns. Further discussion and exploration of these patterns with patients enables us to support their strengths, identify resources, and address identified concerns. Regarding the numerical score of the scale, the authors of the *JAREL Scale* (Hunglemann, et al., 1996) suggest that a low score on one or more items, or on a particular factor, could lead the nurse to explore the patient's perceptions and concerns related to that area. For example, the assessment data might indicate questions about what the patient values, or meaning in the patient's life. Discovering that a person might be experiencing a lack of kinship with others and lack of connection to life provides an opportunity for the nurse to further explore these concerns and plan appropriate interventions. A strong emotional reaction to a particular item would also suggest a potential area of need or concern. Areas in which the patient scores high suggest characteristics or resources the nurse can draw on to support the patient's moving toward even greater realization of his or her spiritual well-being. In whatever way we use the numerical data from assessments, what is most important to remember is that quantitative measures of spirituality should be an adjunct to, not a replacement for, the careful listening of genuine presence.

Within clinical settings, spirituality assessment guides can help us gain a deeper understanding of a person from a holistic perspective. These guides are not checklists that require a response to each item. Rather than considering completion of an instrument to be an end point, these guides are most effective when the questions are used as openings or referent points for discussing spirituality with patients. As we reflect with patients and explore the deeper sense of their responses, we come to better know and understand them in their wholeness. We can adapt the different ways of approaching spirituality assessment to fit the specific situation and person. However we incorporate spirituality into care, our overall assessment of how people understand and express spirituality needs to include exploration of important relationships and their roles and influence in the present circumstances; issues related to meaning and purpose; important beliefs, values, and practices; prayer or meditation styles; and desire for connection with religious groups or rituals.

Each assessment guide mentioned provides a process for exploring the elements of spirituality described earlier in this book. Consider, for example, spirituality as manifested in our connection with others. Each process of spirituality assessment offers a different approach through which a nurse can facilitate the patient's awareness of significant relationships. For example, *The Spiritual Assessment Tool* addresses the area of harmonious interconnectedness; the *Spirituality Assessment Scale* includes questions related to unifying interconnectedness; and the *Spiritual*

Well-Being Assessment asks what relationships are most important to the person. As we become more at home with the concept of spirituality and its language, we become more comfortable in forming our own questions and making our own observations regarding our understanding of another person as a whole being whose essence is spirit.

APPROACHES TO STUDYING SPIRITUALITY

Both qualitative and quantitative methodologies have been used to study spirituality. Qualitative approaches help us flesh out and develop a better understanding of this rather elusive concept. These approaches help us understand the concept from the perspective of the participants. Such studies have helped to further clarify the distinction between spirituality and religion and to further elucidate the many ways people express and experience spirituality. In quantitative research, information about spirituality is gathered through instruments designed to measure the concept. Various instruments reflect different conceptualizations of spirituality depending on how they were developed and the developer's perspective. Because spirituality has so long been associated with religion and religiosity, many scales that claim to measure spirituality seek information primarily about religious beliefs and practices. One difficulty surrounding integrating spirituality into health-care practice is the varied understanding of the concept derived from the many ways it has been conceptualized and measured in research. Although religiosity is an important component of spirituality for many people, instruments that conceptualize spirituality primarily in terms of religious beliefs and practices will exclude people who do not express their spirituality in this way. When choosing an instrument to study spirituality, researchers need to be clear about whether they are measuring spirituality or religiosity. Information regarding each can offer important insights into health and health care; however, using religiosity as the primary indicator of spirituality can be misleading and limit a fuller understanding of the affect of the human spirit on health and healing. Use of spirituality assessment instruments that provide numerical scores might be more useful within the context of a research study than in a clinical setting.

INTEGRATING SPIRITUAL CAREGIVING INTO NURSING AND HEALTH CARE

We recognize that care of the spirit is a professional nursing responsibility. Indeed, within a holistic perspective, providing spiritual care is also an ethical obligation (Wright, 1998). We see spiritual caregiving affirmed in standards for practice reflected in the American Nurses Association Code of Ethics for Nursing, the American Holistic Nurses' Association Standards of Holistic Nursing Practice, the Canadian Nurses' Association Code of Ethics for Registered Nurses, the International Code of Nursing Ethics, and by the Joint Commission for Accreditation of Health Care Organizations. These standards specify that individuals have a right to care that respects individual values, including spiritual values. Developing competence and confidence with spiritual caregiving requires a sound conceptual understanding of spirituality, attentiveness to nurturing our own spirits, and expanding our skills in assessing the spiritual domain and in developing and implementing appropriate interventions. All these areas have been addressed throughout this book. Although we offer some general guidelines and specific suggestions for spirituality assessment and intervention, these processes must be personalized for each patient.

Care planning by health-care practitioners generally follows a fairly standard process in which assessment leads to diagnoses, which engender related interventions, followed by evaluation of outcomes of the process. Because spirituality relates to the wholeness of persons, we need to approach spiritual caregiving somewhat differently, as an integrative rather than a linear process. In spiritual caregiving, assessment and intervention might be the same process. The very act of asking about another's spirituality or inviting another to share her or his story provides an opportunity for that person to be heard, which in and of itself can be very healing. Exploring spirituality with another enables both of us to deepen our awareness of who we are, ponder where we belong, how we fit, where we find meaning, what is important in life, and where we experience significant connections. Beyond merely labeling an experience in terms of a particular diagnosis, our narrative description of the experience might be more useful in developing ways to address expressed concerns. As we identify needs or concerns in the area of spirituality, we appreciate that concerns in this area do not necessarily indicate pathology or impairment. Questions about meaning, difficulties in relationships, feeling strain in our connectedness with God or Sacred Source, and wondering about choices we have made along our journey can all open us to spiritual deepening and greater awareness of who we are. The lives of spiritual teachers and mystics, and indeed, the stories of "ordinary" people shared throughout this book, show us that times of spiritual distress or emptiness, sometimes referred to as the "dark night of the soul," often have a very deep and healing influence on the spiritual journey.

Hall (1997) reminds us how important it is to explore and describe the human spirit in the language of those who are living with particular health care needs and concerns. Through this process of exploration, we begin to understand individual meaning within the context of the values that are part of a person's world. A rather dramatic example is a man who was hospitalized, at the insistence of his children, after being bitten by a poisonous snake during a religious service at his snake-handling church. He had been "treated" at home for several days through prayer and trust in God's healing. Noting that he knew he might die, he refused to have anti-venom, based on the belief that this would indicate lack of trust in

God, which would go against a basic tenet of his religion. As difficult as this might be for those involved in providing care, understanding his choices within the context of his worldview is essential. Ultimately, we recognize that spirituality is an important consideration with all health concerns, both major and minor ones. We address spirituality in the midst of routine care as we collaborate with patients and families in identifying concerns and needs, determining appropriate outcomes, developing plans, and organizing overall care to ensure incorporation of each person's selfhood, values, and worldview. Creating an atmosphere that is accepting and encouraging of spiritual expression in its many and varied forms facilitates this process. As we interact with patients, having an understanding and awareness of our personal spiritual perspective enables us to be alert to how our worldviews influence our relationships and work. This awareness enables us to more readily recognize when we are uncomfortable with a patient's spiritual perspective and either work through our discomfort or involve others who are more able to be with the patient's perspective to provide the needed care.

A basic part of attending to spirit is developing our ability to see and experience the holy in the ordinary, to recognize the sacred in every moment, in every action. Jean Watson's (1999) reflection on the Zen of bedmaking in *Postmodern Nursing, and Beyond,* provides a good example of how to do this. Noting that the Sanskrit roots of the word "Zen" mean "contemplation, meditation," she reflects that when we look at a bed, we can see it as sacred space rather than as a tangential or trivial object. "The bed, or any caring act or nursing art, stands alone in this example as a single statement, symbolizing beauty, simplicity, elegance, wholeness; it is an invitation to comfort, safety, privacy, rest, recovery and a place for healing to occur" (p. 238). She invites us to reframe nursing acts and arts within a new context of meaning and significance in which we see the whole in each part, a "Zen consciousness of each art/act as a sacred act, containing the entire universe of caring-healing practices" (p. 239). Within this consciousness, every act can become a form of meditation, allowing us to pause, center, and contemplate. With this consciousness, the act of handwashing, for example, can "serve as an occasion for clearing one's energy, opening up one's system to be both cleansed and open to receive again" (p. 239).

Medical treatment of Esber's illness included medications with many side effects, including high doses of Prednisone. In reflecting on what helped him counteract what he describes as mind boggling and physically disabling "pharmaceutical moments," he offers the following advice. Note the language that reflects his spiritual orientation and the many spiritual interventions he suggests that we can include in our care with patients.

> The greatest hurdle is making yourself "pick up your bed and walk," as it feels so much better to lie in it. Some form of exercise that is comfortable for your body, without injury or strain, like walking or going to the gym, is a great release. It helps you to focus your attention in a more healthy way . . . Another thought would be meditation and reflection, where one would take

time to lie on a mat with proper pillows and support for the neck, arms, back, and knees. Then put on your favorite music, something very relaxing, rhythmic, and reflective. Shut your eyes and, with your childhood imagination, go to a place that gives you safety, security, harmony, and warmth. See the images that you visualize, listen to the sounds that you hear, feel the emotion that you receive, smell the aromatic fragrances in the air, and taste your favorite flavor on your palate. You may be able to use all of these modalities, or maybe you can just use one, but that's ok. The image can take you back to your youth, or a time before you became ill. Perhaps you can project ahead to a goal you would like to achieve. Another way to meditate might be focusing on something tactile like a stone, a rosary, or beads, prayer ties, or a rainbow reflecting off of a prism on your ceiling and wall. Doing Yoga or T'ai Chi are beautiful resources of rhythm, of body harmony and rootedness. A good body massage gives fantastic results for relaxation and repose.

Last, but not least, the church is open for prayer and spiritual meditation . . . just coming to a service of worship . . . and being present for a moment to the God of all creation, who knows your true nature and respects and appreciates the nature of your soul, gives you the mystery of life beyond all understanding. There are many other facets to overcoming pharmaceutical stresses, from reading, to having a nice lunch with a friend, to sitting in the sun. But one of the most important of all of these is taking time for yourself, for healing, without feeling guilty or responsible for the world. One does not need to be a "Suffering Servant." That has already been given to us. (Tweel, 2000)

Spiritual Care Nursing Diagnoses

The evolving nursing diagnoses of *spiritual well-being* and *spiritual distress* support the importance of including spiritual care in nursing practice. The North American Nursing Diagnosis Association (NANDA) defines *spiritual well-being* as

the process of an individual's developing/unfolding of mystery through harmonious interconnectedness that springs from inner strengths. [Spiritual well-being is the ability to invest meaning, value, and purpose in one's life that gives harmony, peace, and contentment. This provides for life-affirming relationships with deity, self, community, and environment]. (Doenges & Moorhouse, 1998, p. 449)

Desired outcomes and evaluation criteria for this diagnosis include identifying meaning and purpose in one's life, verbalizing a sense of peace and comfort with spirit, acknowledging the stabilizing and strengthening forces in one's life that are needed for balance and well-being, and demonstrating behaviors that provide strength and support for daily living that are congruent with verbalizations. Interventions regarding spiritual well-being relate to (1) nursing priorities for determining spiritual state and motivation for growth, (2) assisting patients in integrating values and beliefs that contribute to a sense of wholeness, and (3) promoting wellness. Examples of specific interventions include: exploring meaning, understanding, and relationship of spirituality, life and death, and illness to one's life journey; discussing patient's understanding of life's or God's plan for them; reviewing religious or spiritual history, activities, rituals, and frequency of participation; exploring how beliefs give meaning and value to daily living; discussing the place of prayer, meditation, spiritual ritual in a person's life; identifying ways to enhance connectedness or harmony with self, others, nature, God or Sacred Source; exploring how religious practices and spirituality have affected one's life; encouraging participation in activities that support and strengthen the inner self.

NANDA defines *spiritual distress* as "disruption in the life principle that pervades a person's entire being and that integrates and transcends one's biological and psychosocial nature" (Doenges & Moorhouse, 1998, p. 445). Desired outcomes and evaluation criteria for this diagnosis include demonstrating the ability to participate in care and in activities with others, verbalizing an increased sense of self-concept and that one is not to blame for illness, discussing values and beliefs regarding spiritual issues, and actively seeking relationships. Interventions regarding spiritual distress relate to (1) nursing priorities for assessing contributing factors, (2) assisting persons to deal with feelings and the situation, and (3) promoting wellness. Examples of specific interventions include noting expressions of inability to find meaning in life; listening to expressions of anger or alienation from God; determining religious or spiritual orientation and influence of both caregiver's and patient's belief systems; conveying acceptance of patient's beliefs and asking how you can be most helpful; providing a quiet setting; developing therapeutic relationship that supports free expression of feelings and concerns; assisting patient in developing goals for dealing with illness and other distressing situations; and assisting patient in identifying spiritual resources and other supports.

Including Prayer and Meditation in Spiritual Caregiving

We recognize that prayer and meditation are spiritual disciplines practiced in one form or another in all spiritual traditions. Indeed, prayer is one of the first things most people think about in relation to spiritual caregiving. As noted previously, many people would like their health-care practitioners to pray both for and with them. Appreciating the personal nature of the disciplines of prayer and meditation, we can, with respect and sensitivity, help patients remember or explore ways in which they reach out to and listen for God or the Sacred. In the clinical setting, the role of prayer and meditation is determined by both the nurse's and the client's understanding of these practices. Recognizing the potentially rich resource offered by prayer or meditation, we might begin by exploring how the patient experiences the presence of and communion with God or the Sacred. We can clarify the patient's understanding of and need for prayer or meditation by inquiring about the place and meaning of prayer in a patient's life. The process of listening for and appreciating the prayer life of another nurtures the spirit and acknowledges the spiritual dimension of that person. The patient might want others to pray with or for her or him, or might not believe in prayer. Exploring as many aspects of the prayer or meditation experience as possible enriches both the patient's and our own understanding of the nature and place of prayer for her or him. Sacred or inspirational readings, music, drumming, movement, light or darkness, aromas, and time of day are among the many factors that could be important considerations in one's practice of prayer or meditation. Our presence and thoughtful inquiry can encourage patients to recognize and express their desire for shared prayer, participation in religious worship, or quiet, uninterrupted periods for personal spiritual practices. We might be able to support the patient's prayer or meditation needs by facilitating changes in the environment or schedule. The patient's requests and needs for prayer or meditation could mean praying with her or him ourselves, or inviting others to take part in various forms of prayer or meditation with and for the patient. By asking patients how they pray or asking them to begin the prayer, we open the opportunity to share prayer together without imposing our own way of praying on them. Of special importance is sensitivity to the patient's name for God or Sacred Source. For example, addressing our prayer to "God" or the "Holy One" would be more appropriate for someone who is Jewish than would addressing our prayer to "our Lord, Jesus, Christ." If we feel uncomfortable verbally praying with patients, we can sit with them, perhaps make physical contact such as touching their hands and suggest that we both pray silently in our own way.

The Interdisciplinary Team for Spiritual Caregiving

Working within an interdisciplinary team is common within all areas of health care, including spiritual caregiving. Although our presence and intentional listening in any situation is a basic way to incorporate spirituality into our care, issues can arise that we feel require more support, skill, time, or energy than we have at the moment. When this occurs, we need to work collaboratively with other members of the health-care team to provide for the patient's needs. We need to know and use the various resources available for providing spiritual support for our patients. Hospitals and other institutions often have pastoral care teams or chaplains who can be called on to provide spiritual care directly or to guide us in attending to patients' needs in this area. Ministerial persons, religious leaders, spiritual advisors, or spiritual healers from a patient's religious congregation or spiritual community can be important members of the healing team. Family members are often the primary spiritual support for some people. Other staff or colleagues who have more comfort and experience dealing with spiritual concerns than we do can guide us and serve as resources for us and our patients. While we use the interdisciplinary team wisely, we remember that we remain an important part of this team and continue to provide spiritual care within our level of competence.

OVERCOMING PERCEIVED BARRIERS TO INCLUDING SPIRITUALITY IN CARE

Nurses acknowledge that, although spirituality is an important component of holistic care, it is often poorly integrated into patient care. We must ask, then, what keeps us from attending to spirituality. Nurses often identify lack of time and feeling insecure or uncomfortable in approaching spiritual concerns as particular barriers. The perceived barrier of time derives from linear thinking, contrasted with having a sense of the whole. Rather than seeing spiritual assessment and care as an "add on," we appreciate that our genuine presence, grounded in and flowing from our own spirits, is at the basis of our spiritual caregiving. From this perspective, we provide spiritual care primarily by *how* we are with patients in every encounter. We also recognize that spirituality assessment is part of our ongoing interaction with patients as we listen for, and invite them to share their stories.

Feeling insecure or uncomfortable with spirituality often reflects a limited understanding of the nature of spirituality. Nurses often associate spirituality with religion and feel uncomfortable addressing spirituality with someone from a different religious perspective, or with someone who claims no religious or spiritual orientation. It is useful to have basic knowledge about practices that influence health and healing within religious traditions common in our area; however, we must take care not to stereotype others based on our understanding of their tradition. Rather than impeding spiritual care, lack of familiarity with practices and beliefs of a particular tradition offers an opportunity to explore what is meaningful and important for the patient. We have learned through our research and clinical experience that people appreciate having a chance to share at the level of spirit with someone who is genuinely interested in hearing about their journeys. Many nurses who feel ill prepared to attend to spiritual needs and concerns reflect that their educational programs have not sufficiently prepared them in this area. Taking responsibility to become more competent in spiritual caregiving through deepening our understanding of ourselves as a spiritual being, reading, self-study, and workshops focused on spirituality and healing helps us develop the confidence in spiritual caregiving that can eliminate this perceived barrier. Sherwood (2000) notes that nurses need assistance and support in being able to respond to patients' spiritual concerns in the midst of an increasingly impersonal health-care delivery system. Her research reflects the benefit of guided reflection as a process that can help practitioners both discover powerful spiritual themes evident in everyday health care interactions and identify practice guidelines for spiritual caring. Through this reflection, nurses can create and clarify the meaning of their experiences and encounters with patients and better recognize the impact of these encounters on the spiritual well-being of both them and their patients.

Barker (1996, 1998) suggests that nurses' attitudes and sense of responsibility can contribute to their viewing spirituality assessment and care as an added burden. For example, nurses might have a "rescue fantasy," thinking that attending to spirituality means they have to solve all the patient's problems, feel responsible for the patient's place in the cosmos, or accept responsibility for the patient's choices. Nurses might also doubt the difference that they can make in the patient's life by merely being with them and providing an opportunity for them to be more conscious of their own spiritual journey. Often, what people really need is a chance to be heard, to share their stories. They are not necessarily asking for answers or solutions but, rather, for someone to be willing to be with them as they reflect, wonder, and question. Spiritual caregiving means providing the space and opportunity to live the questions, to explore unfolding meaning and mystery within our various relationships, rather than needing to have the answers or to fix whatever seems unsettled or disrupted.

Some practitioners note the fear of imposing particular religious values and beliefs on others as a barrier to incorporating spirituality into clinical practice. This is an important consideration because it is inappropriate to impose our perspectives on another. However, we must also recognize that, although we act from and are informed by our own spiritual perspectives, this is not the same as imposing these beliefs and values on another. People who are clear about and comfortable with their own spiritual understandings are less likely to impose their values and beliefs on others. When we are spiritually grounded, we recognize there is nothing to fear in another's perspective. Rather, we appreciate that diverse perspectives help us to clarify and gain appreciation for our own traditions while broadening our understanding of the many expressions of spirit and spirituality.

REFERENCES

Barker, E. R. (1989). *Being whole: Spiritual well-being in Appalachian women: A phenomenological study.* (Unpublished doctoral dissertation, University of Texas, Austin.)

Barker, E. R. (1996, November). *Patient spirituality assessment: A tool that works.* Presented at the Uniformed Nurse Practitioner's Association Meeting.

Barker, E. R. (1998). *How to do research, get finished, and not lose your balance.* Presentation at the Nursing Research Symposium, San Diego, CA. Barnard, D., Dayringer, R., & Cassel, C. (1995). Toward a person-centered medicine: Religious studies in the medical curriculum. *Academic Medicine, 70,* 806–813.

Bruchac, J. (1997). *Tell me a tale.* New York: Harcourt, Brace.

Burkhardt, M. A. (1989). Spirituality: An analysis of the concept. *Holistic Nursing Practice 3*(3), 69.

Burkhardt, M. A., & Nagai-Jacobson, M. G. (2000). Spirituality and health. In B. M. Dossey, L. Keegan, & C. E. Guzzetta (Eds.). *Holistic Nursing: A Handbook for Practice* (3rd ed., pp. 91–121). Gaithersburg, MD: Aspen.

Carr, K. K. (1994). Integration of spirituality of aging into nursing curriculum. *Gerontologic Geriatric Education, 13*(3), 33–47.

Doenges, M. E., & Moorhouse, M. F. (1998). *Nurse's pocket guide: Diagnoses, interventions, and rationales* (6th ed.). Philadelphia: F. A. Davis.

Dossey, B. M., Keegan, L., & Guzzetta, C. E. (2000). *Holistic nursing: A handbook for practice* (3rd ed., pp. 106–107). Aspen.

Fehring, R. J., Miller, J. F., & Shaw, C. (1997). Spiritual well-being, religiosity, hope, depression, and other mood states in elderly people coping with cancer. *Oncology Nursing Forum, 4,* 663–671.

Georgetown Magazine, (2000). Vot? Jewish conversation. *Georgetown Magazine, 32*(2), 10–11.

Hall, B. A. (1997). Spirituality in terminal illness. *Journal of Holistic Nursing, 15,* 82–96.

Hatch, R. L., Burg, M. A., Naberhaus, D. S., & Hellmich, L. K. (1998). The spiritual involvement and beliefs scale: Development and testing of a new instrument. *The Journal of Family Practice, 46,*476–486.

Hill, P. C., & Hood, R. W. (Eds.). (1999). *Measures of religiosity.* Birmingham, AL: Religious Education Press.

Howden, J. W. (1992). *Development and psychometric characteristics of the Spirituality Assessment Scale,* Unpublished doctoral dissertation, Texas Woman's University, Denton, Texas.

Hunglemann, J., Kenkel-Rossi, E., Klassen, L., & Stollenwerk, R. (1997). Focus on spiritual well-being: Harmonious interconnectedness of mind-body-spirit—Use of the JAREL spiritual well-being scale. *Geriatric Nursing, 17,* 262–266.

King, M., Speck, P., & Thomas, A. (1994). Spiritual and religious beliefs in acute illness—Is this a feasible area for study? *Social Science & Medicine, 38*(4), 631–636.

Larson, D. B. (1998). *Health: What does God have to do with it?* Presented at the Third Annual Alternative Therapies Symposium: Creating Integrated Healthcare, San Diego, CA, April 3, 1998.

Larson, D. B., Pattison, M., Blazer, D. G., Omran, A., & Kaplan, B. (1986). Systematic analysis of research on religious variables in four major psychiatric journals 1978–1982. *American Journal of Psychiatry, 143,* 329–334.

Larson, D. B., Lu, F. G., & Swyers, J. P. (1996). *Model curriculum for psychiatry residency training programs: Religion and spirituality in clinical practice.* Rockville, MD: National Institute for Healthcare Research.

Levin, J. S., Larson, D. B., & Puchalski, C. M. (1997). Religion and spirituality in medicine: Research and education. *Journal of the American Medical Association, 278,* 792–793.

Puchalski, C., & Romer, A. L. (2000). Taking a spiritual history allows clinicians to understand patients more fully. *Journal of Palliative Medicine, 3*(1), 129–137.

Shelly, J. A. (1993). *Teaching spiritual care* (2nd ed.). Madison, WI: Nurses Christian Fellowship.

Sherwood, G. (2000). The power of nurse-client encounters: Interpreting spiritual themes. *Journal of Holistic Nursing, 18*(2), 159–175.

Silverman, H. D. (1997). Creating a spirituality curriculum for family practice residents. *Alternative Therapies in Health and Medicine, 3*, 54–61.

Tafoya, T. (1996). *Embracing the shadow: Mending the sacred hoop.* Paper presented at the South Texas AIDS Training (STAT) for Mental Health Providers. The Human, Transcultural, and Spiritual Dimensions of HIV/AIDS, San Antonio, Texas.

Taylor, E. J., Amenta, M., & Highfield, M. (1995). Spiritual care practices of oncology nurses. *Oncology Nursing Forum, 22*(1), 31–39.

Tweel, E. N. (2000). *Unpublished personal journal of illness experience.* Charleston, WV.

Ueland, B. (1992). Tell me more. *Utne Reader* (Nov.–Dec.), 104–109.

Watson, J. (1999). *Postmodern nursing and beyond.* Edinburgh, Scotland: Churchill Livingstone.

Wright, K. B. (1998). Professional, ethical, and legal implications for spiritual care in nursing. *Image: Journal of Nursing Scholarship, 30*, 81–83.

Zorn, C. R., & Johnson, M. T. (1997). Religious well-being in noninstitutionalized elderly women. *Health Care for Women International, 18*, 209–219.

Considerations for the Journey

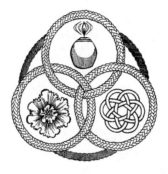

Perhaps life is a spiral of time rather than a circle,

for as we move through each cycle and season,

we are at a different place than we were at the beginning . . .

and in this cycle and season, at once familiar and ever new,

may you know your LIFE to be your true vocation,

and may you live it wide and deep in LOVE.

BURKHARDT AND NAGAI-JACOBSON

Endings are always beginnings. And so, as we bring closure to this book, we invite you to reflect on where you are in your own journey, trusting that you, too, are at a different place than you were at the beginning. Our trust and encouragement is that you follow and deepen your own Soul's path, more consciously living your connectedness. Our goal is not to suggest any particular spiritual path; rather, we invite you to begin or to continue to recognize and experience life as a spiritual journey. What we offer here are some further (though never final) reflections on applying the information in the previous chapters to your life and work.

We live in the eternal NOW. This moment is the place where God, the Holy, the Sacred dwells. Spiritual caregiving is first and foremost about *being* in the present, this moment, *knowing* that this moment is embraced by, held by, sustained by the Life Force (God, Sacred Source) that animates and connects us all. This *knowing* is always alive in us somewhere, even though it might be hidden in our deepest inner being. The processes and reflections included in this book are only pointers to help us connect with and reflect on where we are on our spiritual journeys. These processes and practices, and those found in many of the references we list, are intended as guides and supports to help us discover and recover our deepest knowing, in essence, to help us become more awake and aware so that we can be truly present in this moment. Only in this moment can we encounter the Divine in ourselves and in others.

To be alive means that we are constantly changing in an ever-changing world. Change means opening to the new, often the mysterious and unknown, and this can feel uncomfortable. We so often find our security in that which we know, the familiar, the place of our dwelling. Although it might appear dormant, our spiritual self is never stagnant. The source of our aliveness and of our journey, our spirit or soul recognizes that we find our purpose and meaning in changing . Through change we know we are truly living our lives and not just passing time. Change, in and of itself, does not equate with awareness; we can make all sorts of changes and still not wake up. Awareness enables us to recognize change, both that which we seek and that which seeks us, as a signpost of the spiritual journey. When we are grounded in awareness of our authentic selves, and when our lives reflect this awareness, change becomes a celebration of growth and life, something we can embrace with wonder and trust rather than something to fear and resist.

Being fully alive means consciously living our wholeness, our being/becoming, realizing we are part of the interconnected web of life. We live our lives in an unfinished world, which, like ourselves, is whole and becoming at the same time. And, we are shaped by our bio-psycho-social-spiritual-cultural environment. For all the influences of our environments, however, nothing shapes our lives, our becoming, as much as the questions we ask. As we reflect on where we are in our spiritual journeys, it is worth asking ourselves, "What are the questions that I journey with?," "In how many ways do I ask these questions?" and "How do I seek responses to these questions?" We offer you a space of silence to sit with these questions or just to be with yourself as you honor your questioning. Be open to whatever shows up in your awareness.

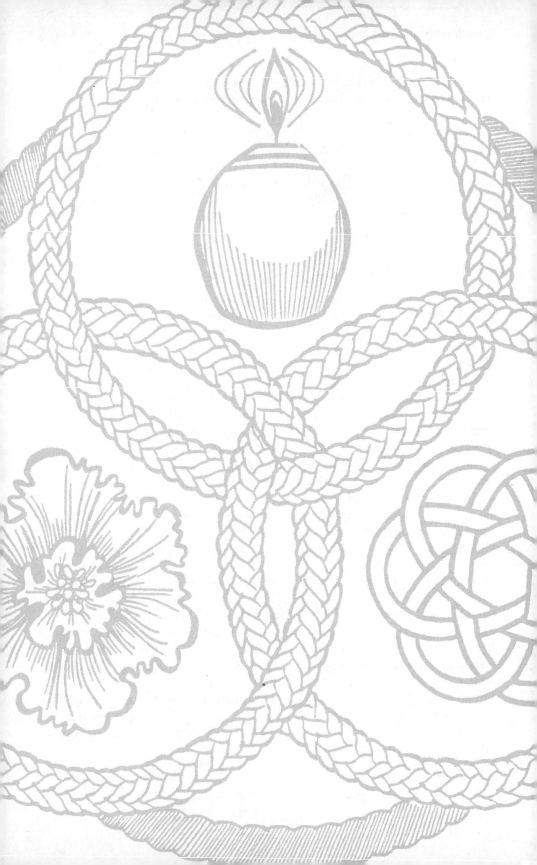

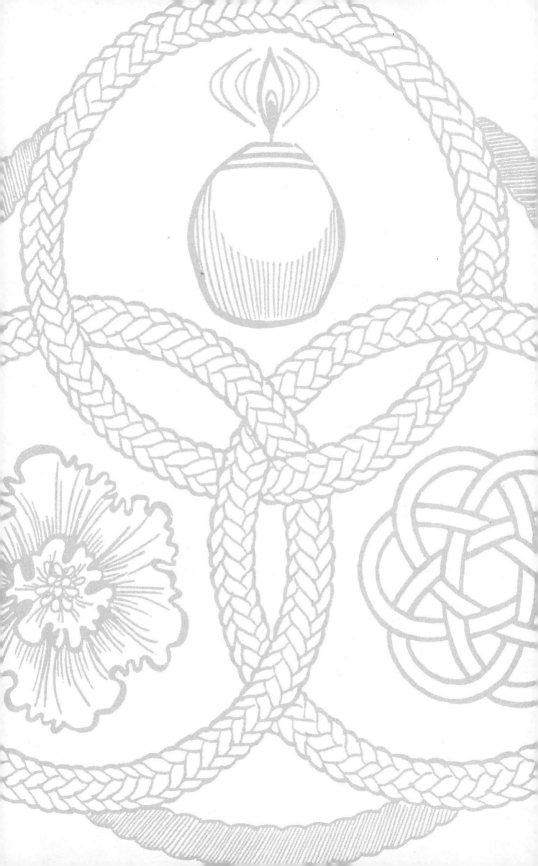

Living fully means paying attention to what truly matters rather than getting caught up in or distracted by issues and concerns that disrupt our connectedness. In this regard, Bernie Siegel (1998) urges us to not wait for a serious illness to become more attuned to our spirituality. As we grow in our understanding of how important our questions are for our spiritual journeys, we learn to ask, not so much "what is wrong?," but "what is important . . . what matters . . . what is our deep concern?" With this in mind, we might ask, not only "who am I?" but "in how many ways might I be myself?" This question opens the door for us to move into new ways of becoming. It prompts us to be and become more fully ourselves in relationship to God or Sacred Source, in relationship to each of the others in our lives, in relationship to nature, and in the various expressions of our physical-mental-emotional-spiritual being. We offer you this space and invite you to reflect on where you are in your spiritual journey at this time, where you feel your path is leading or where you would like to be going, and what is or might be the next step for you in the process. In generosity to yourself, remember that the spiritual path is a life journey, not something to achieve. There is no goal of "enlightenment," no end point to be reached. It is the journey, traveling the path, that is important, one step at a time. Where you see a need for change, start with one thing that you can reasonably do and commit to. We offer some questions to guide your reflection, but encourage you to focus on those questions that speak to you at this time, modify them, or add others as your soul prompts. You may want to record your thoughts and reflections here or in your journal, remembering that your response, needs, and questions might vary each time your revisit a particular question.

CARE AND NURTURE OF THE SPIRITUAL SELF
PERSONAL REFLECTIVE ASSESSMENT

SOURCE: MARGARET A. (PEGGY) BURKHARDT, © 1999

What principles, values, or beliefs guide your life?

How would you describe your life purpose, or where you find meaning in your life at this time? What would you include in a spiritual mission statement for yourself?

How are your life choices congruent with what you consider to be your spiritual path?

(PRA continued)

How and where have you experienced *being* in your life? What helps you to become more aware of who you are, your purpose in being, and your place in the cosmos? Can you become quiet enough to listen to the silence within you, and to attune to your deepest knowing? How might you make this more a part of your life?

What is one thing you are willing to commit to that will honor and nurture your *being* in your life and work?

How do you experience and express your spirit through your physical body? How do you nurture your body? What does your physical self need from you right now? How can you be more nurturing of your physical self? How does your physical being bring you into the present moment?

What one thing are you willing to commit to in order to better care for your physical self?

(PRA continued)

How do you incorporate Sabbath time—balance between activity and rest—into your life? What helps you to re-create? Are there things that usually help you to rest? What is a real vacation like for you? What time of the day (year, season, week) is most restful or peaceful for you? What is play for you? What people help you to relax?

What one thing are you willing to commit to that will enable you create the space you need for re-creation in your life?

How do you nurture your spirit through seeking knowledge and understanding? How has your intuitive knowing supported your spiritual journey? What calls forth gratitude and joy in your life? What helps you to dwell with these experiences? What prompts anger and fear in your life? What helps you when faced with these feelings? How do you nurture your mental and emotional self? What changes are needed to be more nurturing of yourself mentally and emotionally?

What does your mental and emotional being need for nurture and support at the current time? What are you willing to commit to that will nurture you mentally and emotionally?

(PRA continued)

How do you seek and experience relationship with the Divine? What blocks such connection in you life? What do you need to feel more connected to the Divine? What is most sacred for you? How can your relationship with the Sacred be nurtured? What is the role of ritual in your relationship with God or the Sacred? Are particular words or actions important for fostering your relationship with the Sacred? What is the place of formal religion and your own rabbi, priest, imam, shaman, minister, or spiritual leader? What is the place of music, prayer, sacred texts, books, particular objects, foods, or rituals in nurturing your spirit? How can you allow space in your life for nurturing your relationship with the Divine?

As you reflect on your relationship with God or Sacred Source, what is the next thing you need to do to deepen or open more to this connection? How can you make this step real in your life?

How do you incorporate meditation, prayer, mindfulness into your life? What kinds of activities help you find calm in the midst of a busy day? What do you need in order to become more centered and mindful throughout your day? What is prayer for you? What gives you a sense of inner peace? What is the role of ritual in your prayer or meditation?

What is one thing you are willing to commit to that will support and nurture your being more mindful in your life and work?

(PRA continued)

What is sacred space for you? How can you create more sacred space in your work and home environments? How do you attend to your inner sacred space? How do you use your creativity to nurture your spirit? Where and how have you experienced your spirit being enlivened through arts and creativity? How can you include more of these experiences in your life?

What is one thing you are willing to commit to that will honor and nurture your creative self?

Consider the important relationships in your life. How can these be strengthened? What areas need mending? What is needed to mend hurting or discordant relationships? Which relationships allow you to be who you are, and to receive as well as to give? How can you allow more space in your life for such relationships? With what individuals or groups do you feel your spirit most fully alive? How can you foster supportive relationships within your work and home settings? Where is forgiveness needed in your life and relationships—forgiveness of others? from others? of self? How can you begin the process of reconciliation? How do you experience love and intimacy in your life—love of self? for others? from others? for all creation? Divine love? What is needed to increase the energy of love in your daily environments?

What one thing are you willing to commit to that will nurture or heal important relationships in your life?

(PRA continued)

How is your spirit nurtured through receiving from others? What helps you, or makes it difficult for you to receive from others without feeling the need to give something in return? What do you need to help you become a better receiver? How do you nurture your spirit through service to others? How do you share the many aspects of yourself, including your gifts and talents? Where do you find satisfaction and joy in giving of yourself to others? How is your Spirit calling you to service at this time?

What is one thing you are willing to commit to that will support you in receiving or giving more graciously in your relationships?

How is your spirit nurtured through nature? What kinds of connection with nature enliven you—a walk in the woods, fishing, gardening (indoors or out), playing with your pet, watching a sunset, viewing a mountainside of fall colors, feeling the wind? How do you include elements of nature in spiritual worship and ceremony? How does nature speak to you of God or the Sacred? Do your home and workplace have windows with views of nature, or pictures of nature on the walls?

How can you include more spirit-nurturing time in nature into your life?

(PRA continued)

As you reflect on your Soul journey , what is the next thing you wish or need to do to support or attune to your wholeness, your self-becoming? How can you make this step real in your life?

SPIRITUAL CAREGIVING IN PRACTICE

What is true of our own spiritual journey, applies to the spiritual paths of our patients as well. We therefore encourage you to adapt the reflections and suggestions for self-nurture included throughout this book for use in your work setting. The *Personal Reflective Assessment* can also be used as a guide for spirituality assessment in clinical settings. Become familiar with the kinds of questions that facilitate exploration of each area of our connectedness and develop your own way of including these questions in your conversations with patients. You can begin with any section of the assessment based on what seems to be important for the patient or family at a given time. Certainly it is good to revisit areas that are of special or deeper concern for patients.

As we grow in the practice of caring for ourselves as whole beings, spiritual beings, we grow in our understanding of the wholeness of all persons. How then, do we move these understandings into professional practice? Looking at the issue from another perspective provides some guidance for one way of shaping our practice. We might ask: What are the ways in which I can live my wholeness and honor the wholeness of others in all I do? How can I be more conscious of myself as ongoing, unfinished soul story, and thereby see all others in the same light? If I understand that I am a spiritual being, and that all others I meet are spiritual as well, what does that mean for my being and my doing as a nurse? As you think about the contents of this book, we trust that you will find your own questions taking shape as you more consciously bring your spirit, your wholeness into all areas of your life. What are your questions, your puzzlements, your wonderings, as you think about yourself as a spiritual being . . . as you reflect on your soul's journey . . . as you think about yourself as a nurse-person?

We encourage you to see the guidelines and suggestions we offer as a starting place, a place from which you go forth to find your own voice, your own questions, your own unique way of being fully present in your relationships with God or Sacred Source, yourself, others, and the universe in which you live. Honor your personhood, the gifts and graces that are uniquely yours. There are as many ways to say "I want to know more about you, your journey," as there are nurses. "And, what in heck is going on here?" from one nurse in a particular situation is as inviting as "Help me understand this," in another situation. "This is making absolutely no sense to me . . ." can be either invitation or turn-off. So we are reminded again and again that our *presence,* our *being,* and our *perceiving* shape our words and the way they are spoken and received. Listen to what your soul would ask as it seeks to journey with another and listen to your knowing, your personal and professional knowing, to find your words.

SOUL SEARCHING

As nurses caring for patients and families, our roles and functions in physical and psychological care are often more clear than our role in caring for the spirit, the soul. And yet, in offering holistic care we ask, "how can we help you care for your soul as you live with, and through, this health concern, illness, or crisis?" We are reminded of those persons who have lived through tragic happenings and grown stronger, wiser, and more compassionate, into a richer wholeness. We seek to be a part of making each experience a healing one, no matter what the medical outcome.

As you continue to know and nurture your soul, your spirit, you seek to know and understand not only the "presenting" health concerns of others, but also the journeys of their souls through the experience. Your awareness and appreciation of all persons as spiritual beings is reflected in your *being,* and your *perceiving* of others as whole persons, embodied souls.

Take some time when you are with another person to consciously ask yourself: "Who is this person and what do I know of his journey?" Allow those questions to inform the way you listen to and perceive this person.

Think about the ways that you might let another know that you are interested in her as a whole person. How do your body language, your spoken words, your way of being and seeing convey such a message?

Be aware of your whole being as you interact with another person. What is your body doing and saying? What words have you chosen? What are you seeing and experiencing? How is she responding?

What are some words that invite another to share his experience beyond "symptoms"? Become comfortable with the words so that they are *your* words, expressing *your being* in interaction with another, not merely words from a questionnaire.

"I'd like to know more about what this whole experience has been like for you." "Can you tell me more about . . . ?"

How might you be mindful of the opportunity to encourage another to consider or appreciate the place of prayer and meditation in his life? As is so often the case, *listening* for the presence of or interest in such practices gives us further understanding of who this person is, and how we might call attention to existing practices and resources or ask questions that might facilitate consideration of such practices.

"You mentioned that your friends were praying about this." "Sometimes it is helpful to simply be quiet . . . for some people this is prayer, others may call it meditation. Some people don't really have a name for it, but it is like a good quiet, a comfortable silence. Some people call it listening to God, or to their inner being."

How might you encourage another to consider her physical environment? Both the natural world and the creation of sacred space within a home or health care institution are important to the care of the spirit.

"What is going on around us can really make a difference in how we feel. Sometimes just walking outside of the building and taking a deep breath of fresh air and seeing the sky changes the way I am seeing things." (Sharing your own experience and allowing time for their responses often provides the needed encouragement to share their experience of various environments.) "Sometimes having a favorite chair or place in the house where we can really feel at peace can help us to sort things out."

Being aware that our relationships with God or Sacred Source, self, others, and our world or universe are vital to our experience of wholeness, we can help others see the resources within their relationships as well. Sharing our own knowing and experience may be helpful in encouraging others to consider their own relationships.

"I know that sometimes I neglect some of the important relationships in my life, and have to slow down and think about what's important—and make some changes." "I heard John Denver say once that it was in nature that he felt most listened to . . . and it got me thinking about what nature gives to me . . ." "Some mornings I look in the mirror and think 'I really need to spend some time with this gal.'" "Prayer means so many things. At this point in my life it's listening, being quiet. But there are other times when it means sharing what I can't even find words for, somehow just knowing that God is with me." " There have been dry seasons in my soul's life when I walked not really knowing, just having to go forward on faith."

As we grow in our understanding of holistic care, we are each learning that our lives reflect our own relationships with God or Sacred Source, others, ourself, and the universe. We are able to let go of the fear of imposing our understandings and beliefs on another as we live out of our awareness of the sacredness of each person's spiritual journey. Our role becomes one of being a companion to nurture and encourage the other's attention to the journey. The following is an example of being present for the journey:

A chaplain . . . was wonderful . . . I don't even know what faith he is, but he didn't ever try to like impose his faith on me. It wasn't anything like that. He was just there to talk. And it was so neat, because he would say, "well, what are you doing today?" At one point he read what I wrote [about my BMT], and he cried. And I thought , wow, this is really neat. I mean he wasn't afraid to let me see that he was human. And he prayed with me . . . It was like, wow, somebody really cares . . . (Cohen, Headley & Sherwood, 2000, p 43)

THE PERSON IN THE STORY

Take some time to re-read and dwell with the stories in this book. Listen to the "words under the words," and let yourself begin to know the person revealed in each story.

"What has this been like for you?" is a question that conveys your interest in their story and opens the door for them to share.

What questions do you hear in their stories, the questions with which they are journeying? How might you give each of them the opportunity to share those questions with you if you were present and in conversation with them?

"There are a lot of questions about all this, aren't there?" lets them know you hear the questions and offers an opportunity for them to continue. "There's a lot to take in, and to try to make sense of . . ." lets them know you share their wondering.

What do you hear each of them say about where they find meaning in their lives? How might you talk with each of them about how they experience meaning in their lives at this time?

"In all of this, it seems like.. . . . has been important to you," or "I've wondered what it is that gives your life meaning in these difficult times . . ." affords opportunities for consideration of what offers meaning.

Esber Tweel notes that, although some of his parishioners urged him to take some time off, he could not allow himself to do that. What are the ways you might have listened to and spoken with him as he was considering his decision?

"You've mentioned that your parishioners want you to take some time off, but that your aren't ready to do that. Can you tell me more about what makes it difficult for you to take time for yourself right now?" "If you don't feel you can take time off completely, are there ways you can build some larger blocks of time into your schedule for rest and healing?" These questions provide an opportunity to consider the place of rest and healing at this time.

Jean Watson offers glimpses of her relationship with and understanding of the Sacred Source to whom she addresses her psalms. How would you describe her experience of God? Consider what it means to surrender as an active choice, an act of obedience to that which can be trusted, an acceptance rather than a posture of futility or hopeless resignation. How might you have offered her an opportunity to share what was happening in her relationship with God during this time?

"You seem to feel God is distant yet close to you at the same time . . ." or "In the midst of tragedy and pain many people wonder where God is . . ." or "Your trust in God seems to be helping you to have the courage to deal with this," provide an invitation to talk about her experience of God at this time.

Sandra Melville offers a portrait in words of this "Uninvited Guest" in her life. How would you describe this Guest and its impact on her life? What might you have asked to encourage her to share some of her perceptions?

"Tell me more about this 'Uninvited Guest'" or "What more would you like to say to the 'Uninvited Guest'?" uses Sandra's way of referring to the illness and leaves the door open for sharing. More specific questions can be asked to clarify or illuminate her understandings and perceptions: "What do you think this Uninvited Guest has to teach us as nurses?" gives her an opportunity to share from her perspective as a nurse, as well as a patient.

In her story, Jude Fleming relates her experience of finding, through Spirit, the resources not only to endure a difficult work situation, but also to be the catalyst for transformation within the nursing staff. She speaks of her choice to "go to work each day filled with the light and focus of Spirit, to engage all my gifts and intellect to learn, and to learn quickly . . . to return a loving spirit to injustice, trusting Spirit to handle the details . . ." She acknowledges having some pretty ugly thoughts, but "as much as I thought them, I also knew that I had a choice of how 'to be.'"

Remember times when you have consciously chosen how "to be" in a difficult situation. The process of stopping to be aware and to choose is an important one. What guides your choosing? What speaks to your experience and life as you read Jude's story?

Scott reminds us in a powerful way, of the spiritual nature of the physical body as he asks, "What do you do with your body when you pray?" He also points to the disconnect between body and mind in some religious traditions, and urges, "if you want a happy, grateful body, learn to be still."

Consider the ways you use your body to express your spirit. How have you experienced your spirituality through your body sense? As you reflect on your own body-mind-spirit connection, what shapes your understanding of the body's place in the spiritual life? Remember times when your body nurtured or expressed your spirit in a way beyond words.

Listen to Lisa Wayman: "I think now the problem was with the word 'caring,' it is like love, too emotional and fuzzy in general meaning. I mean love with sweat on it, that rock of reality, not the pink emotion . . . My presence includes strong technical skills . . . I think that in the ideal, all my interventions will be done with love, real gritty love for myself and other, and that is what makes it nursing."

What does nursing in the ideal look like for you? Remember a time when you offered or experienced "love with sweat on it."

Re-read Joni Walton's account of her interaction with the spouse of one of the ICU patients. She noticed the woman "hovering at the entrance of her husband's room with an expression of uncertainty." As you read, accompany Joni as she spends time with this particular woman:

What is the effect of Joni's presence in this interaction? Listen as the woman shares her story with Joni, and as Joni listens to the stories of the woman and of her husband. How does she help each person honor and express her and his wishes, and hear the deepest yearnings of each person? And how does she help them hear and reach out to each other?

Beth vividly expressed the power and Presence of nature in her life. As you re-read her description of experiencing Presence at the age of five, although "at that age I had no name for it," think about your own experiences of Presence. How does her description that "Presence had different aspects or flavors—individual trees, the wind, various mossy nooks and crannies, the stream, open fields . . ." fit with your experiences of Presence?

> Some ways of helping another consider her relationship with nature might be "Are there experiences of being in nature that are special for you?" "Tell me about some of your experiences of nature. How do they influence your spirit and how you care for your spirit?" "What is it like for you to be in touch with nature?" "How do you sense God's presence in or through nature?"

What aspects of Tammy's story are also your story, or are familiar to you? She speaks of a journey away from and back to God, and stresses the importance of making "daily, ongoing prayer and meditation . . . a priority . . . I look at the Big Picture and ask what really matters." Words that might help another talk about her story are

> "Someone once described her story as a journey away from and back to God, how would you describe your own soul's journey?" " When you think about your spiritual journey, what are your priorities for taking care of your soul?"

Listen to Lisa Wayman as she tells her story. She describes her "nurse self" standing outside her "mom self." Listen to her descriptions of suffering in many instances and many forms, such as "I could hardly breathe."

> Reflect on experiences when your nurse self has stood outside your other selves on the journey. What was that experience like for you? Remember a time when you were in touch with and connected with another's suffering. What was that experience like for you? Consider how you could "be" with her in her suffering without needing to "fix it." Perhaps acknowledging "I can see and sense your pain, even though I can only imagine what you are going through." Offering just to sit with her for awhile and ask her to tell you some more about her son brings the gift of your presence.

Hear the transformation and healing expressed in Lisa's story.

> Recall a time when you have experienced healing through suffering, a time when you have stood in paradox. Give yourself time to experience again those times of mystery.

Words that can be offered in a time of suffering are highly individual and particular to the persons involved. Simply acknowledging the suffering that you know the other is experiencing and being willing to be present, provide comfort. Nonverbal communication, a gentle touch, conveys wordlessly your connection and caring.

What you are going through is beyond any words I can find. I am here for anything you want to do or ask or say. I am here in your silence too.

Floyd reminds us of the importance of presence and of being able to flow with the patient's story and needs. The nurse who came to be with him that night was able to hear his deep concerns and also to step back and talk of other things, sharing herself with him, letting him know some of her story.

Recall a time when you have been listened to through a difficult time . . . how the listener stayed with you, but gave you the room for silence, changing the subject, and emotion. How do we say to someone, "I want to hear what you want to share . . . I am willing to be here for difficult subjects . . . and for you to set the pace?"

ENDINGS AND BEGINNINGS

And so we conclude—not in the sense of completion but in the sense of ending/beginning. Paraphrasing Henri Nouwen, in his book *Here and Now* (1997, p. 144), one of our discoveries in writing this book is how much more there is to write. This "open ending" encourages us to enter ever more deeply into the Divine Mystery, with knowledge that this mystery is an inexhaustible source of Life and Love. To you who have read this book, we wish to say, do not stop here, journey on! May our words encourage you to find your own words, and our thoughts encourage you to hear and discover your own thoughts. This book reflects our souls paths and spiritual journeys, our personalities, and the many factors that have influenced our lives. Your spiritual journey is unique, with its own form and flow, beauty, boundaries, and boundlessness. Our trust is that this book will be for you both an ever new beginning, and a companion along the way, offering food for thought and reflection, nurturing for your soul, and encouragement for the journey. Journey well!

REFERENCES

Cohen, M. Z., Headley, J., & Sherwood, G. (2000). Spirituality and bone marrow transplantation: When faith is stronger than fear. *International Journal for Human Caring*, 4(2), 40–46.

Nouwen, H. (1997). *Here and now*. New York: Crossroad.

Siegel, B. (1999). *Prescriptions for living*. New York: HarperPerrennial.

Index